Managing Pain in Chil

Uni

Managing Pain in Children:
A Clinical Guide

Edited by

Alison Twycross
Principal Lecturer in Children's Nursing
Kingston University and St George's University of London, United Kingdom

Stephanie J. Dowden
Clinical Nurse Consultant, Paediatric Palliative Care
Princess Margaret Hospital for Children, Perth, Australia

and

Elizabeth Bruce
Lead Clinical Nurse Specialist, Pain Control Service
Great Ormond Street Hospital for Children NHS Trust, London, United Kingdom

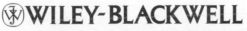
WILEY-BLACKWELL
A John Wiley & Sons, Ltd., Publication

This edition first published 2009
© 2009 Blackwell Publishing Ltd

Blackwell Publishing was acquired by John Wiley & Sons in February 2007. Blackwell's publishing programme has been merged with Wiley's global Scientific, Technical, and Medical business to form Wiley-Blackwell.

Registered office
John Wiley & Sons Ltd, The Atrium, Southern Gate, Chichester, West Sussex, PO19 8SQ, United Kingdom

Editorial offices
9600 Garsington Road, Oxford, OX4 2DQ, United Kingdom
2121 State Avenue, Ames, Iowa 50014-8300, USA

For details of our global editorial offices, for customer services and for information about how to apply for permission to reuse the copyright material in this book please see our website at www.wiley.com/wiley-blackwell.

Library of Congress Cataloging-in-Publication Data

Managing pain in children : a clinical guide / edited by Alison Twycross, Stephanie Dowden, and Elizabeth Bruce.
    p. ; cm.
  Includes bibliographical references and index.
  ISBN 978-1-4051-6894-6 (pbk. : alk. paper) 1. Pain in children--Treatment. I. Twycross, Alison. II. Dowden, Stephanie. III. Bruce, Elizabeth (Elizabeth A.)
  [DNLM: 1. Child. 2. Pain--therapy. WL 704 M2666 2008]

RJ365.M34 2008
618.92'0472--dc22

                        2008028168

A catalogue record for this book is available from the British Library.

Set in 10/11.5 pt Sabon by Newgen Imaging Systems Pvt Ltd, Chennai, India.
Printed and bound in Singapore by C.O.S. Printers Pte Ltd

1 2009

Contents

Foreword

Pain is a common and complicated problem in children and young people. It impacts on the functional and physical aspects of children's lives and their psychological and emotional well-being. Family caregivers suffer a great sense of burden when their children's pain is not adequately relieved and this affects their emotional, social and family functioning. The problem is also exacerbated by the additional financial burdens, which are secondary to increased physician consultation and medication use.

Despite the enormous strides made in this field over the last 30 years, children continue to experience unrelieved pain postoperatively or during procedures. These pains in principle should be easy to manage using multimodal analgesics and non-drug interventions. The consequences of poorly managed acute and postoperative pain can be quite significant. They include an increase in morbidity resulting in longer hospital stays, a slower recovery time, and a delay in resumption of normal life activities for the child. Additionally, ineffective management of acute pain may also increase the risk for chronic pain later in life. It is therefore imperative that parents are given adequate information about treatment options and are included in the decision-making process related to the management of their child's pain.

Chronic pain is a global problem and its impact is significant also in children. It is usually more common in girls and it increases with increasing age in both genders. Children with chronic pain suffer from functional impairments, which have significant impacts on their growth and development. Headache prevalence in school children, for example, is on the increase in the Netherlands and stress is seen as its major trigger. These children usually report the lowest quality of life and the lowest quality of health, as well as problems related to physical functioning, daily and leisure activities, and social functioning at home, which are depicted in low levels of family support, poor relationships at home and a disorganised daily family life. Most of these children miss school due to pain. Follow-up studies report persistence of chronic pain after several years, reaching early adulthood and affecting several domains in life. The impact of chronic pain on parents is also as significant. Parents usually struggle for control and adherence and they suffer when their child's pain cannot be diagnosed. They have a sense of being disbelieved by family and society. They also experience helplessness and distress whenever there is uncertainty about pain prognosis, and powerlessness because they are not able to help their child. They may lead a very different life; major changes in family relationships may result secondary to their child's condition.

Fortunately, infant and child mortality has significantly decreased in the last decades. Children, who had in the past little or no chance of surviving, are now living longer. Many of these children regain their health but a large group continues to suffer from life-threatening problems. These children need support and long-term care in palliative settings. As children approach death their symptoms change and their needs and those of their parents intensify. However, and despite treatment at end of life, children's suffering is never adequately relieved. Parents and children need particular types of help at this stage and the healthcare system must be responsive enough to accommodate their requirements.

This book covers the above topics among many others and provides solutions for improvement. The authors are to be commended for this comprehensive and cutting-edge compendium on pain in children and for providing the reader with evidence-based knowledge on pain assessment and management in children. The content of this book provides a road map towards understanding the various aspects of pain in children including palliative care and is essential reading for all those involved in this field. Nurses and other healthcare professionals working with children in different healthcare settings will benefit from the state-of-the-art work provided in this book.

Huda Abu-Saad Huijer RN, PhD, FEANS
Professor of Nursing Science
Director, School of Nursing
American University of Beirut
Beirut, Lebanon

List of Contributors

Elizabeth Bruce, Lead Clinical Nurse Specialist, Pain Control Service, Great Ormond Street Hospital for Children NHS Trust, London, United Kingdom

Stephanie J. Dowden, Clinical Nurse Consultant, Paediatric Palliative Care, Princess Margaret Hospital for Children, Subiaco, Perth, Australia (Formerly Clinical Nurse Consultant, Children's Pain Management Service, Royal Children's Hospital, Melbourne, Australia)

Joanna Smith, Lecturer, Child Health Nursing, School of Healthcare Studies, University of Leeds, United Kingdom

Jennifer Stinson, CIHR Post-Doctoral Research Fellow and Advanced Practice Nurse, Chronic Pain Program, Department of Anesthesia and Pain Medicine, The Hospital for Sick Children, Toronto, Ontario, Canada

Alison Twycross, Prinicipal Lecturer in Children's Nursing, Kingston University and St George's University of London, Faculty of Health and Social Care Sciences, London, United Kingdom

CHAPTER 1
Why Managing Pain in Children Matters
Alison Twycross

Introduction

Despite the ready availability of evidence to guide practice, the management of pain in children is often suboptimal. This chapter will start by providing a definition of pain and pain management and will highlight the consequences of unrelieved pain. Children's views about the effectiveness of their pain management will be discussed, and the commonly held misconceptions about pain in children identified. The factors thought to influence nurses' pain management practices will be outlined. Information about pain management standards published in several countries will be provided and how well nurses currently manage children's pain will be considered alongside the issue of professional accountability. Finally the ethical imperative for managing children's pain effectively will be identified.

1.1 What is Pain?

> **Pain** is whatever the experiencing person says it is, existing wherever they say it does (McCaffery 1972).
>
> '**Pain** is an unpleasant sensory and emotional experience associated with actual or potential tissue damage, or described in terms of such damage. Pain is always subjective. Each individual learns the application of the word through experiences related to injury in early life' (International Association for the Study of Pain [IASP] 1979, p. 249).

These two well-known definitions of pain illustrate that the experience of pain is both a subjective and an individual phenomenon. This is particularly clear in the IASP definition, which explains how the many facets of pain interrelate and affect pain perception. Although supporting the concept of pain as a subjective phenomenon, the original IASP definition fell short in relation to those unable to communicate verbally, including neonates, young children and disabled children. This was addressed in 2001 when the following amendment was made:

> 'The inability to communicate in no way negates the possibility that an individual is experiencing pain and is in need of appropriate pain relieving treatment.' (IASP 2001, p. 2)

> **Pain management** means applying the stages of the nursing process – assessment, planning, implementation and evaluation – to the treatment of pain.

Pain management therefore involves:

- assessing the child's pain;
- selecting appropriate pain relieving interventions;
- implementing these interventions;
- evaluating the effectiveness of these interventions.

1.2 Consequences of Unrelieved Pain

Painful experiences are part of life for every child (Fearon et al. 1996; Van Cleve et al. 1996; Perquin et al. 2000; McGrath and Hillier 2003). Pain has an important purpose, serving as a warning or protective mechanism, and people who are unable to feel pain often suffer extensive tissue damage (Melzack and Wall 1996). However, unrelieved pain has a number of undesirable physical and psychological consequences (Box 1.1). When these are considered, the need to manage children's pain effectively is clear.

BOX 1.1

Consequences of unrelieved pain

Physical effects

- Rapid, shallow, splinted breathing, which can lead to hypoxaemia and alkalosis
- Inadequate expansion of lungs and poor cough, which can lead to retention of secretions and atelectasis
- Increased heart rate, blood pressure and myocardial oxygen requirements, which can lead to cardiac morbidity and ischaemia
- Increased stress hormones (e.g. cortisol, adrenaline, catecholamines), which in turn increase the metabolic rate, impede healing and decrease immune function
- Slowing or stasis of gut and urinary systems, which leads to nausea, vomiting, ileus and urinary retention
- Muscle tension, spasm and fatigue, which lead to reluctance to move spontaneously and refusal to ambulate, further delaying recovery

Psychological effects

- Behavioural disturbances – fear, anxiety, distress, sleep disturbance, reduced coping, developmental regression

---

Poor pain management in early life can affect children when older. The results of studies demonstrating this are outlined in Box 1.2.

1.3 Children's Views about the Effectiveness of Pain Management

Pain is a bio-psycho-social experience (see Chapter 3). One individual cannot predict what another person will feel during a painful episode. When considering children's painful experiences it is, therefore, essential to explore children's views. Indeed the United Nations Convention of the Rights of the Child states that:

'Children's views must be taken into account in all matters affecting them, subject to children's age and maturity.'

BOX 1.2

Examples of research demonstrating the effects of poor pain management

Taddio et al. 1997

- Data from a clinical trial studying the use of EMLA® during routine vaccinations at 4 or 6 months was used to ascertain whether the effect of having a circumcision impacted on boys' pain response.
- Boys, who had been circumcised without anaesthesia as neonates, were observed to react significantly more intensely to vaccinations than uncircumcised boys ($p > 0.001$).
- Supported findings from a previous study (Taddio et al. 1995).

Grunau et al. 1998

- Examined the pain-related attitudes in two groups of children, aged 8–10 years: extremely low birthweight children ($n = 47$) and full birthweight children ($n = 37$).
- The very low birthweight group of children had been exposed to painful procedures as neonates, the other group had not.
- Children were shown the *Pediatric Pain Inventory*, which comprises 24 line drawings, each depicting a potentially painful event (Lollar et al. 1982).
- The two groups of children did not differ in their overall perceptions of pain intensity. However, the very low birthweight children rated medical pain intensity significantly higher ($p < 0.004$) than psychosocial pain, suggesting that their early experiences affected their later perceptions of pain.

Saxe et al. 2001

- Investigated the relationship between the dose of morphine administered during a child's hospitalisation for an acute burn and the course of post-traumatic stress disorder (PTSD) symptoms over the 6-month period following discharge.
- Children ($n = 24$) admitted to the hospital for an acute burn were assessed twice with the Child PTSD Reaction Index: while in the hospital and 6 months after discharge. The Colored Analogue Pain Scale was also administered during the hospitalisation. All patients received morphine while in the hospital. The mean dose of morphine (mg/kg/day) was calculated for each subject.
- There was a significant association between the dose of morphine received while in the hospital and a 6-month reduction in PTSD symptoms. Children receiving higher doses of morphine had a greater reduction in PTSD symptoms.

Rennick et al. 2002

- A prospective cohort study of patients ($n = 120$) in paediatric intensive care units and medical-surgical wards.
- 17.5% of patients expressed significant medical fears 6 weeks after discharge.
- 14% continue to express these fears 6 months later.

Taddio et al. 2002

- A prospective cohort study of babies ($n = 21$) born to mothers with diabetes and babies ($n = 21$) born to mothers with an uneventful pregnancy. Infants of diabetic mothers had repeated heel sticks in the first 24–36 hours of life.
- Babies of diabetic mothers demonstrated significantly greater pain behaviours at venepuncture for newborn blood screening ($p = 0.04$).

Further information about the long-term consequences of pain in neonates can be found in Grunau (2000) and Goldschneider and Anand (2003).

The effects of poorly managed pain on older children are discussed in McGrath and Hillier (2003).

This is supported by current policy (for example, Department of Health [DH] 2004). Children's views about how well their pain has been managed have been explored in three studies (Box 1.3). Despite the limited number of studies in this area it is evident that from the child's perspective there is need to evaluate practices. (Further discussion about undertaking research with children can be found in Chapter 11.)

BOX 1.3

Studies exploring children's views about pain management

Alex and Ritchie (1992)

- Children ($n = 24$), aged 7–11 years, were asked about their pain postoperatively following ortho-paedic, abdominal or neurological surgery.
- Children rated their pain three times a day for the first three postoperative days using a vertical visual analogue scale and were then interviewed about their pain.
- Children felt that nurses needed to take a more active role in pain management. They suggested, for example, that nurses need to communicate with children about their pain.

Doorbar and McClarey (1999)

- Data collected from several sources to obtain a picture of children's perceptions and experiences of pain – all participants had had recent experience of acute pain.
- Children ($n = 61$) gave in-depth interviews; children ($n = 45$) drew pictures or completed sentence and/or picture sheets; and children ($n = 67$), took part in a *pain conference*. The pain conference used several data collection methods including drama, art and video workshops, graffiti wall, post boxes and a short questionnaire.
- The children indicated that they felt that pain was poorly managed in hospital and that healthcare professionals needed to listen to what children were saying about their pain. Children, again, felt that nurses needed to communicate with children about their pain and felt that better explana-tions about what to expect were needed. Some children found it difficult to convince others that they were in pain.

Polkki et al. (2003)

- Children ($n = 52$), aged 8–12 years, were asked about their postoperative pain experiences and to suggest what nurses could do to improve postoperative pain management.
- Children indicated that they wished the nurses had given them more or stronger analgesic drugs, as soon as they asked for them, and that they would like nurses to ask them about their pain on an hourly basis. Children would also like nurses to provide them with *meaningful things to do* to distract them from their pain.

Further insight into children's experiences of pain in hospital can be found in Kortesluoma and Nikkonen (2004).

1.4 Misconceptions About Pain

Children's pain is clearly not being managed adequately; one reason for this could be the perceptions of the nurses caring for the child. A number of misconceptions about children's pain have been identified. A comprehensive summary of these is provided by Twycross (1998). The key misconceptions and a summary of the evidence demonstrating their myth-ological status can be seen in Table 1.1. (Other misconceptions are discussed in Chapters 2, 4 and 9.) These misconceptions have all been shown to have no scientific basis.

Table 1.1 Key misconceptions about pain in children

Misconception	Evidence
Infants do not feel as much pain as adults	Pain pathways (although immature) are present at birth and pain impulses are able to travel to and from the pain centres in the brain (Wolf 1999; Coskun and Anand 2000; Fitzgerald 2000) Neonates exhibit behavioural, physiological and hormonal responses to pain (Franck 1986; Hogan and Choonara 1996; Carter 1997; Abu-Saad et al. 1998; Stevens 1999).
Infants cannot feel pain because of an immature nervous system	Complete myelination is not necessary for pain to be felt (Volpe 1981) Painful stimuli are transmitted by both myelinated and unmyelinated fibres (Volpe 1981; Craig and Grunau 1993) Incomplete myelination implies only a slower conduction speed in the nerves, which is offset by the shorter distances the impulse has to travel (Volpe 1981; Anand and Hickey 1987) Noxious stimuli have been shown to produce a cortical pain response in preterm babies (Bartocci et al. 2006; Slater et al. 2006).
Young children cannot indicate where pain is located	Children as young as 4 years old can demonstrate on a body chart where they hurt without knowing the names of body parts (Van Cleve and Savedra 1993) Children are able to report the intensity of pain by the age of 3–4 years (Harbeck and Peterson 1992)
Active children are not in pain A child engaged in playing activities cannot be in pain	Increased activity is often a sign of pain (Eland 1985) Children are particularly gifted in the use of distraction and use play as a diversion and as a coping mechanism (Eland 1985; McCaffery and Beebe 1989)
Sleeping children cannot be in pain	Sleep may be the result of exhaustion because of persistent pain (Hawley 1984)

1.5 Factors Affecting Nurses' Perceptions of Pain

The results of several studies provide an indicator of the factors, relating to both the child and the nurse, which may affect pain management practices (Table 1.2). This research has been conducted over the past two decades and the results are contradictory.

Other suggestions as to why pain management practices remain poor include:

- nurses distancing themselves from their patients because of the stressful nature of caring for people in pain (Atchison et al. 1986; Choiniere et al. 1990; Glass and Knight 1996; Nagy 1999);
- nurses managing patients' pain behaviours rather than managing their pain (Burokas 1985; Gadish et al. 1988; Ross et al. 1991; Woodgate and Kristjanson 1996; Byrne et al. 2001);
- nurses becoming desensitised to patients' pain over time (Davitz and Davitz 1981; Allcock and Standen 1999, 2001).

Table 1.2 Factors that influence nurses' perceptions of pain in children

Factor	Burokas (1985)	Wallace (1989)	Gadish et al. (1988)	Ross et al. (1991)	Hamers et al. (1994)	Hamers et al. (1996)	Twycross (2004)
Age of child	X		√		√	X	
Child's temperament		√			√	√	
Child's gender	X						
Diagnosis/type of surgery	X		√	√	√	X	
Time since surgery			√	√			
Type of unit	√						
Priority nurse gives to pain relief/their attitude to analgesic drugs			X	√	√		X
Nurse having a child of their own who has had a painful experience	√						
Nurses' educational level/knowledge of nurse			√		√		X
Nurses' workload/ lack of time				√	√		X
Nurses' past experiences of pain management	√			√			

√ = significant difference found; X = no significant difference found

1.6 Pain Management Standards

Pain management standards have been published in several countries to promote best practice. In England, the *National Service Framework for Children, Young People and Maternity Services* (NSF) (DH 2004) includes six pain standards (Box 1.4), making it clear that pain management is an essential component of quality care for children in hospital.

Within the USA the Joint Commission for the Accreditation of Healthcare Organisations (JCAHO) published standards for pain management in 2001 (Box 1.5). These standards are not specific to children but mean that, to be accredited, each hospital in the USA needs to demonstrate that it is meeting these standards. The JCAHO standards reflect the standards from the English NSF. Whether the implementation of these standards improves pain management needs to be evaluated.

Pain management standards have also been produced in other countries. Some of those published in the last 10 years are listed in Box 1.6. These guidelines and standards provide us with the knowledge about how pain should be managed.

BOX 1.4

Pain standards from the English *National Service Framework*

Standard 4.28

- Pain is unpleasant, delays recovery, and adds to the trauma of illness, injury and clinical procedures
- Historically, pain has been underestimated and undertreated
- There is evidence that pain remains inadequately dealt with for children in hospital

Standard 4.29

- Where procedures are planned, children should be prepared through play and education, pain relief should be planned for use during the procedure
- The use of psychological therapies, including distraction, coping skills and cognitive-behavioural approaches should be used for procedural pain and for pain from illness or trauma

Standard 4.30

- To treat children's pain effectively, a thorough pain assessment is necessary, and a number of guides are available to do this
- These guides offer different options for communication, and can be completed in different ways by the child, family or professionals
- Particular attention should be given to children who cannot express their pain because of their level of speech or understanding, communication difficulties, and those with altered consciousness or serious illness

Standard 4.31

- The treatment of children's pain using medicines requires appropriate choice of drug, dose, frequency and route
- Research has found that some hospital staff may be reluctant to prescribe at all, and they tend to use a dose that is too small to address the child's pain adequately
- Protocols, education and training can support staff in their management of children's pain, which should be reviewed regularly through audit
- The involvement of pharmacists in the development of pain management guidelines is encouraged

Standard 4.32

- Children with long-term pain need a similar approach, spanning prevention, assessment and treatment
- Special consideration should be given to children recovering from trauma and burns, and children with cancers, joint conditions, sickle cell disease, and those needing palliative care

Standard 4.33

- Hospital policies for managing children's pain should apply to all children in every hospital department, including newborns in neonatal units
- Special focus should be given to children in accident and emergency departments, postoperative pain, pain related to procedures, and long-term pain in cancer

Source: DH (2004)

An international consensus document relating to the assessment and management of pain in neonates was published by Anand and the International Evidence-Based Group for Neonatal Pain in 2001. This document identified general principles for the prevention and management of pain in newborns. These recommendations are outlined in Box 1.7.

BOX 1.5

JCAHO Pain management standards

Standard

RI.1.2.9 Patients have the right to appropriate assessment and management of pain.

Intent of RI.1.2.9

Pain can be a common part of the patient experience; unrelieved pain has adverse physical and psychological effects. The patient's right to pain management is respected and supported. The healthcare organisation plans, supports, and coordinates activities and resources to assure the pain of all patients is recognised and addressed appropriately. This includes:

(a) initial assessment and regular assessment of pain;
(b) education of all relevant providers in pain assessment and management;
(c) education of patients, and families when appropriate, regarding their roles in managing pain as well as the potential limitations and side effects of pain treatments; and
(d) after taking into account personal, cultural, spiritual, and/or ethnic beliefs, communicating to patients and families that pain management is an important part of care.

BOX 1.6

Other pain standards and guidelines

Australia and New Zealand

Australian and New Zealand College of Anaesthetists and Faculty of Pain Medicine (2007) *Acute Pain Management: Scientific Evidence*, Updated 2nd edition, Australian and New Zealand College of Anaesthetists, Melbourne. Available from: http://www.anzca.edu.au/resources/books-and-publications/acutepain_update.pdf

Australian and New Zealand College of Anaesthetists and Faculty of Pain Medicine (2005) *Acute Pain Management: Scientific Evidence*, 2nd edition, Australian and New Zealand College of Anaesthetists, Melbourne. (Pain in children addressed in Chapter 10 Section 1). Available from: http://www.anzca.edu.au/resources/books-and-publications/acutepain.pdf

Royal Australasian College of Physicians, Paediatrics and Child Health Division (2005) *Guideline Statement: Management of Procedure-Related Pain in Children and Adolescents,* Royal Australian College of Physicians, Sydney. Available from: http://www.racp.edu.au/index.cfm?objectid=A4268489–2A57–5487-DEF14F15791C4F22

Royal Australasian College of Physicians (2006) Management of Procedure-Related Pain in Neonates (Guideline Statement), *Journal of Paediatrics and Child Health*, 42: 531–539. Available from: http://www.racp.edu.au/index.cfm?objectid=A4268489–2A57–5487-DEF14F15791C4F22

United Kingdom

Howard, R., Carter, B., Curry, J., Morton, N., Rivett, K., Rose, M., Tyrrell, J., Walker, S. and Williams, G. (2008) Good Practice in Postoperative and Procedural Pain Management, *Pediatric Anesthesia*, 18: 1–81.

Procedural pain guidelines for the newborn in the United Kingdom: McKechnie, L. and Levene, M., J (2007) Perinatal advance online publication, doi:10.1038/sj.jp.7211822. Available from: http://www.nature.com/jp/journal/vaop/ncurrent/index.html#13092007

Scottish Intercollegiate Guidelines Network (SIGN) (2004) Safe Sedation of Children Undergoing Diagnostic and Therapeutic Procedures. A National Clinical Guideline. Available from: http://www.apagbi.org.uk/docs/sign58.pdf

NHS Quality Improvement Scotland (2004) Safe Sedation of Children Undergoing Diagnostic and Therapeutic Procedures: A National Clinical Guideline, NHS Quality Improvement Scotland, Edinburgh. Available from: http://www.sign.ac.uk/pdf/sign58.pdf

---

BOX 1.6 Continued

Royal College of Nursing (2000) *The Recognition and Assessment of Acute Pain in Children: Technical Report*, RCN Publishing, London. Available from: http://www.rcn.org.uk/publications/pdf/guidelines/cpg_contents.pdf

Royal College of Paediatrics and Child Health (1997) *Prevention and Control of Pain in Children: A Manual for Healthcare Professionals*, BMJ Publishing Group, London

USA

American Academy of Pediatrics and American Pain Society (2001) The assessment and management of acute pain in infants, children and adolescents, *Pediatrics*, 108(3): 793–797. Available from: http://www.ampainsoc.org/advocacy/pediatric2.htm

World Health Organization

World Health Organization (1998) *Cancer Pain Relief and Palliative Care in Children*, World Health Organisation, Geneva

---

BOX 1.7

General principles for the prevention and management of pain in newborns

- Pain in newborns is often unrecognised and undertreated. Neonates do feel pain, and analgesia should be prescribed when indicated during their medical care
- If a procedure is painful in adults, it should be considered painful in newborns, even if they are preterm
- Compared with older groups, newborns may experience a greater sensitivity to pain and are more susceptible to the long-term effects of painful stimulation
- Adequate treatment of pain may be associated with decreased clinical complications and decreased mortality
- The appropriate use of environmental, behavioural and pharmacological interventions can prevent, reduce or eliminate neonatal pain in many clinical situations
- Sedation does not provide pain relief and may mask the neonate's response to pain
- Healthcare professionals have the responsibility for assessment, prevention and management of pain in neonates
- Clinical units providing healthcare to newborns should develop guidelines and protocols for the management of neonatal pain

Source: Anand et al. (2001)

1.7 How Effective are Current Pain Management Practices?

Few studies have focused on exactly how healthcare professionals manage children's pain. The results of key studies examining nurses' practices over the past 10 years are summarised in Box 1.8. The results of these studies indicate that nursing practice does not always conform to current best practice guidelines. There is very little information regarding the perceptions of other healthcare professionals about children's pain. It is likely that suboptimal practices would also be evident among other professional groups.

BOX 1.8

Studies examining nurses' pain management practices

Jacob and Puntillo (1999)

- Nurses ($n = 260$) in the USA completed a questionnaire about their pain management practices.
- Nurses were not consistently assessing pain in children, and pain management practices were not based on systematic assessment.
- The most frequently reported tool for assessing pain was the numerical rating scale.
- Nurses reported that they were not consistently administering analgesics for painful procedures.
- Nurses rarely used distraction and relaxation techniques (these were the most frequently reported non-drug methods used).

Byrne et al. (2001)

- Observational data were collected of the verbal interaction of nurses ($n = 13$) with children ($n = 16$). Standardised open-ended interviews were also carried out with the nurses, children and parents. Data was analysed using discourse analysis.
- Children were required to conform to ward routines and schedules of recovery.
- Rather than asking the child how much pain they were in, nurses appeared to manage pain using a set of behavioural milestones.

Polkki et al. (2001)

- Nurses ($n = 162$) completed a questionnaire about their use of non-drug methods of pain relief in five Finnish hospitals.
- Distraction and preparatory information were reported as being used frequently and imagery was only used occasionally.
- Almost all nurses indicated that they used positioning. Massage and the application of heat/cold were used less frequently.
- TENS was hardly ever used when managing children's postoperative pain.

Twycross (2007)

- Registered nurses ($n = 13$) on a children's surgical ward in the English Midlands were each observed for a period of five hours per shift for two to four shifts. The role of the *observer as participant* was adopted, whereby the researcher could shadow the nurse and act primarily as an observer.
- Although nurses administered analgesic drugs when a child complained of pain, in most other areas practices did not conform to current recommendations and were in need of improvement. Nurses did not, for example, routinely assess a child's pain, nor use non-drug methods of pain relief on a regular basis.

1.8 Professional Accountability

Registered nurses are accountable for their actions. In the UK nurses' professional conduct must conform to the Nursing and Midwifery Council's (NMC) Code (2008). The code states that nurses must use the best available evidence and keep their knowledge and skills up to date (Box 1.9).

Current healthcare policy across the UK recognises the need for evidence-based practice (DH 1999, 2000; Scottish Executive Health Department (SEHD) 2000; SEHD 2001; DH 2004). Indeed, the (English) *National Service Framework for Children, Young People and Maternity Services* (DH 2004) states that children and young people should receive high quality evidence-based hospital care.

BOX 1.9

What the NMC Code (2008) says in relation to using evidence in practice and keeping knowledge and skills up to date

Use the best available evidence
- You must deliver care based on the best available evidence or best practice.
- You must ensure any advice you give is evidence based if you are suggesting healthcare products or services.
- You must ensure that the use of complementary or alternative therapies is safe and in the best interests of those in your care.

Keep your skills and knowledge up to date
- You must have the knowledge and skills for safe and effective practice when working without direct supervision.
- You must recognise and work within the limits of your competence.
- You must keep your knowledge and skills up to date throughout your working life.
- You must take part in appropriate learning and practice activities that maintain and develop your competence and performance.

Evidence-based practice is:
- the conscientious, explicit and judicious use of current best evidence in making decisions about the healthcare of patients (Sackett et al 1997);
- doing the right things right (Muir-Grey 1997).

Everyone is responsible for pain management. The bedside nurse is as responsible as the analgesia prescriber or the member of the specialist pain management team. If any of these clinicians do not fulfil their role, the patient suffers. Thus all healthcare professionals have a responsibility to:

- learn and be educated about pain;
- know about pain management strategies (pharmacological strategies and non-drug methods);
- assess and respond to patients in pain.

Pain management practices should be based on **scientific facts** or agreed best practice, not personal beliefs or opinions. The burden of proof lies with the healthcare professional, **not** the patient.

The aim of this book is to provide healthcare professionals with knowledge about current research and best practice guidelines in relation to managing children's pain. Each practitioner is accountable and responsible for evaluating their practices to ensure they conform to current best practice guidelines.

1.9 Managing Pain in Children is an Ethical Imperative

The United Nations, in its *Declaration on the Rights of the Child*, states that:

'children should in all circumstances be among the first to receive protection and relief, and should be protected from all forms of neglect, cruelty and exploitation.' (United Nations 1989)

This principle can be applied to the management of pain, particularly as good practice guidelines are available (Box 1.6). Further, the UNICEF Child-Friendly Hospital Initiative highlights the importance of pain management, stating that:

> 'A team will be established in the hospital whose remit is to establish standards and guidance in the control of pain and discomfort (psychological as well as physical) in children.' (UNICEF 1999, p. 8)

Yet there is evidence that children still experience moderate to severe unrelieved pain (Polkki et al. 2003; Vincent and Denyes 2004; Johnston et al. 2005). Failing to provide children with satisfactory pain relief can be considered a violation of their human rights. Indeed, when the consequences of unrelieved pain are taken into account, managing children's postoperative pain effectively is an ethical imperative (Kachoyeanos and Zollo 1995; Franck 1998; Rich 2000).

Summary

- Pain is an individual and subjective phenomenon.
- Unrelieved pain has a number of undesirable physical and psychological consequences.
- Children's reports of how well their pain is managed indicate that practices are suboptimal.
- The continuing belief in misconceptions about children's pain by some healthcare professionals may account, at least in part, for suboptimal practices.
- Other reasons for suboptimal practices include nurses distancing themselves from patients in pain; nurses managing patients' pain behaviours rather than their pain; and nurses becoming desensitised to patients' pain.
- Clinical guidelines and best practice standards have been produced in several countries to promote good pain management practices.
- Healthcare professionals' practices in some areas need evaluating to ensure that they conform to current best practice guidelines.
- Every healthcare professional is responsible for managing pain.
- Pain management practices should be based on scientific facts, not personal beliefs or opinions.
- Managing children's pain effectively is an ethical imperative.

Useful web resources

The IASP Special Interest Group on Pain in Childhood: http://childpain.org/
International Association for the Study of Pain (IASP): http://www.iasp-pain.org
Pain Resource Book: www.painsourcebook.ca/index.html provides information about standards and guidelines relating to pain management from across the world

---

References

Abu-Saad, H.H., Bours, G.J., Stevens, B. and Hamers, J.P. (1998) Assessment of pain in the neonate, *Seminars in Perinatology*, 22(5): 402–16.
Alex, M. and Ritchie, J. (1992) School-aged children's interpretation of their experience with acute surgical pain, *Journal of Pediatric Surgery*, 7(3): 171–188.

Allcock, N. and Standen, P. (1999) The effect of student nurses' experiences over the Common Foundation Programme on their inferences of suffering, *International Journal of Nursing Studies*, 36(1): 65–72.

Allcock, N. and Standen, P. (2001) Student nurses' experiences of caring for patients in pain, *International Journal of Nursing Studies*, 38(3): 287–95.

Anand, K.J.S., Hickey, P.R. (1987) Pain and its effects in the human neonate and fetus, New England *Journal of Medicine*, 317: 1321–1329.

Anand, K.J.S. and the International Evidence-Based Group for Neonatal Pain (2001) Consensus statement for the prevention and management of pain in the newborn, *Archives of Pediatrics and Adolescent Medicine*, 155: 173–180.

Atchison, N., Guercio, P. and Monaco, C. (1986) Pain in the pediatric burn patient: Nursing assessment and perception, *Journal of Pediatric Nursing*, 9: 399–409.

Bartocci, M., Bergqvist, L.L., Lagercrantz, H. and Anand, K.J.S. (2006) Pain activates cortical areas in the preterm newborn brain, *Pain*, 122: 109–117.

Burokas, L. (1985) Factors affecting nurses' decisions to medicate pediatric patients after surgery, *Heart and Lung*, 14(4): 373–378.

Byrne, A., Morton, J. and Salmon, P. (2001) Defending against patients' pain: a qualitative analysis of nurses' responses to children's postoperative pain, *Journal of Psychosomatic Research*, 50: 69–76.

Carter, B. (1997) Pantomimes of pain, distress, repose and lability: the world of the preterm baby, *Journal of Child Healthcare*, 1(1): 17–23.

Choiniere, M., Melzack, R., Girard, N., Rondeau, J. and Paquin, M. (1990) Comparisons between patients' and nurses' assessment of pain and medication efficacy in severe burn injuries, *Pain*, 40: 143–151.

Coskun, V. and Anand, K.J.S. (2000) Development of supraspinal pain processing. In Anand K.J.S., Stevens B.J. and McGrath P.J. (eds.) *Pain in Neonates*, 2nd edition, Elsevier, Amsterdam, pp. 23–54.

Craig, K.D. and Grunau, R.V.E. (1993) Neonatal pain perception and behavioural measurement. In Anand, K.J.S. and McGrath, P.J. (eds.) *Pain in Neonates*, Elsevier, Amsterdam, pp. 67–105.

Davitz, J. and Davitz, L. (1981) *Influences on Patients' Pain and Distress*, Springer, New York.

Department of Health (1999) *Making a Difference*, The Stationery Office, London.

Department of Health (2000) *The NHS Plan*, The Stationery Office, London.

Department of Health (2004) *National Service Framework for Children, Young People and Maternity Services*, The Stationery Office, London.

Doorbar, P. and McClarey, M. (1999) *Ouch! Sort It Out: Children's Experiences of Pain*, London, RCN Publishing.

Eland, J. (1985) Myths about pain in children, *The Candlelighters Childhood Cancer Foundation*, V(1).

Fearon, I., McGrath, P.J. and Achat, H. (1996) 'Booboos': the study of everyday pain among young children, *Pain*, 68: 55–62.

Fitzgerald, M. (2000) Development of the peripheral and spinal pain system. In Anand K.J.S., Stevens B.J. and McGrath P.J. (eds.) *Pain in Neonates*, 2nd edition, Elsevier, Amsterdam, pp. 9–22.

Franck, L. (1986) A new method to quantitatively describe pain behavior in infants, *Nursing Research*, 35(1): 28–31.

Franck, L.S. (1998) The ethical imperative to treat pain in infants: are we doing the best we can? *Neonatal Intensive Care*, 11(5): 28–34.

Gadish, H., Gonzalez, J. and Hayes, J.S. (1988) Factors affecting nurses' decisions to administer pediatric pain medication postoperatively, *Journal of Pediatric Nursing*, 3(6): 383–389.

Glass, D.C. and Knight, J.D. (1996) Perceived control, depressive symptomatology and professional burnout: A review of the evidence, *Psychological Health*, 11: 23–48.

Goldschneider, K.R. and Anand, K.J.S. (2003) Long-term consequences of pain in neonates. In Schechter, N.L., Berde, C.B. and Yaster, M. (eds.) *Pain in Infants, Children and Adolescents*, 2nd edition, Lippincott, Williams & Wilkins, Baltimore, pp 58–70.

Grunau, R.E. (2000) Long-term consequences of pain in human neonates. In Anand, K.J.S., Stevens, B.J., McGrath, P.J. (eds.) *Pain in Neonates*, 2nd edition, Elsevier, Amsterdam, pp 55–76.

Grunau, R.V.E., Whitfield, M.F. and Petrie, J. (1998) Children's judgements about pain at aged 8–10 years: Do extremely low birthweight children differ from their full birthweight peers? *Journal of Child Psychology and Psychiatry*, 39(4): 587–594.

Hamers, J., Abu-Saad, H., Halfens, R.J.G. and Schumacher, J.N.M. (1994) Factors influencing nurses' pain assessment and interventions in children, *Journal of Advanced Nursing*, 20: 853–860.

Hamers, J.P.H., Abu-Saad, H.H., van den Hout, M.A., Halfens, R.J.G. and Kester, A.D.M. (1996) The influence of children's vocal expressions, age, medical diagnosis and information obtained from parents on nurses' pain assessments and decisions regarding interventions, *Pain*, 65: 53–61.

Harbeck, C. and Peterson, L. (1992) Elephants dancing in my head: a developmental approach to children's concepts of specific pains, *Child Development*, 63: 138–149.

Hawley, D. (1984) Postoperative pain in children: misconceptions, descriptions and interventions, *Pediatric Nursing*, 10(1): 20–23.

Hogan, M. and Choonara, I. (1996) Measuring pain in neonates: an objective score, *Paediatric Nursing*, 8(10): 24–27.

International Association for the Study of Pain (1979) Pain terms: a list with definitions and notes on usage, *Pain*, 6: 249–252.

International Association for the Study of Pain (2001) IASP Definition of Pain, *IASP Newsletter*, 2: 2.

Jacob, E. and Puntillo, K.A. (1999) A survey of nursing practice in the assessment and management of pain in children, *Pediatric Nursing*, 25(3): 278–286.

Johnston, C.C., Gagnon, A.J., Pepler, C.J. and Bourgault, P. (2005) Pain in the emergency department with one-week follow-up of pain resolution, *Pain Research and Management*, 10(2): 67–70.

Joint Commission for the Accreditation of Healthcare Organizations (2000) *Pain Assessment and Management Standards*, JCAHO, Oakbrook Terrace, Illinois.

Kachoyeanos, M. and Zollo, M. (1995) Ethics in pain management of infants and children, *American Journal of Maternal/Child Nursing*, 20: 142–147.

Kortesluoma, K-L. and Nikkonen, M. (2004) 'I had this horrible pain': the sources and causes of pain experiences in 4- to 11-year-old hospitalized children, *Journal of Child Health Care*, 8(3): 210–231.

Lollar, D.J., Smits, S.J. and Patterson, D.L. (1982) Assessment of pediatric pain: An empirical perspective, *Journal of Pediatric Psychology*, 7: 267–77.

McCaffery, M. (1972) *Nursing Management of the Patient in Pain*, Lippincott, Philadelphia.

McCaffery, M. and Beebe, A.B. (1989) *Pain: Clinical Manual for Nursing Practice*, C V Mosby, St Louis.

McGrath, P.A. and Hillier, L.M. (2003) Modifying the psychological factors that intensify children's pain and prolong disability. In Schechter, N.L., Berde, C.B. and Yaster, M. (eds.) *Pain in Infants, Children and Adolescents*, 2nd edition, Lippincott, Williams & Wilkins, Baltimore, pp 85–104.

Melzack, R. and Wall, P. (1996) *The Challenge of Pain*, Updated 2nd edition, Penguin, London.

Muir-Gray, J. (1997) *Evidence-Based Healthcare: How to Make Health Policy and Management Decisions*, Churchill Livingstone, New York.

Nagy, S. (1999) Strategies used by burns nurses to cope with the infliction of pain on patients, *Journal of Advanced Nursing*, 29(6): 1427–1433.

Nursing and Midwifery Council (2008) *The Code: Standards of Conduct, Performance and Ethics for Nurses and Midwives*, NMC, London.

Perquin, C.W., Hazebroek-Kampschreur, A.A.J.M., Hunfield, J.A.M., Bohen, A.M., van Suijlekom-Smit, L.W.A., Passchier, J. and van der Wouden, J.C. (2000) Pain in children and adolescents: a common experience, *Pain*, 87: 51–58.

Polkki, T., Vehvilamen-Julkunen, K. and Pietila, A-M. (2001) Nonpharmacological methods in relieving children's postoperative pain: a survey on hospital nurses in Finland, *Journal of Advanced Nursing*, 34(4): 483–492.

Polkki, T., Pietila, A-M. and Vehvilamen-Julkunen, K. (2003) Hospitalized children's descriptions of their experiences with postsurgical pain-relieving methods, *International Journal of Nursing Studies*, 40: 33–44.

Rennick, J.E., Johnston, C.C., Dougherty, G., Platt, R. and Ritchie, J.A. (2002) Children's psychological responses after critical illness and exposure to invasive technology, *Journal of Developmental & Behavioral Pediatrics*, 23(3):133–144.

Rich, B.A. (2000) An ethical analysis of the barriers to effective pain management, *Cambridge Quarterly of Healthcare Ethics*, 9: 54–70.

Ross, R.S., Bush J.P. and Crummette B.D. (1991) Factors affecting nurses' decisions to administer PRN analgesic medication to children after surgery: an analog investigation, *Journal of Pediatric Psychology*, 16(2): 151–167.

Sackett, D., Richardson, W.S., Rosenberg, W. and Haynes, R.B. (1997) *Evidence-Based Medicine: How to Practice and Teach EBM*, Churchill Livingstone, New York.

Saxe, G., Stoddard, F., Courtney, D., Cunningham, K., Chawla, N., Sheridan, R., King, D. and King, L. (2001) Relationship between acute morphine and the course of PTSD in children with burns, *Journal of the American Academy of Child & Adolescent Psychiatry*, 40(8):915–21.

Scottish Executive (2000) *Our National Health. A Plan for Action. A Plan for Change*, The Stationery Office, Edinburgh.

Scottish Executive (2001) *Caring for Scotland: The Strategy for Midwifery and Nursing in Scotland*, The Stationery Office, Edinburgh.

Slater, R., Cantarella, A., Gallella, S., Worley, A., Boyd, S., Meek, J. and Fitzgerald, M. (2006) Cortical pain response in human infants, *Journal of Neuroscience*, 26(14): 3662–3666.

Stevens, B. (1999) Pain in infants. In McCaffery, M. and Pasero, C. (eds.) *Pain: Clinical Manual*, 2nd edition, Mosby, St Louis, pp. 626–673.

Taddio, A., Goldbach, M., Ipp, M., Stevens, B. and Koren, G. (1995) Effect of neonatal circumcision on pain responses during vaccination in boys, *Lancet*, 345: 291–292.

Taddio, A., Katz, J., Ilersich, A.l. and Koren, G. (1997) Effect of neonatal circumcision on pain response during subsequent routine vaccination, *Lancet*, 349: 599–603.

Taddio, A., Shah, V., Gilbert-MacLeod, C. and Katz J. (2002) Conditioning and hyperalgesia in newborns exposed to repeated heel lances, *Journal of the American Medical Association*, 288(7):857–61.

Twycross A. (1998) Perceptions about paediatric pain. In Twycross, A., Moriarty, A. and Betts, T (eds.) *Paediatric Pain Management: A Multi-disciplinary Approach*, Radcliffe Medical Press, Oxford, pp. 1–24.

Twycross, A. (2004) *Children's Nurses' Pain Management Practices: Theoretical Knowledge, Perceived Importance and Decision-Making*, Unpublished PhD Thesis, University of Central Lancashire.

Twycross, A. (2007) What is the impact of theoretical knowledge on children's nurses' postoperative pain management practices? An exploratory study, *Nurse Education Today*, 27(7): 697–707.

United Nations (1989) *Convention on the Rights of the Child*, United Nations, New York.

UNICEF (1999) Global millennium targets: UNICEF child-friendly hospital initiative, *Paediatric Nursing*, 11(10): 7–8.

Van Cleve, L.J. and Savedra, M.C. (1993) Pain location: validity and reliability of body outline markings by 4- to 7-year-old children who are hospitalized, *Pediatric Nursing*, 19(3): 217–220.

Van Cleve, L., Johnson, L. and Pothier, P. (1996) Pain responses of hospitalised infants and children to venipuncture and intravenous cannulation, *Journal of Pediatric Nursing*, 11(3): 161–168.

Vincent, C.V.H. and Denyes, M.J. (2004) Relieving children's pain: nurses' abilities and analgesic administration practices, *Journal of Pediatric Nursing*, 19(1): 40–50.

Volpe J. (1981) *Neurology of the Newborn*, Saunders, Philadelphia.

Wallace, M. (1989) Temperament: a variable in children's pain management, *Pediatric Nursing*, 15(2): 118–121.

Wolf, A.R. (1999) Pain: nociception and the developing infant, *Paediatric Anaesthesia*, 9: 7–17.

Woodgate, R. and Kristjanson L. (1996) A young child's pain: how parents and nurses 'take care', *International Journal of Nursing Studies*, 33(3): 271–284.

CHAPTER 2
Anatomy and Physiology of Pain
Joanna Smith

Introduction

This chapter will provide an overview of the anatomy and physiology of the nervous system in relation to pain. Understanding the anatomical and physiological processes about pain is essential to:

- appreciate how the structure and function of the nervous system results in pain being a bio-psycho-social phenomenon;
- understand that different types of pain exist and are a result of different pathologies;
- challenge misconceptions relating to the pathophysiology of pain in children;
- select appropriate pain management strategies.

Pain is a multifaceted and complex phenomenon that is still not well understood. This is illustrated by the definitions of pain provided in Chapter 1 and the factors affecting an individual's pain perception discussed in Chapter 3. There is an ever-increasing amount of research into pain; as more is learned about pain the level of complexity becomes more apparent.

Within this chapter the misconceptions relating to the physiology of pain in children will be discussed. An overview of the anatomy of the nervous system in the context of pain management will then be provided. The different types of pain will be described. The physiology of nociceptive and neuropathic pain will be outlined. The gate control theory of pain will be used to explain individual variations in pain perception. The consequences of unrelieved pain are discussed in Chapters 1 and 7.

2.1 Misconceptions Relating to the Physiology of Pain in Children

Within Chapter 1 general misconceptions about pain in children are highlighted. These misconceptions are often related to a lack of understanding of the development/physiology of the nervous system and perceptions about the physiological processes relating to pain in children. The misconceptions relating to the physiology of pain in children are outlined in Table 2.1.

2.2 Overview of the Anatomy of the Nervous System

Although the nervous system functions as a whole, for descriptive purposes it is divided into the **central nervous system** and the **peripheral nervous system**.

- The central nervous system consists of the brain and spinal cord, with the brain being the control centre for the entire nervous system.

Table 2.1 Misconceptions about the physiology of pain in children

Misconception	Facts
Pain pathways in young infants are not developed sufficiently for them to experience pain	Neural pathways are in place in utero and maturation continues into adulthood, consequently pain responses exist even in the very premature neonate Immature synapses within the spinal cord may cause activation of nerve impulses below the normal threshold increasing the pain response Immature *gating mechanisms* in the neonate result in an inability to distinguish between some types of stimuli, which may result in an exaggerated pain response
Lack of myelination prevents young infants from feeling pain	Myelin does not influence the generation of a nerve impulse The presence of myelin increases the speed of the impulse The process of myelination begins at about twenty-two weeks gestation
A young child's lack of previous experiences limits their ability to experience pain	Emotional processing and cognitive abilities develop over time, which may influence pain coping mechanisms Infants and young children have not yet developed these coping strategies and therefore they express pain differently

Source: Fitzgerald and Howard (2003)

- The spinal cord is the link between the brain and other organs of the body.
- The peripheral nervous system consists of all the sensory and motor nerve networks that link the central nervous system with the periphery, for example, the skin, muscles, glands and organs.

The two cell types unique to the nervous system are the **neurone** (nerve cell) and the **dendrite** (glial cell), which support the functions of neurones. The neurone has a highly specialised structure that enables information to be received from sensory receptors and transmitted to effector organs such as muscles. Neurones consist of a cell body from which several processes appear (Figure 2.1). Dendrites receive information, which is transmitted to the cell body. The axon or nerve fibre carries information away from the cell body to the effector organ.

There are three types of neurones:

1. Afferent or sensory neurones transmit nerve impulses from peripheral receptors to the central nervous system.
2. Efferent or motor neurones transmit nerve impulses away from the spinal cord to the effector organs.
3. Interneurones integrate information within the central nervous system.

The most important feature of a neurone is the ability to generate and conduct nerve impulses, which enables information to travel around the central nervous system. Before a sensory signal can be relayed to the nervous system it must be converted into a nerve impulse in an axon. This involves a process of opening ion channels in the neurone's cell membrane in response to stimuli. The disruption of the ion concentration outside and inside the cell membrane causes an ionic current flow, creating a nerve impulse (Waugh and Grant 2006; Longstaff 2005; Swenson 2006).

Once activated, the speed of a nerve impulse is independent of the stimulus strength and is determined by the presence or absence of myelin, the diameter of the nerve fibre and body temperature. Myelin is a fatty substance that wraps round the axons of certain neurones and speeds up the nerve impulse. Nerve myelination begins from about

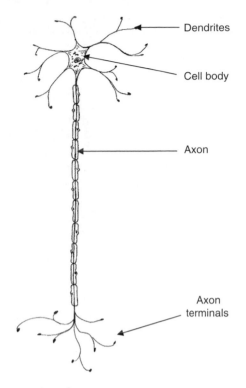

Figure 2.1 Schematic representation of a neurone.

22 weeks of gestation in the spinal cord and slightly later in the brain. The process continues postnatally and is thought not to be complete until adult life (Padgett 2006).

There are two types of nociceptive fibres: A-delta fibres and C fibres, which are primarily responsible for pain transmission:

- **A-delta fibres** have a large diameter, are myelinated, have fast impulse speeds and produce sensations that are well localised and sharp.
- **C fibres** have a smaller diameter, are unmyelinated, have slower impulse speeds and produce sensations that are poorly localised, diffuse, aching and dull.

A series of actions occur when a neurone receives a painful stimuli, which are outlined in Box 2.1.

BOX 2.1

Neurone response to painful stimuli

- Free sensory nerve endings are located in the skin, muscle, glands and internal organs
- When a sensory nerve is stimulated sufficiently a nerve impulse is generated
- If these impulses are transmitted to the brain, they are perceived as sensations such as touch, pressure, temperature and pain
- Free nerve endings that respond to painful stimuli are known as **nociceptors**
- Most nociceptors are polymodal, thus they can respond to a range of stimuli such as touch, pressure, heat and cold
- If these stimuli are of sufficient intensity they will be perceived as a painful sensation

---

Stimuli of nociceptors by non-painful stimuli can also be perceived as pain if the level of stimulation is sufficient. This is one of the characteristics of neuropathic pain (Charlton 2005).

Each neurone is a separate entity. Information can only pass between neurones if their membranes are in close proximity. The junctions between neurones are known as synapses. Impulses are transmitted across synapses chemically by substances known as neurotransmitters. Many substances in the body can function as neurotransmitters. Box 2.2 outlines the main neurotransmitters that are important in pain pathways. Unlike nerve impulses, which once initiated must proceed along the entire length of the neurone, a stimulus arriving at a synapse can continue or be inhibited. The ability for nerve impulses to be inhibited or be allowed to proceed is an important function of neurotransmitters found at synapses. Indeed, several analgesic drugs work by inhibiting the production of certain neurotransmitters, outlined in Chapter 4.

BOX 2.2

Neurotransmitters important in pain pathways

- **Acetylcholine** is the main neurotransmitter at neuromuscular and neuroglandular junctions and causes *excitation* of neurones in muscles and endocrine glands
- **Glutamate** causes *excitation* of neurones in the central nervous system
- **γ-aminobutyric acid (GABA)** causes *inhibition* of neuronal receptors in the central nervous system
- **Substance P** causes *excitation* of neurones and is the main neurotransmitter within the dorsal horn of the spinal cord
- **Noradrenaline** is concentrated in the brainstem and causes either *inhibition* or *excitation* of neurones
- **Serotonin** is concentrated in the brainstem and is involved in the regulation of temperature, sensory perception, sleep and mood and causes *inhibition* of neurones
- **Dopamine** is concentrated in the midbrain and is involved in the regulation of emotional responses and subconscious movements of the skeletal muscles and causes *inhibition* of neuronal receptors in dendrites

---

Impulses pass between sensory neurones, interneurones and the nerves of the spinothalmic tract via synapses. The main neurotransmitter at the synapses in the dorsal horn of the spinal cord is substance P.

There does not appear to be a specific cluster of neurones that act as a *pain centre* within the brain. However, there are specific regions of the brain that are actively involved in perceiving stimuli as a painful sensation and coordinating a response to these stimuli. Areas of particular importance are the postcentral gyrus, reticular formation, pons, limbic system, midbrain, thalamus and sensory cortex (Heuther and Defriez 2006).

2.3 Types of Pain

A range of sensory experiences can potentially manifest as pain. Pain can be broadly divided into two groups: **protective pain sensations** and abnormal **non-protective pain sensations** (Cervero and Laird 1991). Protective and non-protective pain sensations are described in Box 2.3.

BOX 2.3

Protective and non-protective pain sensations

Protective pain sensations are referred to as normal, sensory or **nociceptive pain**

- This reflects the basic understanding that this type of pain is a normal response to the sensory stimulation of nociceptors
- Being sensitive to both painful and tissue damaging stimuli and responding appropriately are essential to prevent or minimise further injury

Non-protective pain sensations are referred to as abnormal, aberrant or **neuropathic pain**

- This reflects the view that this type of pain is a consequence of damage to peripheral nerves or the central nervous system
- Neuropathic pain may be persistent or chronic in nature, having no defined time limit, often no apparent cause and serves no apparent biological purpose

It is now postulated that acute and persistent or chronic pain are a continuum, rather than separate entities, for example, in some situations neuropathic pain may be a component of acute pain, that is, due to postoperative pain, cancer pain or trauma (Australian and New Zealand College of Anaesthetists and Faculty of Pain Medicine [ANZCA] 2005). An overview of nociceptive pain and neuropathic pain is provided in Table 2.2.

Table 2.2 An overview of nociceptive pain and neuropathic pain

Type of pain	Pathology	Divisions
Nociceptive pain	If nociceptors are stimulated sufficiently, e.g. following injury or tissue damage, a nerve impulse is generated and conveyed by neurones to the brain where it is interpreted as pain	Somatic pain arises from bone, joints, muscles, skin and connective tissues. • The pain is usually well defined and well localised Visceral pain arises from internal organs such as those of the gastrointestinal system. • This pain is usually less well defined and poorly localised or may be referred to another body area
Neuropathic pain	Abnormal processing of nerve impulses caused by a lesion or dysfunction within the nervous system	Centrally generated pain due to processing abnormalities within the central nervous system, for example, Central Pain Peripherally generated pain, for example, Complex Regional Pain Syndrome • Complex regional pain syndrome type 1 (CRPS 1; also known as reflex sympathetic dystrophy, RSD) is the result of abnormalities in processing of peripheral pain sensations with no clear nerve injury or lesion • Complex regional pain syndrome type 2 (CRPS 2; also known as causalgia) occurs as a result of damage to a peripheral nerve

For further information about the management of CRPS see Chapter 8.
Source: McCaffery and Pasero (1999); Pickering (2002)

2.4 Physiology of Nociceptive (Acute) Pain

For a stimulus to be perceived as *pain* the noxious stimulus must be of sufficient intensity to generate a nerve impulse and the impulse must be transmitted via the many nerve pathways to the brain. There are many sites that can potentially enhance or inhibit the progression of the impulse. This results in a unique and specific experience for each individual, explaining why pain is a bio-psycho-social phenomenon (see Chapter 3). The physiological processes involved in perceiving pain are traditionally described in four stages: transduction, transmission, perception and modulation (Figure 2.2).

2.4.1 Transduction

The detection of a stimulus by a nociceptor is known as transduction. Stimuli can be internal, such as the chemical mediators of local cell damage, which include bradykinins, serotonin, prostaglandins, histamines and substance P; or external, such as heat, cold and mechanical forces. If strong enough these stimuli generate a nerve impulse.

2.4.2 Transmission

Once a nerve impulse is generated, it needs to reach the brain to be interpreted. This process is known as transmission. The process of transmission has three stages:

1. The transmission of the impulse from the nociceptor to the spinal cord.
2. The transmission of the impulse from the spinal cord to the brainstem and thalamus.
3. The transmission of the impulse from the thalamus to the cerebral cortex.

The nerve impulse travels to the spinal cord without interruption and terminates in an area of the spinal cord known as the substantia gelatinosa. The substantia gelatinosa is a collection of neuronal bodies and interneurones situated in the dorsal (posterior) horn of the spinal cord. The substantia gelatinosa contains cells that have an *inhibitory* effect at synaptic junctions (inhibitory SC cells) and cells that have an *excitatory* effect at synaptic junctions (T cells). If impulses are allowed to proceed across the synaptic junctions of the interneurones in the substantia gelatinosa they terminate in the brain.

Ascending and descending spinal pain pathways
The white matter of the spinal cord contains the ascending and descending nociceptive pathways that form connections between the spinal cord and the brain. The ascending pathway is further separated into three columns or tracts. The two most significant tracts for nociceptive transmission are:

1. The spinothalamic tract – carrying information on the site and type of the pain stimulus;

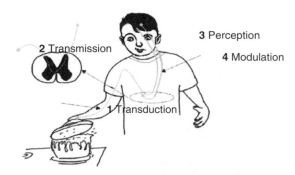

Figure 2.2 Schematic representation of the stages of pain pathways.

2. The spinoreticular tract – carrying information on the emotional/affective components of the pain.

(Almeida et al. 2004; ANZCA 2005)

The spinothalamic tract

Most of the axons cross the spinal cord and ascend the spinothalamic tract, which terminates in the brain stem and thalamus (Figure 2.3) (Heuther and Defriez 2006). The thalamus acts as the main *relay station* for sensory information before redistributing it to different areas of the somatosensory cortex for processing (McCaffery and Pasero 1999; Almeida et al. 2004; ANZCA 2005).

Nerve axons of the spinothalamic tract pass through the brainstem, medulla, hypothalamus and limbic system before reaching the thalamus. All these brain structures play an important part in the pain experience, being responsible for aspects of pain localisation and intensity, emotional aspects of pain, and psychomotor, autonomic and affective responses to pain (Almeida et al. 2004).

The spinoreticular tract

The spinoreticular tract also originates in the dorsal horn of the spinal cord, although it involves different types of neurones. The spinoreticular tract ascends to the reticular formation in the brainstem, before ascending further to the cerebral cortex. The reticular formation consists of a complex matrix of nerve cells in the core of the brainstem. It is primarily involved in integrating ascending and descending information between the spinal cord and higher cortical centres. The areas of the reticular formation reached by the spinoreticular tract are primarily involved with the affective or mood response to pain and also activate brain stem areas responsible for suppression of the pain response by the descending pain pathway (Almeida et al. 2004; Swenson 2006; Waugh and Grant 2006).

2.4.3 Modulation

The processes involved in modifying or inhibiting pain impulses are known as modulation. The descending pain pathway is primarily responsible for modulation of pain transmission in the spinal cord. This pathway originates from higher cortical areas such as the amygdala (within the limbic system, responsible for processing and memory of emotions) and hypothalamus, passing through the brainstem and terminating in the dorsal horn of the spinal cord (ANZCA 2005). Multiple mechanisms contribute to modulation, with the two main effects on pain transmission being inhibitory or excitatory.

Descending inhibitory effects

- Inhibition of ascending neurones from transmitting nociceptive inputs to the brain
- Inhibition or suppression of the release of pain-producing neurotransmitters (e.g. substance P, NMDA, glutamate)

Descending excitatory effects

- Stimulation of neurotransmitters that produce analgesia (e.g. endogenous opioids, noradrenaline, serotonin, GABA, dopamine)

Source: ANZCA (2005)

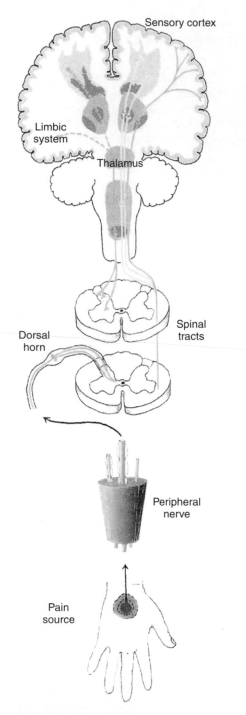

Sensory cortex

Limbic
system

Thalamus

Dorsal
horn

Spinal
tracts

Peripheral
nerve

Pain
source

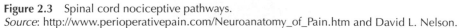

Figure 2.3 Spinal cord nociceptive pathways.
Source: http://www.perioperativepain.com/Neuroanatomy_of_Pain.htm and David L. Nelson.

The body contains endogenous opioids (enkephalins, dynorphins and endorphins), which are natural analgesics and have the ability to inhibit or enhance the action of neurotransmitters at specific neurone receptor sites and therefore modulate pain pathways. Endogenous opioids bind with neuronal receptor sites blocking the action of substance P and other excitatory (pain producing) neurotransmitters causing an analgesic effect.

2.5 Perception of Pain

When a nociceptive nerve impulse reaches the brain it is interpreted as a painful sensation and becomes a conscious experience. This is where the factors identified as affecting pain perception, discussed in Chapter 3, probably contribute to the perception of pain. A range of theories has been postulated in an attempt to explain the pathophysiology that results in the experience of pain being unique for every individual. These theories include specificity theory, intensive theory, pattern theory and gate control theory.

Specificity theory

Pain sensations are mediated through the activation of specific peripheral pain receptors that link via specific pain pathways to a defined pain centre in the brain

Intensive theory

Any sensory stimulus of sufficient intensity can be interpreted as pain

Pattern theory

Pain is a learned process triggered by spatial and temporal patterns of activation

Gate control theory

Stimuli entering the spinal cord can be manipulated through a process of opening and closing *gates* allowing impulses to proceed or not

Several decades after it was first proposed by Melzack and Wall in 1965, the *gate control theory* still commands universal support (Weisenberg 2000). The gate control theory provides the most likely physiological explanation for the complexity of the processes involved in the perception of pain. The gate control pain theory will now be discussed in relation to the modulation of pain.

The gate control pain theory proposes:

- A *gating mechanism* exists in the substantia gelatinosa.
- The degree to which the *gate* is opened or closed determines whether impulses are inhibited or allowed to proceed (Wall and Melzack 1989).
- The *gating mechanism* consists of two types of cells: inhibitory SG cells and excitatory T cells.
- There appear to be two interactive systems that influence the *gating* mechanism: competitive peripheral input and modulation from descending nerve pathways from the brain.
- Figure 2.4 provides further explanation of the gate control theory.

There are a number of factors that can open or close the pain gate (Table 2.3).

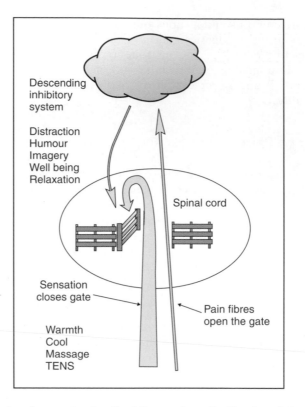

When nerve impulses from nociceptor stimulation reach a critical level, excitatory T cells in the substantia gelatinosa are activated and the *gate* opens, allowing information to progress to the thalamus and sensory cortex resulting in the perception of pain (Wall and Melzack 1989).
There are situations where the *gate* remains closed despite stimulation by a nerve impulse, for example, by activation of the inhibitory SG cells from competing non-painful peripheral nerve input (Wall and Melzack 1989).

The classic example of this is the *mummy rubbing it better* scenario:

- A kick on the knee would activate nociceptors and if the stimulus were large enough a nerve impulse via A-beta fibres would be initiated, arriving in the spinal cord and activating the excitatory T cells.
- The *gate* would open and activate interconnections in the spinal cord enabling the impulse to proceed to the brain.
- However, if the knee is vigorously rubbed non-painful sensory fibres would be activated and transmission of a nerve impulse via A-delta fibres would compete to *open* or *close* the gate.
- The sensory stimulation that is stronger will influence whether the gate remains closed or not.
- In addition, descending tracts have the potential to stimulate the inhibitory SG cells or the excitatory T cells, depending on the type of neurotransmitter released, which can *open* or *close* the gate (Wall and Melzack 1989).

Figure 2.4 Explanation of the gate control theory.
Source: Carr and Mann (2000).

2.6 Physiology of Neuropathic Pain

The pathophysiology of neuropathic pain, which is often associated with chronic pain, is less clearly understood than nociceptive (acute) pain and reflects the difficulty in managing this type of pain. Neuropathic pain probably occurs due to a combination of nociceptive pain and abnormal processing of sensory inputs by the nervous system (McCaffery and Pasero 1999; Gilron et al. 2006). The effect of this repeated

Table 2.3 Factors that close or open the gate

	Physical/sensory	Emotional/behavioural	Cognitive
Close	Analgesic drugs Adjuvant analgesic drugs Counter-stimulation, e.g. massage, TENS, heat, acupuncture, acupressure Exercise	Positive thoughts Relaxation Biofeedback Controlled breathing techniques Distraction	Hypnosis/imagery Meditation Psychotherapy
Open	Severity of illness or injury Excessive activity Re-injury	Anxiety, fear or worry Tension Depression	Focusing on the pain Catastrophising

nociceptive activity is sensitisation of the nervous system (Schwartzman et al. 2001). Repetitive nociceptive stimulation of peripheral nerves lowers the threshold for pain transmission (known as '*wind-up*') and contributes to the process of central sensitisation, which may have a crucial role in chronic pain (Eide 2000). *Central sensitisation* results in hyper-excitability and hypersensitivity to all incoming nerve impulses, thus innocuous non-painful stimuli may be perceived as pain. This sensitisation can lead to long-term physiological changes occuring in the peripheral nervous system and at the dorsal horn of the spinal cord, which may further generate abnormal nerve impulses (Schwartzman et al. 2001).

> Healthcare professionals need to understand that neuropathic pain intensity can appear to be disproportionate to the likely cause of the pain.

Neuropathic pain in children can occur following damage to the peripheral or central nervous system (for example, from trauma or surgery, chemotherapy or radiotherapy, infection or inflammation).

Key components of neuropathic pain include (Gilron et al. 2006):

- continuous or paroxysmal pain that increases rather than improves over time;
- burning or electric shock-like, stabbing or aching, throbbing or cramping qualities;
- pain that is disproportional to the injury or disease process;
- increased response to a stimulus that is normally painful (*hyperalgesia*);
- pain that can be evoked by a non-painful stimulus (*allodynia*);
- unpleasant abnormal sensations, either spontaneous or evoked (*dysaesthesia*).

The medical treatment of neuropathic pain includes adjuvant analgesic drugs, which are discussed in Chapters 4 and 8.

Summary

- Pain is a complex phenomenon that is not well understood.
- There are several misconceptions relating to the physiology of pain in children.
- Pain can be classified as nociceptive or neuropathic.
- Nociception is a normal response to both painful and tissue damaging stimuli.
- There are four stages involved in perceiving nociceptive pain: transduction, transmission, perception and modulation.
- Several theories have attempted to explain the subjectivity of pain. The *gate control pain theory* is accepted as providing the best explanation.

- An individual's perception of pain can be modified by several factors that cause the gate to *open* or *close*.
- Neuropathic pain is the consequence of damage to peripheral nerves or the central nervous system and is often difficult to treat.
- See Chapter 8 for detailed discussion about diagnosis and management of neuropathic pain.

Useful web resources

Dartmouth Medical School, *Review of Clinical and Functional Neuroscience* http://www.dartmouth.edu/~rswenson/NeuroSci/

University of Utah, Pain Research Center: http://www.painresearch.utah.edu/cancerpain/neuro-movMenu.html

University of the West of England, Faculty of Health and Social Care: http://hsc.uwe.ac.uk/manacuteill/links.asp

---

References

Almeida, T.F., Roizenblatt, S. and Tufik, S. (2004) Afferent pain pathways: a neuroanatomical review, *Brain Research*, 1000: 40–56.

Australian and New Zealand College of Anaesthetists and Faculty of Pain Medicine [ANZCA] (2005) *Acute Pain Management: Scientific Evidence*, 2nd edition, Australian and New Zealand College of Anaesthetists, Melbourne.

Carr, E.C.J. and Mann, E.M. (2000) *Pain: Creative Approaches to Effective Pain Management*, Macmillan Press Ltd., Basingstoke.

Cervero, F. and Laird, J. (1991) One pain or many pains? A new look at pain mechanisms, *News in Physiological Sciences*, 6: 268–273.

Charlton, J.E. (ed.) (2005) *Core Curriculum for Professional Education in Pain*, 3rd edition, IASP Press, Seattle.

Eide, P.K. (2000) Wind-up and the NMDA receptor complex from a clinical perspective, *European Journal of Pain*, 9: 5–17.

Fitzgerald, M. and Howard, R.F.M. (2003) The neurobiologic basis of pediatric pain. In Schechter, N.L., Berde, C.B. and Yester, M. (eds) *Pain in Infants, Children and Adolescents,* 2nd edition, Philadelphia, Lippincott Williams and Wilkins, pp. 19–42.

Gilron, I., Watson, P. and Cahill, C. (2006) Neuropathic pain: a practical guide for the clinician, *Canadian Medical Association Journal*, 175(3): 265–275.

Heuther, S.E. and Defriez C.B. (2006) Pain, temperature regulation, sleep and sensory function. In McCance, K.L. and Huether, S.E. (eds) *Pathophysiology: The Biological Basis for Disease in Adults and Children, 5th* edition, St Louis Mosby, pp. 447–487.

Longstaff, A. (2005) *Instant Notes: Neuroscience*, 2nd edition, Taylor & Francis, Abingdon, UK.

McCaffery, M. and Pasero, C. (1999) *Pain: Clinical Manual*, 2nd edition, Mosby, St Louis.

Padgett. K. (2006) Alterations of neurological function in children. In McCance, K.L. and Huether, S.E. (eds.) *Pathophysiology: The Biological Basis For Disease In Adults And Children*, 5th edition, St Louis Mosby, pp. 623–654.

Pickering, A.E. (2002) An overview of neuropathic pain, *British Journal of Anaesthesia (CPED Reviews)*, 2(3): 65–68.

Schwartzman. R., Grothusen, J. and Kiefer, T. (2001) Neuropathic central pain: epidemiology, etiology and treatment options. *Archives of Neurology*, 58(10): 1547–1550.

Swenson, R.S. (2006) Review of Clinical and Functional Neuroscience, online version. Dartmouth Medical School, http://www.dartmouth.edu/~rswenson/NeuroSci/ [accessed 18th September 2007].

Wall, P.D. and Melzack. R. (1989) *Textbook of Pain*, Churchill Livingstone, London.

Waugh, A. and Grant, A. (2006) *Ross and Wilson: Anatomy and Physiology in Health and Illness.* 10th edition, Churchill Livingstone, Edinburgh, UK.

Weisenberg, M. (2000) Cognitive aspects of pain. In Wall, R.D. and Melzack, R. (eds.) Textbook of Pain, 4th edition, Churchill Livingstone, Edinburgh, pp. 345–358.

CHAPTER 3
Pain: A Bio-Psycho-Social Phenomenon
Alison Twycross

Introduction

There are many factors that influence a child's perception of pain and the way they behave when in pain. These include age, level of cognitive development, culture, family learning, previous experiences of pain, and the child's personality and temperament. These can be classified as biological, psychological and social factors (Figure 3.1). This chapter will discuss each of these in turn. Factors affecting nurses' perceptions of and response to pain in children are discussed in Chapters 1 and 11.

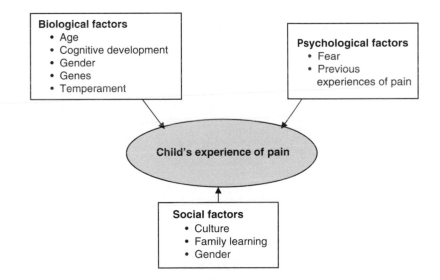

Figure 3.1   Pain as a bio-psycho-social phenomenon.

3.1 Biological Factors

3.1.1 Age

The effect of a child's age on their perception of pain has been examined in a few studies. Children recognise at an early age that pain is unpleasant. Their understanding and descriptions of pain depend on their age and also on their level of cognitive development and previous experiences of pain (McGrath and Hillier 2003). Several studies have examined children's perceptions of procedural pain, which have demonstrated age-related differences in pain intensity (Fradet et al. 1990; Lander and Fowler-Kerry 1991; Manne et al. 1992; Goodenough et al. 1997). Children's ratings of pain during painful procedures seem to decrease with age. This is attributable to several factors. Older children may have:

- a greater understanding of what is happening to them and thus feel less anxious;
- developed coping strategies and methods to distract themselves from procedural pain.

However, in relation to the effect of age on the experience of postoperative pain, the research evidence is contradictory. Bennett-Branson and Craig (1993) found that for children ($n = 60$) aged 7–16 years, postoperative pain increased with age, while Palmero and Drotar (1996) found that for children ($n = 28$) aged 7–17 years, postoperative pain decreased with age. No age-related differences were found by Gidron et al. (1995) among young people ($n = 67$) aged 13–20 years.

> Younger children may experience more procedure-related pain than older children. In relation to postoperative pain it is unclear whether age influences children's perception of pain. Further research is needed in this area.

3.1.2 Cognitive development

The impact of a child's level of cognitive development on their perception of pain has been explored in a number of studies over the past 30 years (Scott 1978; Ross and Ross 1984; Jeans and Gordon 1981; Hurley and Whelan 1988; Gaffney 1993; Crow 1997). The results of these studies indicate that children's perception about the cause and effect of pain develops in line with Piaget's stages of cognitive development (Table 3.1). The implications for nursing practice can be seen in Box 3.1. It is important to note that a child's experiences of illness and hospitalisation may change their perception of and their ability to cope with pain; for example, they may regress to an earlier stage of development. Conversely, children with chronic illness often develop an understanding of concepts associated with a later stage of development.

> Children develop an understanding about pain, which mirrors the stages of development described by Piaget.

Although his theories are widely accepted, Piaget is not without his critics. The area of most debate seems to be Piaget's preoperational stage. During this stage Piaget believes that a child is not capable of conscious thought and is unable to grasp the concept of reality. However, in a review of the literature on cognitive development Hauck (1991) suggests that Piaget underestimates pre-school age children's ability to think logically. Hauck cites research by other experts in the field of cognitive development, which suggests that if they are given information in the appropriate way children as young as three are capable of greater logic than Piaget's theories suggest. Hauck suggests that these findings have important implications for nurses working with children. They are strengthened by the findings of Harbeck and Peterson (1992) who interviewed children as young as three and concluded that even at this early age a child is able to describe their pain if the questions asked are appropriate to their level of understanding.

Table 3.1 How children perceive the cause and effect of pain (adapted from Hurley and Whelan 1988)

Piaget's stage of development	Perception of pain
Preoperational (2–7 years)	• Pain is primarily a physical experience – i.e. children focus on the physical sensations of pain • Children think about the magical disappearance of pain • Children are not able to distinguish between cause and effect of pain • Pain is often perceived as punishment for a wrong doing or bad thought, particularly if the child did something they were told not to do immediately before they started experiencing pain • Children's egocentricity means that they hold someone else responsible for their pain and, therefore, are likely to strike out verbally or physically when they have pain • Child is apt to tell a nurse who gave them an injection, 'you are mean'
Concrete-operational (7–11 years)	Children: • relate to pain physically • are able to specify location in terms of body parts • have an increased awareness of the body and internal organs; their fear of bodily harm is a strong influence in their perception of painful events • have a fear of total annihilation (body destruction and death)
Transitional-formal (10–12 years)	• Children's perception of pain that is not quite as sophisticated as formal-operational children • Children's perception of pain is not as literal as would be expected in children who are in the concrete-operational stage of development • Children in the transitional-formal stage are beginning to understand the concept of *if … then* propositions
Formal-operational (12 years and above)	Children: • begin to solve problems • do not always have required coping mechanisms to facilitate consistent mature responses • imagine the sinister implications of pain

---

BOX 3.1

Implications for nursing practice

• Nurses need knowledge regarding a child's level of development and their understanding of cause and effect of pain.
• Age appropriate explanations about pain and treatment are required.
• A preoperational child:
  • needs reassurance that pain is not a punishment;
  • may 'hate' the nurse who appears to be inflicting pain;
  • cannot see the connection between treatment and relief of pain.
• A concrete operational child needs:
  • reassurance about their fears regarding bodily annihilation;
  • appropriate explanations about their pain and treatment.
• A formal operational child needs:
  • opportunities to discuss their fears;
  • information about their condition and treatment.

Source: Adapted from Twycross (1998)

3.1.3 Genes

The results of one research study indicate that a single gene affects how people tolerate pain (Zubieta et al. 2003). The gene produces an enzyme which regulates endorphin production in the body. A person's genes can, therefore, influence their perception of pain.

3.1.4 Temperament

> **What is temperament?**
>
> Temperament refers to the general nature, behavioural style or characteristic mood of the individual (Chess and Thomas 1986).
>   Temperament is largely determined by an individual's genetic makeup, but is also considerably influenced by social and psychological factors.

Several studies have demonstrated that children of different temperaments behave differently when in pain (Box 3.2).

> A child's temperament appears to influence how they behave when they are in pain.

> **Practice point**
>
> A child's personality will affect how they behave when in pain (that is, whether they cry and complain or withdraw and feign sleep).

3.2 Psychological Factors

3.2.1 Fear

Fear has a huge impact on a child's perception of pain. The International Association for the Study of Pain (1979) definition of pain provided in Chapter 1 describes pain as both a *sensory* and an *emotional* experience. Fear and distress are common negative emotions experienced by children in pain. The greater the level of fear, the more likely a child is to feel pain and distress. (The use of play, preparation and information to manage the *emotional* component of pain is discussed in Chapter 10.)

> **Practice point**
>
> Treating only the sensory component of a painful and frightening procedure is rarely effective. The most effective interventions combine preparation, explanation and drug and non-drug interventions. (See Chapter 5 for a discussion of non-drug methods of pain relief and Chapter 10 for further information about managing procedural pain.)

3.2.2 Previous experiences of pain

A child's previous experiences of pain will influence how they react to subsequent painful events (see Chapter 1). Frequent exposure to painful stimuli does not desensitise the subject but, rather, increases their sensitivity to the pain (Fowler-Kerry 1990; Weisman et al. 1998; McGrath and Hillier 2003). The perception of pain is not a learned response

BOX 3.2

Summary of research about the effects of temperament on children's pain

Wallace (1989)

- Examined the correlation between the temperament of children ($n = 31$), aged 3–7 years, having elective surgery and the number of analgesic medications administered postoperatively.
- Prior to surgery parents completed the *Behavioural Style Questionnaire* (BSQ) and children were grouped as low, medium or high anxiety.
- Children rated as high intensity received a significantly greater amount of analgesia than children rated as low intensity ($p = 0.05$).

Schechter et al. (1991)

- Parents of children ($n = 65$) receiving preschool immunisations completed the BSQ and a pain questionnaire exploring attributes and parental beliefs about the children's ability to cope with pain 2–4 weeks before the immunisation. Parents were also asked to predict the amount of discomfort their child would experience during the immunisation. Data were also collected from the children using a semi-structured interview.
- During the immunisation children's responses were assessed by collecting data about: muscular rigidity, crying, screaming and facial gestures. The researcher also gave an overall global pain score of the child's discomfort using the *Procedure Rating Scale – Revised* (PRS-R).
- At the end of the procedure the child was asked to rate their discomfort using the Oucher (see Chapter 6).
- The results indicated that children rated by their parents as having temperaments at the *difficult* end of the scale had PRS-R scores 2–3 higher than the other children.

Lee and White-Traut (1996)

- Children ($n = 126$), aged 3–7 years, requiring a preoperative blood test were asked to report their pain prior to the blood test.
- The blood-taking was videotaped and the child's pulse and oxygen saturation recorded throughout the procedure.
- When the procedure was completed children reported their pain during venepuncture.
- The parents completed a questionnaire prior to the procedure, which provided information about the child's temperament.
- Children rated by their parents as having temperaments at the *difficult* end of the scale displayed more distress than other children ($p = 0.05$).

Chen et al. (2000)

- Explored the relationship between sensitivity to pain (measured using the *Sensitivity Inventory for Pain*) and pain intensity during a lumbar puncture with children ($n = 55$), aged 3–18 years, with leukaemia.
- Higher levels of pain sensitivity were associated with greater pain ($p < 0.05$).

Kleiber et al. (2007)

- Set out to describe the relationship between pain-sensitive temperament and self-report of pain intensity following surgery.
- Adolescents and young adults ($n = 59$) (average age 14 years) completed the *Sensitivity Inventory for Pain, Child Version* prior to admission.
- Pain intensity information was gathered from the computerised medical record.
- There was a small but significant correlation between the perceptual sensitivity and reporting subscales of the Sensitivity Inventory for Pain and pain intensity on the third postoperative day.

(Anand and Craig 1996), but the experience of pain is modified by previous exposure to painful situations. It follows that the way a child's pain has been managed in the past will affect how they perceive subsequent painful experiences.

> How well a child's pain has been managed in the past will affect their response to future painful experiences. Children experiencing frequent painful experiences become more sensitive to pain.

3.3 Social Factors

3.3.1 Culture

> **What is culture?**
>
> Culture can be defined as the way of life of people. It consists of conventional patterns of thought and behaviour, including values, beliefs, rules of conduct, political organisation and economic activity, which are passed from one generation to the next by learning and not by inheritance (Hatch 1985).
>   Culture is a framework for learning behaviour and communication, which might shape a child's perspective of health and illness (Craig 1986).

A child's cultural background is, thus, likely to influence how they perceive and react to pain. This is probably attributable to *social learning*. Social learning occurs when an individual learns something by observing another person doing it; in other words it is learning by modelling (Bandura 1977). Several studies have explored the impact of culture on children's pain experiences (Box 3.3).

> **BOX 3.3**
>
> **Summary of research about the impact of culture on children's pain experiences**
>
> *Abu-Saad (1984a, b)*
>
> - Arab-American ($n = 27$) and Chinese-American ($n = 24$) children, aged 9–12 years, were interviewed to ascertain whether there were differences in descriptions of pain experiences.
> - No statistical differences were found between the groups.
> - Participants were first-generation American and may have adopted the cultural characteristics of the predominant American culture.
>
> *Pfefferbaum et al. (1990)*
>
> - Examined the influence of culture on pain in white American and Hispanic-American children.
> - Children ($n = 78$), aged 3–15 years, being treated for leukaemia or lymphoma participated in the study, were observed during a spinal tap or bone marrow aspiration.
> - Little difference was observed between the two groups.
>
> *Fritz et al. (1991)*
>
> - Vietnamese refugees ($n = 14$) who had recently immigrated to the USA were interviewed about their expectations of children's reactions to pain.
> - Most participants were unfamiliar with western medicine and relied on traditional techniques to treat pain.
> - Sickness, evil spirits and imbalance in life's elements were identified as causes of pain.
> - Crying and complaints about pain were acceptable for young children but children over the age of eight years were expected to respond stoically to pain.

Culture does have some impact on children's perception of pain. However, once children have been in a new country for a period of time they may become socialised into the behavioural norms of the dominant culture.

3.3.2 Family learning

The reaction of the family to the child in pain will teach the child how to behave in a manner that is acceptable to the family. If the child receives minimal attention they will learn to cope with their pain. However, if the child receives a great deal of attention they will learn that it is appropriate (and worthwhile) to express their pain. Indeed, the results of several studies indicate that children in families where one of the parents suffers from chronic pain are more likely to experience chronic and recurrent pain themselves (Mikail and von Baeyer 1990; Armistead et al. 1995; Kotchick et al. 1996; Aromaa et al. 2000; Saunders et al. 2007). These familial patterns can also be explained by Bandura's (1977) social learning theory.

How a family responds to a child when they are in pain impacts on how the child behaves in future painful situations.

3.3.3 Gender

There has been limited research on the differences in pain perceptions and behaviour between boys and girls (Box 3.4).

BOX 3.4

Summary of research about the effects of gender on children's pain experiences

Fearon et al. (1996) found differences in the ways girls and boys behaved when in pain.
300 painful incidents were observed for children, aged 3–7 years, in day care. Girls responded more frequently at the higher end of the distress scale ($p = 0.03$).
Girls also responded to painful events with verbal complaints, sobbing, crying or screaming more often than boys. In the majority of incidents no adult response was offered but when an adult did respond girls were given physical comfort more often than boys were.

Perquin et al. (2000) found that, among children ($n = 5424$) aged 4–18 years, girls reported severe pain more often than boys ($p < 0.001$).
Girls also reported chronic pain (pain lasting for more than three months) more often than boys ($p < 0.001$).

Roth-Isigkeit et al. (2005) found that, for children ($n = 619$) aged 10–18 years, the prevalence of restrictions attributable to pain was significantly higher for girls than boys of the same age ($p < 0.05$).
Self-reported triggers also differed between girls and boys.

Lynch et al. (2007) examined sex and age differences in coping strategies among children with chronic pain. Pain intensity (*Visual Analogue Scale*), pain coping strategies (*Pain Coping Questionnaire*), and coping efficacy were assessed in children (aged 8–12 years) and adolescents (aged 13–18 years), presenting to a paediatric chronic pain clinic ($n = 272$).
Significant sex differences in coping strategies were found ($p < 0.001$). Girls used social support-seeking more than boys, while boys used more behavioural distraction techniques. For girls, pain coping efficacy was also significantly negatively correlated with internalising/catastrophising.

Martin et al. (2007) interviewed children (95 females; 48 males) three years after their last appointment at a paediatric pain clinic. They found that females may be at higher risk for continuing pain and report greater use of healthcare, medication and non-drug methods of pain relief.

A review of research examining gender variation in clinical pain experiences demonstrated that women were more likely than men to experience a variety of recurrent pains (Unruh 1996).

Gender differences in pain behaviours have in the past been attributed to social factors such as parents responding differently in the same situation, depending on the gender of the child, or to the fact that it is more socially acceptable for girls to express pain than it is for boys. However, recent research has found that females may be more susceptible to pain than males because of hormonal and other factors (Fillingim and Ness 2000; Kuba and Quinones-Jenab 2005).

A child's gender may impact on how much pain they experience.

Summary

- Pain is a bio-psycho-social phenomenon.
- A wide range of factors affect children's perception of pain and help to explain why different children behave differently when experiencing similar painful situations.
- Biological factors include the child's age, gender and genetic makeup.
- Psychological factors include fear, knowledge and previous experiences of pain.
- Social factors include culture and learning.
- Healthcare professionals must take all these factors into account when assessing and managing children's pain.

References

Abu-Saad, H. (1984a) Cultural components of pain: the Asian-American child, *Child Health Care*, 13: 11–14.

Abu-Saad, H. (1984b) Cultural group indicators of pain in children, *Maternal and Child Nursing*, 13: 187–193.

Anand, K.J.S. and Craig, K.D. (1996) New perspectives on the definition of pain, *Pain*, 67: 3–6.

Armistead, L., Klein, K. and Forehand, R. (1995) Parental physical illness and child functioning, *Clinical Psychology Review*, 15: 409–422.

Aromaa, M., Sillanpaa, M., Rautava, P. and Helenius, H. (2000) Pain experience of children with headache and their families: a controlled study, *Pediatrics*, 106(1): 270–275.

Bandura, A. (1977) *Social Learning Theory*, Prentice-Hall, New Jersey.

Bennett-Branson, S.M. and Craig, K.D. (1993) Postoperative pain in children: developmental and family influences on spontaneous coping strategies, *Canadian Journal of Behavioral Sciences*, 25: 355–383.

Chen, E., Craske, M.G., Katz, E.R., Schwartz, E. and Zeltzer, L.K. (2000) Pain-sensitive temperament: does it predict procedural distress and response to psychological treatment among children with cancer? *Journal of Pediatric Psychology*, 25(4): 269–278.

Chess, S. and Thomas, A. (1986) *Temperament in Clinical Practice*, Guildford Press, New York.

Craig, K. (1986) Social modelling influences. In Strenbach, R.A. (ed.) *The Psychology of Pain*, Raven Press, New York, pp. 67–95.

Crow, C.S. (1997) Children's pain perspectives inventory (CPPI): developmental assessment, *Pain*, 72: 33–40.

Fearon, I., McGrath, P.J. and Achat, H. (1996) 'Booboos': the study of everyday pain among young children, *Pain*, 68: 55–62.

Fillingim, R.B. and Ness, T.J. (2000) Sex-related hormonal influences on pain and analgesic responses, *Neuroscience & Biobehavioral Reviews*, 24(4): 485–501.

Fowler-Kerry, S. (1990) Adolescent oncology survivors' recollection of pain. In Tyler, D.C. and Krane, E.J. (eds.) *Advances in Pain Research Therapy*, New York, Raven Press Ltd, pp. 365–371.

Fradet, C., McGrath, P.J., Kay, J., Adams, S. and Luke, B. (1990) A prospective survey of reactions to blood tests by children and adolescents, *Pain*, 40: 53–60.

Fritz, K.J., Schechter, N.L. and Bernstein, B. (1991) Cultural components of pain in Vietnamese refugee children (Abstract), *Journal of Pain and Symptom Management*, 6: 205.

Gaffney, A. (1993) Cognitive development aspects of pain in school-age children, In: Schechter NL, Berde, C.B. and Yaster, M. (eds.) *Pain in Infants, Children and Adolescents*, Baltimore, Williams & Wilkins, pp. 75–86.

Gidron, Y., McGrath, P.J. and Goodday, R. (1995) The physical and psychosocial predictors of adolescents' recovery from oral surgery, *Journal of Behavioral Medicine*, 18: 385–399.

Goodenough, B., Addicoat L., Champion G.D., McInerney M., Young B., Juniper K. and Ziegler J.B. (1997) Pain in 4–6 year old children receiving intramuscular injections: a comparison of the Faces Pain Scale with other self-report and behavioural measures, *Clinical Journal of Pain*, 13(1): 60–73.

Harbeck, C. and Peterson, L. (1992) Elephants dancing in my head: a developmental approach to children's concepts of specific pains, *Child Development*, 63: 138–149.

Hatch, E. (1985) Culture. In Kuper, A. and Kuper, J. (eds.) *The Social Science Encyclopaedia*, Routledge & Kegan Paul, London.

Hauck, M. (1991) Cognitive abilities of preschool children: implications for nurses working with young children, *Journal of Pediatric Nursing*, 6: 230–235.

Hurley, A. and Whelan, E.G. (1988) Cognitive development and children's perception of pain, *Pediatric Nursing*, 14(1): 21–24.

International Association for the Study of Pain (1979) Pain terms: a list with definitions and notes on usage, *Pain*, 6: 249–252.

Jeans, M.E. and Gordan, D. (1981) *Developmental characteristics of the concept of pain*, Paper presented at the 3rd world congress on pain, Edinburgh, Scotland.

Kleiber, C., Suwanraj, M., Dolan, L.A., Berg, M. and Kleese, A. (2007) Pain-sensitive temperament and postoperative pain, *Journal of the Society of Pediatric Nursing*, 12(3): 149–158.

Kotchick, B.A., Forehand, R., Armistead, L., Klein, K. and Wierson, M. (1996) Coping with illness: interrelationships across family members and predictors of psychological adjustment, *Journal of Family Psychology*, 10: 358–370.

Kuba, T. and Quinones-Jenab, V. (2005) The role of female gonadal hormones on behavioural sex differences in persistent and chronic pain: clinical versus preclinical studies, *Brain Research Bulletin*, 66: 179–188.

Lander, J. and Fowler-Kerry, S. (1991) Age differences in children's pain, *Perceptual and Motor Skills*, 73(2): 415–418.

Lee, L.W. and White-Traut, R.C. (1996) The role of temperament in pediatric pain response, *Issues in Comprehensive Pediatric Nursing*, 19: 49–63.

Lynch, A.M., Kashikar-Zuck, S., Goldschneider, K.R. and Jones, B.A. (2007) Sex and age differences in coping styles among children with chronic pain, *Journal of Pain and Symptom Management*, 33(2): 208–216.

Manne, S., Jacobsen, P. and Redd, W.H. (1992) Assessment of acute paediatric pain: do child self-report, parent ratings and nurse ratings measure the same phenomenon? *Pain*, 48: 45–52.

Martin, A.L., McGrath, P.A., Brown, S.C. and Katz, J. (2007) Children with chronic pain: impact of sex and age on long-term conditions, *Pain*, 128: 13–19.

McGrath, P.A. and Hillier, L.M. (2003) Modifying the psychologic factors that intensify children's pain and prolong disability. In Schechter, N.L., Berde, C.B. and Yaster, M. (eds.) *Pain in Infants, Children and Adolescents*, 2nd edition, Lippincott, Williams & Wilkins, Baltimore, pp. 85–127.

Mikail, S.F. and von Baeyer, C.L. (1990) Pain, somatic focus and emotional adjustment in children of chronic headache sufferers and controls. *Social Science and Medicine*, 31(1): 51–59.

Palmero, T.M. and Drotar, D. (1996) Prediction of children's postoperative pain: the role of presurgical expectations and anticipatory emotions, *Journal of Pediatric Psychology*, 21: 683–698.

Perquin, C.W., Hazebroek-Kampschreur, A.A.J.M., Hunfield, J.A.M., Bohen, A.M., van Suijlekom-Smit, L.W.A., Passchier, J. and van der Wouden, J.C. (2000) Pain in children and adolescents: a common experience, *Pain*, 87: 51–58.

Pfefferbaum, B., Adams, J., and Aceves, J. (1990) The influence of culture on pain in Anglo and Hispanic children with cancer, *Journal of the American Academy of Child and Adolescent Psychiatry*, 29(4): 642–647.

Roth-Isigkeit, A., Thyen, U., Stoven, H., Schwarzenberger, J. and Schumaker, P. (2005) Pain among children and adolescents: restrictions in daily living and triggering factors, *Pediatrics*, 115(2): 152–162.

Ross, D.M. and Ross, S.A. (1984) Childhood pain: the school-aged child's viewpoint, *Pain*, 20:179–191.

Saunders, K., Von Korff, M., LeResche, L. and Mancl, L. (2007) Relationship of common pain conditions in mothers and children, *Clinical Journal of Pain*, 23(3): 204–213.

Schechter, N.L., Bernstein, B.A., Beck, A., Hart, L. and Scherzer, L. (1991) Individual difference in children's responses to pain: role of temperament and parental characteristics, *Pediatrics*, 87(2): 171–177.

Scott, R. (1978) 'It hurts red': a preliminary study of children's perceptions of pain, *Perceptual and Motor Skills*, 47:787–791.

Twycross, A. (1998) Children's cognitive level and their perceptions of pain. In Twycross, A., Moriarty, A. and Betts, T. (eds.) *Paediatric Pain Management: A Multi-disciplinary Approach*, Radcliffe Medical Press, Oxford, pp. 25–37.

Unruh, A. (1996) Gender variations in clinical pain experience, *Pain*, 65: 123–167.

Wallace, M. (1989) Temperament: a variable in children's pain management, *Pediatric Nursing*, 15(2): 118–121.

Weisman, S.J., Bernstein, B. and Schechter, N.L. (1998) Consequences of inadequate analgesia during painful procedures in children, *Archives of Pediatric Adolescent Medicine*,152: 147–149.

Zubieta, J-K., Heitzeg, M.M., Smith, Y.R., Bueller, J.A., Xu, K., Xu, Y., Koeppe, R.A., Stohler, C.S. and Goldman, D. (2003) COMT val158met genotype affects [mu]-opioid neurotransmitter responses to a pain stressor, *Science*, 299(5610): 1240–1243.

CHAPTER 4
Pharmacology of Analgesic Drugs
Stephanie J. Dowden

Introduction

This chapter will provide an overview of the pharmacology of the commonly used analgesic drugs and some adjuvant medications. Although the range of analgesic drugs is increasing, many of these medications have not been tested in children and are not licensed for use in children under 12 years or are administered off-label (outside recommended guidelines), due to a lack of paediatric clinical trials (Berde and Sethna 2002; Kanneh 2002a; WHO 2007). In practical terms this means that clinicians have to rely on best practice principles and/or opinions and recommendations from leading paediatric institutions rather than clinical data from high-quality paediatric pharmacological research (Kanneh 2002a). Measures are being taken to address this issue, with the European Union and North America taking a lead by legislating new frameworks to ensure best practice in pharmaceutical products for children (WHO 2007).

Having a greater knowledge about the pharmacology of analgesic drugs is likely to enhance nurses' pain management practice; a lack of understanding of this area has been postulated as a one reason for the poor management of pain in children. This is discussed in detail in Chapter 11.

While analgesic drugs have a significant role in pain management their combined effect with non-drug strategies for better pain management outcomes should not be underestimated (Berde and Sethna 2002). Conversely, Berde and Sethna (2002) caution that the use of non-drug strategies should not be a reason to withhold analgesia.

4.1 Misconceptions

Several misconceptions about pain in children exist (see Chapters 1, 2 and 9). There are many and varied reasons for misconceptions about pain in childhood. Some of these are due to a lack of knowledge, inaccurate education or a poor understanding of the similarities and differences between children and adults. The key misconceptions about the use of analgesic drugs for children are outlined in Table 4.1.

4.2 Addiction, Dependence and Tolerance

Confusion exists among many nurses, and other healthcare professionals, about tolerance and physical dependence and the terminology relating to substance abuse (Australian and New Zealand College of Anaesthetists and Faculty of Pain Medicine [ANZCA] 2005;

Table 4.1   Misconceptions about the use of analgesic drugs for children

Misconception	Facts
All children are sensitive to analgesic drugs	• Infants and children require the same categories of analgesic drugs as adults, however age-appropriate dosing must be considered
Children are at greater risk (than adults) of addiction from opioids	• The fear of opioid addiction in children has been greatly exaggerated with the incidence <1%
Opioids are not safe to use for infants and children	• Opioids are no more dangerous to infants and children than they are to adults • The risk of respiratory depression is no greater for infants and children provided the dose is appropriate

Source: Charlton (2005)

Charlton 2005). Unfortunately this misinformation is passed on to colleagues, patients and their families, leading to further confusion, unnecessary anxiety and suboptimal pain management (ANZCA 2005). To diminish confusion and encourage uniformity of practice a number of lead clinical organisations including the American Pain Society, the American Academy of Pain Medicine and the American Society of Addiction Medicine developed consensus statements and agreed definitions. ANZCA (2005) outlines a summary of these statements and definitions in Box 4.1.

BOX 4.1

Definitions of opioid terminology

Tolerance

• Decreased effectiveness of a drug over time, thus a higher dose of the drug is needed to achieve the same effect.
• Tolerance develops to desired (*analgesia*) and undesired (*sedation, itch,* etc.) effects of opioids at different rates.

Physical dependence

• A physiological response to the abrupt discontinuation (or dose reduction or reversal) of a drug that leads to a withdrawal (abstinence) syndrome.

Addiction

• Psychological dependence on drugs with drug-seeking and drug-using behaviour that is characterised by cravings, compulsion, loss of control and lack of concern for social or health consequences.

Withdrawal syndrome

• A cluster of physiological signs and symptoms that occur following the abrupt discontinuation of an opioid (Box 4.2).

Source: ANZCA (2005)

Practice point

Opioid withdrawal is not considered a life-threatening condition compared to benzodiazepine or alcohol withdrawal. However, the infants and children at greatest risk of opioid withdrawal are those who have experienced a prolonged intensive care unit (ICU) admission, with administration of high doses of opioids, benzodiazepines and other sedative agents.

Many of these infants or children have pre-existing or acquired cardiovascular instability. This, in combination with the autonomic instability caused by acute opioid withdrawal, can have profound physiological effects and may be a cause of unplanned re-admissions to ICU.

Fears of addiction related to the use of opioids for severe and short-term pain are unsupported, with the incidence of addiction considered to be very low (<1%) (Bryant et al. 2003; Jovey et al. 2003; Ballantyne and LaForge 2007). However, signs of both tolerance and physical dependence can occur in patients following administration of opioids and other drugs, (e.g. benzodiazepines and other sedative agents) for more than 5–10 days (Yaster et al. 1997). Although tolerance and physical dependence (withdrawal) are two components of addiction, a person cannot be defined as having addiction without *also* having the behavioural factors associated with addiction (e.g. cravings, compulsive drug seeking, loss of control and lack of concern). The key issue is to ensure that all opioid-tolerant patients (including those with *and* without problematic opioid use) are identified and steps are taken to ensure abstinence syndrome is avoided or minimised (Box 4.2).

BOX 4.2

Pain management for opioid-tolerant patients

Who are opioid-tolerant patients?

- Patients with a history of illicit drug use; either using opioids or on a treatment programme
- Patients with chronic cancer pain or non-cancer pain being treated with opioids
- Patients with acute opioid tolerance due to recent high opioid requirements e.g. following ICU admission or major trauma *(This group is the most commonly seen in paediatric clinical practice)*

Key principles

- Ensure effective analgesia
- Do *not* withhold opioids (this places the patient at risk of acute opioid withdrawal)
- Usual opioid regimens will need to be maintained (often used as a baseline for other analgesia)
- Be aware that opioid requirements may be several times higher than for opioid-naïve patients
- Opioid-tolerant patients may report higher pain scores and have lower levels of adverse opioid effects than opioid-naïve patients
- Adjuvant medications may assist with analgesia, e.g. tramadol, ketamine, NSAIDs and/or regional analgesia.
- Be alert to signs of opioid withdrawal, that is, sweating, nausea and/or vomiting, agitation, diarrhoea, yawning, dilated pupils, anxiety, restlessness, insomnia, tachycardia, hypertension, cramping abdominal pain.

Source: ANZCA (2005)

Undertreatment of pain and consequential drug-seeking behaviour (also referred to as **pseudo-addiction**) is far more common than addiction, and perhaps should be considered an iatrogenic condition. These behaviours are commonly caused by clinicians with a poor understanding of the risk of addiction withholding or minimising access to analgesia for patients with chronic or recurrent painful conditions (e.g. haemophilia, renal calculi, back pain and sickle cell disease). This, in turn, can lead to blaming, stigmatisation and ongoing punitive clinical management, rather than a more balanced approach or referral to pain specialists. The key characteristic of pseudo-addiction is that it ceases when adequate analgesia is given.

4.3 How Drugs Work

This section will summarise the main points about drugs and how they work, with particular emphasis on analgesic drugs. Additional reading of key pharmacology texts such as Rang et al. (2003), Neal (2002) and Bryant et al. (2003) will assist understanding further.

- A drug is a bioactive molecule that is not normally a part of the body. It may be a therapeutic agent, a poison or a food component.
- The action of a drug is the chemical interaction between the drug and body tissue.
- Each drug affects the body in a specific way. However, no drug is completely specific in its action, which is why adverse effects can occur (Rang et al. 2003).
- The aim of drug therapy is to give the right dose of a drug, that is, enough to achieve a useful effect but not so much as to be toxic (Begg 2003).
- The two key pharmacological actions are pharmacodynamics (the study of drug action) and pharmacokinetics (the study of drug movement).

Commonly used pharmacology definitions are outlined in Table 4.2.

4.3.1 Pharmacodynamics

Pharmacodynamics is the mechanism of drug actions and their biochemical and physiological effects on body systems, that is, *what the drug does to the body* (Kanneh 2002a; Begg 2003).

- Drug molecules must be bound to a body substance to reach the target tissue and produce a physiological response (Rang et al. 2003).
- There are four types of substances that drugs are bound to: receptors, ion channels, carriers and enzymes.

Receptors are proteins that perform an action in response to recognising another substance. Some drugs must combine with receptors to achieve an effect, like a key being inserted into a lock. Drugs bind to receptors in response to the concentration of the drug and their ability to bind (affinity) to a receptor. The higher the affinity of the drug the lower the dose needed to produce an effect. Drugs can be agonists (that bind with the receptors and activate them) or antagonists (that bind at the receptor without activation, or block their usual action).

Practice point

Morphine is a *full agonist* at the μ (mu) opioid receptor. It has strong *affinity* for the mu receptor, thus even a small dose will exert an effect. Morphine is a *partial agonist* at the δ (delta) and κ (kappa) opioid receptors.

Naloxone is an *antagonist* at the mu opioid receptor. This means it blocks the binding of morphine to the mu receptor, which in turn blocks the action of morphine.

Ion channels are pores in the cell wall that allow passage of ions. Some ion channels require a receptor to be bound by an agonist before they open, with other ion channels being directly targeted by drugs (Rang et al. 2003).

Table 4.2 Pharmacology definitions

Term	Definition
Adverse drug reaction (ADR)	Undesired effect of the drug or consequences of the drug–receptor interaction occurring at usual or desired doses of the drug
Adverse effect	*See adverse drug reaction*
Affinity	The attraction between the drug and the receptor (described as high or low)
Agonist	A drug that binds to a receptor and activates it (fully or partially)
Antagonist	A drug that binds to a receptor without activating it, but blocking agonist access
Bioavailability	The rate and extent of drug absorbed into systemic circulation after administration. Bioavailability is 100% after intravenous administration
Ceiling effect	When a dose higher than recommended will not produce a greater effect
Clearance	The rate at which a drug is eliminated from the body over time
Dose interval	Time needed between drug doses to keep the drug within the therapeutic index
Drug action	The action between the drug and receptor
Drug:drug interaction	When the effects of one drug are increased or decreased by another drug
Duration of action	Time the drug action lasts at an effective concentration
Enzymes	Proteins that regulate the rate of chemical reactions in the body
First-pass metabolism	Drugs that are taken orally enter the portal (hepatic) circulation and are partly metabolised prior to entering the systemic circulation
Half-life (t½)	Time (in hours) it takes for the drug concentration in blood to fall by half its value
Hormones	Chemicals produced in the body that regulate activity of some cells and organs
Ion channels	Pores in the cell membrane that allow passage of ions into and out of the cell
Loading dose	Administering a higher dose to achieve early therapeutic plasma levels
Maintenance dose	Dose required to maintain plasma drug levels at a steady state
Onset of action	Time it takes for the drug to begin working
OTC	Over the counter (drugs that are able to be purchased without a prescription)
Prodrug	A drug that is metabolised in the body to another form before it becomes active
Receptors	Protein molecules activated by transmitters or hormones
Side effect	*See adverse drug reaction*
Steady state	The drug at a uniform level in the body, where the administration rate of the drug equals the elimination rate of the drug
Time to steady state	How long it takes the drug to reach a steady state (usually $4 \times t1/2$)
Therapeutic index (sometimes referred to as the 'therapeutic window')	The variance between the therapeutic dose and the toxic dose of a drug: Narrow or low therapeutic index drugs have a high risk of toxicity Wide or high therapeutic index drugs have a low risk of toxicity
Volume of distribution	How and where the drug is distributed around the body

Source: Kanneh (2002a, b); Neal (2002); Begg (2003)

Practice point

Local anaesthetics directly target sodium ion channels in nerve fibres.
  By blocking the sodium channels, conduction along the nerve fibre is prevented, thus blocking transmission of sensations such as pain and touch.

Carriers are protein molecules that help to *carry* or transport substances across cell membranes (Rang et al. 2003). Some carriers work at nerve terminals and are involved with the movement of neurotransmitters, e.g. serotonin, noradrenaline, γ-aminobutyric acid (GABA) and glutamate. These carriers are specifically targeted by some drugs, which can reduce or enhance the amount of neurotransmitter at the synapse.

Practice point

Tramadol inhibits the reuptake of serotonin and noradrenaline from nerve synapses, thus leading to higher levels of these pain-modulating neurotransmitters.

Enzymes are biological catalysts that control biochemical reactions of a cell (Bryant et al. 2003). Some drugs can inhibit the action of an enzyme and thus alter the physiological response.

Practice point

Non-steroidal anti-inflammatory drugs (NSAIDs), such as ibuprofen and diclofenac, inhibit the action of the enzyme cyclo-oxygenase, which in turn stops the synthesis of prostaglandins and thus reduces pain and the inflammatory response.

4.3.2 Pharmacokinetics

Pharmacokinetics is the process of the movement of drugs through the body involving absorption, distribution, metabolism and elimination (Kanneh 2002b). Begg (2003) describes pharmacokinetics more simply as *what the body does to the drug*.

Absorption involves entrance of the drug into the circulatory system from the site of entry. Absorption is dependent on factors such as the drug formulation, the route of administration, the blood flow at the site of administration and the surface area exposed to the drug (Kanneh 2002b).

Practice point

- The rectal route of administration can lead to erratic drug absorption due to drug placement issues, rectal blood flow and faecal loading.
- With the oral route of administration liquid preparations are absorbed faster than tablet or capsule formulations.
- Intravenous administration of drugs provides the fastest onset of action.

Distribution of the drug around the body occurs once the drug enters the circulatory system and from there reaches the drug's target tissue. Drugs are mostly bound to plasma proteins and *piggy-back* on them to get to their destination. Drug distribution is affected by cardiac output, total amount of body water (infants and children have greater body water compared to adults) and the concentration of plasma proteins (decreased in infants compared to older children and adults) (Kanneh 2002b).

Metabolism is when the drug is broken down into active and/or inactive components (metabolites) prior to elimination. This process is mostly carried out by enzymes and occurs predominantly in the hepatic system. One of the major enzyme groups involved in metabolism is the cytochrome p450 (also known as CYP) family of enzymes (Begg 2003; Bryant et al. 2003). There are about 18 groups of CYP enzymes, which are separately coded into various subfamilies, for example CYP2D6 (Cytochrome P450 2D6) is involved in tramadol, amitriptyline and codeine metabolism (Bryant et al. 2003). A basic knowledge of CYP enzymes can help nurses understand why giving drugs metabolised by the same P450 system might be problematic, for example giving tramadol and codeine together can reduce their efficacy.

The liver metabolises some drugs so efficiently that the amount reaching the systemic circulation is less than the amount first absorbed. This is known as *first-pass metabolism* and means that larger doses are needed orally than via other routes. Morphine, which has a high first-pass effect, has significant dosing difference when administered orally versus intravenously, with the oral dose being three times greater than the intravenous dose. Some drugs (e.g. lignocaine and glyceryl trinitrate) have such high first-pass metabolism they are almost inactive when administered orally and must be given by other routes (Neal 2002).

Practice point

Some drugs (pro-drugs) are inactive when administered and need to undergo metabolism to be converted from an inactive form to an active form. For example, diamorphine (heroin) and codeine are converted to morphine.

Elimination is the process of removal of the drug from the body. It occurs most commonly via renal excretion, with lesser amounts removed via the gastrointestinal system, expiration, saliva, sweat and tears. Drugs that are removed from the body primarily by renal excretion can cause toxicity when renal function is impaired.

Practice point

If a patient has hepatic dysfunction they will have decreased rates of drug metabolism, thus increased circulating drug levels and an increased risk of toxicity.

If a patient has renal dysfunction they will have decreased drug elimination with reduced clearance of the drug and thus increased circulating drug levels and increased risk of toxicity.

Neonates have reduced hepatic metabolism and renal excretion abilities due to their organ immaturity, thus they too are at risk of high circulating drug levels and drug toxicity.

Consequently, patients with hepatic and/or renal dysfunction (and neonates) may need lower doses of drugs, or decreased dosing frequency or have drugs prescribed with fewer renal or hepatic effects.

4.4 Routes of Drug Administration

The route of drug administration affects the speed of onset and the amount of therapeutic response (Bryant et al. 2003). The effect that is desired from the drug will also influence the route chosen. For example, a topical route would be chosen for a drug that is required to act on the skin, but for a rapid systemic effect the parenteral or inhalation route would be more appropriate. There are four main routes of drug administration: enteral, parenteral, inhalation and topical (Box 4.3).

BOX 4.3

Four main routes of drug administration

Enteral

(via the gastrointestinal system)
This is the most common route of drug administration

- oral (PO)
- sublingual/buccal
- rectal (PR)
- nasogastric (NG)
- gastrostomy
- nasojejunal (NJ)

Parenteral

(via the circulatory system)

- intravenous (IV)
- intra-arterial (IA)
- intramuscular (IM)
- subcutaneous (SC)
- intrathecal (spinal) (IT)
- epidural
- intraosseous (IO)

Inhalation

(via the respiratory system)

- gas
- mist/aerosol
- nebuliser/puffer

Topical

(via the skin or mucous membranes)

- skin
- transdermal (TD)
- eyes
- ears
- nose

Source: Bryant et al. (2003)

Other aspects to consider are the advantages and disadvantages of using different routes of analgesic drug administration, some of which are specific to children. All these factors need to be considered when deciding the best route to use (Table 4.3).

Table 4.3 Routes of analgesic drug administration for children: advantages and disadvantages

Route	Advantages	Disadvantages
Oral	Painless Large drug choice Preferred by children	Slow acting Some children dislike oral analgesic drugs Problem if nausea/vomiting
Nasogastric	Useful if children can't/won't take oral medication Large drug choice Useful for high volume/noxious tasting medication Preferred by some children	Slow acting Invasive/painful to insert NG tube Additional nursing care required Some children dislike NG tubes
Rectal	Useful if nausea/vomiting Not reliant on gut function Useful if no IV, avoids IM injections	Wide variability in drug levels/absorption Slowest acting Limited drug choice Generally disliked by children
Intravenous	Fast acting, allows rapid analgesia Useful for intermittent bolus, infusion and patient-controlled analgesia (PCA)	Invasive/painful to insert IV Additional nursing care required More risks/side effects from IV and analgesic drugs
Intramuscular	Easy insertion Fewer side effects compared to IV	Painful Disliked by children Slower analgesic onset Wide variability in drug levels/absorption
Subcutaneous	Easy insertion Fewer side effects compared to IV and IM Avoids need for IV Useful in community settings Useful for intermittent bolus, infusion and patient-controlled analgesia (PCA)	May be painful to insert Slower analgesic onset compared to IV
Epidural	Fast acting Extremely effective, allows total analgesia	Invasive, needs highly skilled clinicians Inserted under sedation/anaesthesia Intensive nursing care required More risks/side effects
Buccal Nasal Inhalation	Avoids first-pass metabolism, not reliant on gut function Fast acting and short acting Less invasive	Variable acceptability by children Limited drug availability
Topical (e.g. creams, transdermal patches)	Least invasive Painless	Slowest acting Very limited drug availability

Source: Adapted from WHO (1998)

4.5 Selection of Analgesic Drugs

In addition to deciding the most appropriate route of administration it is also important to consider the most appropriate type of analgesic drug to give.

Practice point

For optimal analgesic drug selection:

- assess pain (see Chapter 6);
- identify the type and severity of pain;
- select the most appropriate analgesic drug considering route, adverse effects, benefits, risks and safety.

4.5.1 WHO analgesic ladder

The World Health Organization (WHO) *analgesic ladder* (Figure 4.1) was developed as a model for providing guidelines to clinicians about cancer pain management (WHO 1996). The analgesic ladder was designed for oral cancer pain management but is also applicable to acute pain management, and can be used in reverse for weaning. It offers a 3-step approach to pain management, which suggests as the pain increases the analgesic drugs should be adjusted accordingly.

Step 1 (mild pain)
- Administer a non-opioid, i.e. paracetamol and/or NSAID (e.g. ibuprofen or diclofenac).

Step 2 (moderate pain)
- Continue Step 1 medications and add a simple opioid, e.g. codeine or dihydrocodeine.

Step 3 (severe pain)
- Continue steps 1 and 2 medications and add a strong opioid (e.g. morphine or fentanyl or hydromorphone or oxycodone or diamorphine).
- Consider the addition of regional anaesthesia (e.g. epidural or nerve block).

Other medications, such as the adjuvants ketamine, tramadol, clonidine, amitriptyline or nortriptyline and gabapentin may be added at different steps of the ladder according to the type and quality of the pain. Eisenberg et al. (2005) suggest if step 1 is ineffective or if the pain is severe to begin with to avoid step 2 and go directly to step 3. Thus one should select the *starting* step according to current pain severity. Eisenberg et al. (2005) also suggest that weak opioids have little role in acute pain management (except in countries with no access to strong opioids) and that small doses of strong opioids are more efficacious.

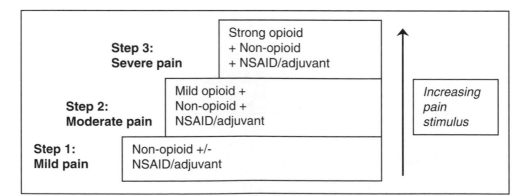

Figure 4.1   WHO Analgesic Ladder (adapted from WHO 1996).

4.5.2 Analgesic drugs

The following sections will provide details of the main analgesic drugs in three categories: non-opioids, opioids and adjuvant analgesic drugs.

4.6 Non-opioid analgesic drugs

4.6.1 Paracetamol (acetaminophen)

Overview
Paracetamol:

- is the most commonly used analgesic drug for children;
- has antipyretic (fever reducing) activity, but minimal anti-inflammatory effects (unlike NSAIDs);
- is highly effective as a sole analgesic for mild to moderate pain;
- enhances analgesia when used in combination with NSAIDs or tramadol (Remy et al. 2006);
- also has opioid sparing effects (reduces the amount of opioid required) of up to 20% in adults when given in combination with opioids (Remy et al. 2006);
- is probably underused in patients with moderate to severe pain, when many clinicians rely heavily on opioids (Harrop 2007).

Action
- Paracetamol selectively inhibits prostaglandin synthesis (probably by inhibiting cyclo-oxygenase-3; COX-3) in the central nervous system, which is why it has antipyretic and analgesic effects but no anti-inflammatory effects or unwanted gastrointestinal effects (Chandrasekharan et al. 2002; Remy et al. 2006; Harrop 2007; Morton 2007).
- Normal gastrointestinal function is required for oral paracetamol administration, thus if the child has an ileus the intravenous or rectal routes are more efficacious, with some authors suggesting the intravenous route is superior (Anderson and Palmer 2006; Henneberg and Nilsson 2007).

Metabolism/elimination
Paracetamol is metabolised in the liver. Glucuronide and sulfate are the main metabolites, which are excreted via the kidneys. Another metabolite, N-acetyl-p-benzo-quinone-imine (NAPQI), is responsible for the toxic effects of paracetamol. NAPQI is normally metabolised to a harmless compound by glutathione (an antioxidant enzyme). However, with excessive paracetamol levels (>150 mg/kg) glutathione is unable to metabolise NAPQI fast enough and liver toxicity results. In some clinical groups (nutritionally compromised, hepatic disease or abnormal gastrointestinal function) glutathione levels are depleted, leaving these patients at greater risk of paracetamol toxicity (Bryant et al. 2002; Remy et al. 2006; Rose 2007).

Practice point

Paracetamol toxicity is most likely to occur: (i) following a paracetamol overdose; (ii) with chronic paracetamol use; (iii) in patients who already have some degree of liver malfunction; (iv) in neonates.

Liver toxicity and subsequent fulminant liver failure present at least two to three days following a paracetamol overdose.

Unfortunately, early symptoms of paracetamol poisoning are non-specific (nausea or vomiting, anorexia and abdominal pain). Thus if the paracetamol overdose is unsuspected or unreported the consequences can be fatal.

With early intervention NAPQI is neutralised by administration of N-acetylcysteine, to form a non-toxic compound that is excreted renally.

Adverse effects

There are very low rates of adverse drug effects with paracetamol, but the potential for hepatotoxicity still exists (Remy et al. 2006). Acute hepatotoxicity is considered to be very unlikely when therapeutic dose regimes are followed. Minor adverse effects from paracetamol are uncommon and include gastrointestinal upset and skin reactions.

Dose, onset time, peak effect and half-life

- Paracetamol can be administered via oral, rectal and intravenous routes (Table 4.4).
- For greatest efficacy a loading dose is suggested.
- Due to their immature liver function, neonates require reduced doses.

Table 4.4   Paracetamol doses

Drug	*Route*	*Dose*	*Onset/Peak/t1/2*
Paediatric paracetamol doses			
Paracetamol	Oral	Loading dose: 20 mg/kg Then: 15 mg/kg 4 to 6 hourly (maximum dose: 90 mg/kg/day) For prolonged use the maximum dose should be 75 mg/kg/day	Onset time: 30–60 min Peak effect: 1–2 h t1/2: 1–3 h
Paracetamol	Rectal	Loading dose: 30 mg/kg Then: 20 mg/kg 6 hourly (maximum dose: 90 mg/kg/day)	Onset time and peak effect: longer and more variable than oral dosing (peak effect up to 2.5 h)
Perfalgan® (intravenous paracetamol)	Intravenous	Loading dose: 15 mg/kg Then: 15 mg/kg 6 hourly (maximum dose: 60 mg/kg/day)	Onset time: 15–30 min Peak effect: 1 h t1/2: 1.5–3 h
Neonatal paracetamol doses			
Paracetamol *Term neonates*	Oral	Loading dose: 20 mg/kg Then: 10–15 mg/kg 8 hourly (maximum dose: 60 mg/kg/day)	Onset time: 30–60 min Peak effect: 1–3 h
Perfalgan® *Term neonates*	Intravenous	7.5 mg/kg 8 hourly (maximum dose: 30 mg/kg/day)	Onset time: 15–30 min Peak effect: 1 h
Paracetamol *Term neonates*	Rectal	Loading dose: 30 mg/kg Then: 20 mg/kg 8 hourly (maximum dose: 60 mg/kg/day)	Onset time and peak effect: longer and more variable than oral dosing (peak effect up to 2.5 h)
Preterm Neonates			
Paracetamol *>32 weeks post-conception age*	Oral	Loading dose: 20 mg/kg Then: 10–15 mg/kg 8–12 hourly (maximum dose: 60 mg/kg/day)	
Paracetamol *28–32 weeks post-conception age*	Oral	Loading dose: 20 mg/kg Then: 10–15 mg/kg 12 hourly (maximum dose: 35 mg/kg/day)	

There is very limited safety and efficacy data for the use of Perfalgan® in preterm neonates

Source: Anderson and Palmer (2006); Henneberg and Nilsson (2007); Morton (2007); Rose (2007)

4.6.2 Non-steroidal anti-inflammatory drugs

Overview
Non-steroidal anti-inflammatory drugs (NSAIDs):

- are used for the treatment of mild to moderate pain, especially inflammatory-mediated conditions;
- in children are used mainly in the postoperative setting, following trauma or for home-based pain and fever management;
- are also used for chronic inflammatory diseases (e.g. arthritis) and for bone pain caused by cancer;
- have antipyretic activity as well as anti-inflammatory and analgesic activity;
- have a significant opioid-sparing effect and may reduce morphine requirements by up to 30–40% (Morton 2007); this has the added benefit of reducing opioid-related adverse effects, as lower doses of opioids are needed.

Action
NSAIDs act by inhibiting the synthesis of prostaglandins by inhibiting the production of (cyclo-oxygenase-1) COX-1 and (cyclo-oxygenase-2) COX-2 enzymes. This in turn reduces inflammatory pain-inducing chemicals and thus decreases the response of peripheral and central pain receptors. Older NSAIDs (e.g. ibuprofen, diclofenac, indomethacin, aspirin) are less selective and block both COX-1 and COX-2, hence their incidence of adverse effects. Newer NSAIDs (e.g. celecoxib, parecoxib) selectively block COX-2 rather than COX-1, which reduces their adverse effects. The effects of COX-1 and COX-2 are compared in Table 4.5.

Table 4.5   Comparing the effects of COX-1 and COX-2

COX-1	COX-2
Present in most body tissues.	Present in inflammatory cells when activated.
Involved in cell/tissue homeostasis, e.g. maintain gastric acid balance, maintain protective mucous lining in gastrointestinal tract, maintain renal blood flow, platelet function and bronchodilation.	Responsible for many mediators of inflammation leading to: vasodilation, oedema, hyperalgesia and pyrogenesis (fever production).
Blocking COX-1 causes gastric irritation/gastric ulceration, renal impairment or renal failure, platelet dysfunction (bleeding) and bronchospasm.	Blocking COX-2 causes analgesia, anti-inflammatory and antipyretic actions.

Practice point

A new class of NSAIDs, cyclo-oxygenase-2 selective inhibitors (COX-2 inhibitors), was introduced onto the market in the late 1990s.

It was thought that the COX-2 inhibitors would be safer and gentler than existing NSAIDs by selectively inhibiting COX-2 inflammatory prostaglandins without affecting COX-1.

Worldwide sales were huge and a new generation of drugs for treating arthritis pain was heralded. Unfortunately the level of selectivity was not as great as first thought, with large numbers of patients suffering adverse COX-1 effects.

Consequently rofecoxib (Vioxx) and valdecoxib (Bextra) were withdrawn from the market in 2004/5 and clinical indications for the use of COX-2 inhibitors revised.

Metabolism/elimination
- Most NSAIDs undergo hepatic metabolism (Kokki 2003).
- Two-thirds of the drug or its metabolites are excreted renally, with the remainder excreted in the faeces (Kokki 2003).

Adverse effects

> **Reye's syndrome**
>
> Use of aspirin in children with viral illnesses is associated with an increased risk of developing Reye's Syndrome (acute encephalopathy with liver damage), although the degree of causality is questioned.
>
> **Thus it is not recommended that aspirin be used in children under 16 years in the UK.**
>
> *This age recommendation varies in different countries.*

- Due to their inhibition of COX-1 production, NSAIDs have the potential for serious side effects: bleeding, gastrointestinal mucosal damage, asthma and renal impairment.
- The risk of bleeding following surgery (mainly tonsillectomy) has been overstated but is still present (Kokki 2003; Lonnqvist and Morton 2005; Anderson and Palmer 2006).
- NSAIDs may cause bronchoconstriction and induce acute episodes of asthma in *aspirin-sensitive* asthmatics, especially those with multiple allergies or nasal polyp disease (Anderson and Palmer 2006).
- Renal blood flow may be reduced and renal failure may result, particularly in children with pre-existing renal impairment or hypovolaemia or dehydration.
- NSAIDs have been shown to decrease osteoblast activity in animal studies, thus they may slow bone healing, particularly following bone grafting; however, the benefits of short-term use may outweigh the risks (Kokki 2003; Lonnqvist and Morton 2005).
- Less serious adverse effects include skin reactions, diarrhoea, nausea and vomiting.

> **Practice point**
>
> It is important to note that the adverse effects of NSAIDs can occur with *all* routes of administration, not just the oral route.

NSAIDs should be avoided or used with caution in patients with:

- bleeding disorders or at risk of haemorrhage;
- renal impairment;
- dehydration or hypovolaemia;
- moderate to severe asthma with nasal polyp disease;
- known aspirin or NSAID allergy;
- history of gastrointestinal ulceration or bleeding.

Dose, onset time, peak effect and half-life
- NSAIDs can be administered via oral, rectal and intravenous routes (Table 4.6).
- Due to infants' immature renal function, NSAIDs are not generally prescribed to children under the age of six months.

Table 4.6 NSAID doses

Drug	Route	Dose	Onset/Peak/t1/2
Diclofenac	Oral or rectal	0.5–2 mg/kg 8–12 hourly (maximum 3 mg/kg/day)	Onset time: 20–30 min Peak effect: 1–2 h t1/2: 1–2 h
Ibuprofen	Oral	5–10 mg/kg 6–8 hourly (maximum 600 mg/dose)	Onset time: 20–30 min Peak effect: 1–2 h t1/2: 1–2 hours
Ketorolac	Oral or intravenous	0.2–0.4 mg/kg 6–8 hourly (maximum 2 mg/kg/day) *IV = maximum 20 doses or 5 days duration*	Onset time: 20–30 min Peak effect: 1–2 h t1/2: 4–6 h (oral) t1/2: 4 h (IV)
Naproxen	Oral	5–7.5 mg/kg 12 hourly (maximum 500 mg/dose)	Onset time: 20–30 min Peak effect: 2–4 h t1/2: 12–15 h
Piroxicam	Oral	0.2–0.5 mg/kg Daily dose (maximum 15 mg/day)	Onset time: 60–90 min Peak effect: 3–5 h t1/2: 30–50 h

Source: Kokki (2003); Lonnqvist and Morton (2005); Anderson and Palmer (2006); Rose (2007)

Practice point

Most non-opioid analgesic drugs have a *ceiling effect*, which means that doses higher than the recommended dose will not produce greater pain relief.

Most opioids (except codeine) do not have a ceiling effect other than that imposed by side effects; therefore, larger doses can be given for increasing severity of pain.

4.7 Opioid analgesic drugs

Overview
Opium:

- was discovered in pre-biblical times and is extracted from the opium poppy;
- was widely used from the Middle Ages in a medicine known as *tincture of opium* or laudanum;
- contains about 20 alkaloids (compounds), two of which, morphine and codeine, have analgesic action.

Opioid or opiate or narcotic?

Opioid: refers to *any* substance with morphine-like actions including natural, semi-synthetic and synthetic opioids. (***This is the preferred term***.)

Opiate: refers to *only* those drugs derived from the opium poppy, for example, morphine (thus excluding synthetic opioids such as fentanyl).

Narcotic: an obsolete term for opioids because governments, law enforcement and media use the term to refer to drugs of addiction and other illicit drugs including opioids, cocaine and amphetamines, thus it has no place in medical terminology about analgesic drugs.

Opioids:

- are used for treating moderate to severe pain;
- come in different levels of potency and efficacy, referred to as weak opioids (e.g. codeine) or strong opioids (e.g. morphine, hydromorphone);
- can be given in reduced doses without loss of analgesic effect when used in combination with non-opioids such as paracetamol and NSAIDs;
- have no ceiling dose for severe pain, with dosing only limited by adverse effects;
- for acute pain management, one opioid is not superior over others but some opioids are better tolerated by some patients, thus they may benefit from changing to another opioid if they have adverse effects (ANZCA 2005).

Action

- All opioids bind to opioid receptors located in the peripheral nervous system, central nervous system and spinal cord.
- Opioid receptors are distributed variably in the CNS with higher concentrations of receptors in areas most involved with nociception, e.g. the cerebral cortex, amygdala, thalamus and spinal cord.

> There are three main opioid receptors:
>
> **mu (μ)** primary action site for most opioid effects, except dysphoria;
> **delta (δ)** contributes to spinal analgesia, reduced gut motility and dysphoria;
> **kappa (κ)** contributes to peripheral analgesia, sedation and dysphoria.

The mu receptor has a principal role in analgesia:

- it is subtyped into mu-1 and mu-2 receptors;
- the mu-1 receptor is responsible for analgesia;
- the mu-2 receptor is responsible for most adverse effects of opioids: respiratory depression, cardiovascular depression, decreased gastrointestinal motility, miosis (pupil constriction), sedation, euphoria, urinary retention and physical dependence;
- the opioid action of all known natural and synthetic opioids at mu receptors is *nonspecific*;
- no opioid has yet been found or developed that acts *only* on the mu-1 receptor.

The two main cellular actions of opioid receptors (Rang et al. 2003):

1. They *close* calcium ion channels on presynaptic neurones, thus reducing the release of neurotransmitters that contribute to pain (e.g. substance P).
2. They *open* potassium ion channels, which inhibits postsynaptic neurones by reducing release of neurotransmitters that contribute to pain.

Metabolism/elimination

- Opioids are converted into metabolites (active and inactive) in the liver then excreted via the renal system.
- All opioid metabolites may accumulate in patients receiving long-term infusions or patients with renal impairment.
- Morphine has two main metabolites: morphine-3-glucuronide (M3G), which has no analgesic effects, but causes neurotoxic effects (including myoclonus and tremor); and morphine-6-glucuronide (M6G), which is a powerful analgesic three to four times stronger than morphine.

- Hydromorphone has one main metabolite, hydromorphone-3-glucuronide (H3G), which can cause neurotoxic effects (including confusion, tremor and agitation).
- Pethidine has one main metabolite, nor-pethidine, which can cause neurotoxic effects (including nervousness, confusion, tremor and seizures), it rapidly accumulates with pethidine infusions and patients with renal dysfunction are at higher risk of nor-pethidine toxicity, as they clear the drug more slowly.
- Fentanyl has no active metabolites, although prolonged fentanyl infusions may result in drug accumulation and potential increase in adverse effects.
- Codeine and oxycodone are metabolised by the CYP enzyme system (CYP2D6).

Practice point

For many years codeine has been considered a safer option than other opioids for children, largely due to the lower incidence of respiratory depression, but it has also been viewed as ineffective by many pain management clinicians.

In a study by Williams et al. (2002) up to 47% of children under 12 years were found to lack the enzyme to convert codeine to morphine, thus receiving little or no analgesic effect. This is the most likely explanation for the ineffectiveness of codeine and is why many pain management services now prefer to prescribe oral morphine or oxycodone as alternatives.

Adverse effects

Most adverse effects of opioids are dose-related (Table 4.7). By titrating the dose to the desired analgesic effect, ensuring vigilant nursing observation (particularly assessing sedation level, see Chapter 7) and the use of opioid-sparing drugs (e.g. paracetamol and NSAIDs) most significant adverse effects can be avoided (ANZCA 2005).

Table 4.7 Opioid adverse effects

Opioid adverse effect	Causes
Respiratory depression	Suppression of the brain stem respiratory centre leads to sedation, decreased tidal volume, reduced respiratory rate and reduced oxygen saturation, resulting in hypoxia and raised carbon dioxide levels, which leads to further sedation and further respiratory depression
Sedation	Central nervous system effect but may be due to accumulation of metabolites if renal impairment or receiving high doses of opioids
Nausea and vomiting	Stimulation of the chemoreceptor trigger zone (vomiting centre) in the CNS, stimulation of the vestibular system (middle ear) and decreased gastric motility
Constipation	Decreased gastrointestinal motility, especially large intestine peristalsis
Miosis (pupil constriction)	Central nervous system effect on the 3rd cranial nerve (oculomotor)
Euphoria	Central nervous system effect, causes altered perception of pain and a sense of well-being
Dysphoria	Central nervous system effect, but may be due to accumulation of metabolites if renal impairment or receiving high doses of opioids
Urinary retention	Increased muscle tone of ureters, bladder and sphincter
Pruritus	Histamine release

Source: Rang et al. (2003)

It should also be noted that:

- tolerance develops to respiratory depression, sedation, euphoria, dysphoria, nausea, vomiting, pruritus and urinary retention;
- minimal tolerance develops to miosis and constipation.

Dose, onset time, peak effect and half-life

- Opioids can be administered by almost all routes: oral, intravenous, subcutaneous, epidural and intrathecal, intranasal, inhaled and transdermal (Table 4.8).
- Requirements vary widely between individuals, thus opioids should *always* be titrated to effect.
- Pethidine should be avoided due to its higher rate of adverse effects.
- Due to their immature hepatic, renal and respiratory systems, neonates require reduced doses of opioids.
- Infants remain sensitive to opioids and at risk of apnoea for the first three months of life.

Table 4.8   Opioid doses

Drug	Route	Dose	Onset/Peak/t1/2
Buprenorphine	Oral/SL	3–5 microgram/kg 6–8 hourly	Onset time: 30 min Peak effect: 30–60 min t1/2: 3 h
Codeine	Oral or PR	0.5–1 mg/kg 4 hourly (Maximum 60 mg/dose)	Onset time: 15–20 min Peak effect: 30–60 min t1/2: 3 h
Diamorphine (Heroin)	Intranasal	0.1 mg/kg (Single dose, over 3 years)	Onset time: 20–30 min Peak effect: 30–45 min t1/2: 3 h
Dihydrocodeine	Oral	0.5–1 mg/kg 4–6 hourly	Onset time: 30 min Peak effect: 30–60 min t1/2: 3 h
Fentanyl	IV	IV bolus: 0.5–1 microgram/kg 1–2 hourly	Onset time: 1–3 min Peak effect: 10 min t1/2: 0.3–0.5 h
Hydromorphone	Oral or IV	Oral: 40–80 microgram/kg 3–4 hourly IV bolus: 10–20 microgram/kg 2–4 hourly	Onset time: 20 min (oral) Peak effect: 30–60 min (oral) t1/2: 3–4 h (oral)
Methadone	Oral	0.1–0.2 mg/kg 12–36 hourly	Onset time: 30–60 min Peak effect: 0.5–2 h t1/2: 15–80 h
Morphine	Oral or IV	Oral: 0.2–0.4 mg/kg 3–4 hourly (immediate [normal] release) IV bolus: 0.05–0.1 mg/kg 2–4 hourly	Onset time: 2–5 min (IV) Peak effect: 30–60 min (oral) Peak effect: 5–20 min IV t1/2: 2–4 h
Oxycodone	Oral	0.1–0.2 mg/kg 4 hourly (immediate [normal] release)	Onset time: 20–30 min Peak effect: 1–2 h t1/2: 3–4 h
Pethidine	IV	IV bolus: 0.5–1 mg/kg 2–4 hourly	Onset time: 2–5 min Peak effect: 1–2 h t1/2: 2–4 h

For details of opioid boluses and infusions and patient-controlled analgesia (PCA) regimes see Chapter 7
Source: Brown and Fisk (1992); ANZCA (2005); Brislin and Rose (2005); Greco and Berde (2005); Harrop (2007); Morton (2007); Rose (2007)

Practice point

A number of other opioids (e.g. ketobemidone, sufentanil, alfentanil, remifentanil) are used in paediatric practice. However, as they are mainly used in very specialised situations (e.g. during anaesthesia or in the ICU context) the doses are not discussed here.

4.7.1 Naloxone

Naloxone:

- is a pure opioid antagonist, which occupies and displaces opioids from all opioid receptors;
- has the greatest affinity to the mu-opioid receptor;
- is used to manage opioid-induced adverse effects, e.g. respiratory depression, sedation, nausea and vomiting, itch and urinary retention.

Metabolism/elimination
- Naloxone is metabolised in the liver then excreted via the renal system.

Dose, onset time, peak effect and half-life
- Naloxone can be administered by a number of routes, however the preferred route is intravenous (Table 4.9).
- Many patients achieve rapid reversal of adverse opioid effects following very small doses of naloxone, thus doses should be titrated to effect if possible to avoid inducing severe pain.
- The duration of action is 45 minutes, which is shorter than most opioids, thus repeated intravenous bolus doses or an infusion may be required.

4.8 Adjuvant analgesic drugs

Adjuvant analgesic drugs are a diverse group of drugs that work in a variety of ways to enhance analgesia (Knotkova and Pappagallo 2007), although some were originally developed for indications other than pain. They may:

- work to assist analgesia (co-analgesics) (e.g. muscle relaxants or antispasticity drugs).
- be used to counter the effect of an analgesic drug (e.g. laxatives or antiemetics).
- be analgesics in their own right (e.g. ketamine, gabapentin or amitriptyline).

Table 4.9 Naloxone doses

Drug	Route	Dose	Onset/Peak/t1/2
Naloxone	IV	Pruritus/urinary retention: 0.25–1 microgram/kg Sedation: 2–4 microgram/kg Respiratory depression: 5–10 microgram/kg	Onset time: 1–2 min Peak effect: 5 min t1/2: 1h

For details about managing opioid-induced respiratory depression see Chapter 7
Source: Brislin and Rose (2005); Greco and Berde (2005)

4.8.1 Tramadol

Overview
Tramadol:

- is a synthetic analgesic;
- is used for mild to moderate pain;
- is useful when combined with other analgesic drugs;
- has a lower risk of respiratory depression and impairs gastrointestinal function less than other opioids at equi-analgesic doses (ANZCA 2005);
- has effects on both acute nociceptive and neuropathic pain.

Action
Tramadol has both opioid and non-opioid properties and is either not considered a true opioid or it is classified as a weak opioid. It is a partial agonist at the mu-opioid receptor but has no affinity for the delta or kappa opioid receptors (Bozkurt 2005). Its main action occurs centrally where it inhibits reuptake of the neurotransmitters noradrenaline and serotonin at the nerve synapse.

Adverse effects
- Tramadol causes nausea and vomiting at similar or reduced rates to opioids (Bozkurt 2005).
- It has minimal effects on the cardiovascular or respiratory systems and does not cause sedation (Bozkurt 2005).
- Tramadol may have a reduced effect if given with codeine as it is partly metabolised by the same P450 enzyme system.
- Tramadol should be used with caution or avoided in patients with seizure disorders or on psychiatric medications (e.g. MAOI antidepressants and antipsychotic agents) as it can lower the seizure threshold (Bozkurt 2005).

Dose, onset time, peak effect and half-life
- Tramadol can be administered via oral or intravenous routes (Table 4.10).
- For optimal analgesia a loading dose is recommended.
- Concurrent administration with codeine may reduce efficacy.

4.8.2 Local anaesthetics

Overview
- Local anaesthetics are drugs that *reversibly* block transmission of pain along nerve fibres (Neal 2002).
- Unlike most other analgesic drugs, local anaesthetics can give complete pain relief without affecting conscious state.

Table 4.10 Tramadol doses

Drug	Route	Dose	Onset/Peak/t1/2
Tramadol	Oral or IV	Loading dose: 2 mg/kg Then 1–2 mg/kg 8–12 hourly (maximum 8 mg/kg/day)	Onset time: 30–60 min (oral) Peak effect: 2 h t1/2: 6 h

Source: Bozkurt (2005); Brislin and Rose (2005)

Action

Local anaesthetics:

- work by blocking transmission in sensory, motor and autonomic nerve fibres (see Chapter 2 for further details);
- are more effective on smaller diameter nerve fibres (pain and autonomic) than larger diameter (motor and proprioceptive) nerve fibres;
- can be used topically (e.g. skin anaesthesia);
- can be administered by subcutaneous infiltration (e.g. wound infiltration);
- can be administered by direct injection to a peripheral nerve (e.g. ring block or femoral nerve block);
- can be injected adjacent to the spinal cord (e.g. caudal, epidural or intrathecal) (Bryant et al. 2002).

Practice point

The degree, duration and efficacy of the local anaesthetic block depend on the drug used, the dose administered and nature of the drug.

There are two main types of local anaesthetic, amides and esters.

Amides:

- are the most common injected anaesthetics;
- have a longer duration of action;
- are metabolised by the liver;
- have a low incidence of allergy and more stable in solution;
- examples include lignocaine (lidocaine), prilocaine, bupivacaine, ropivacaine, levobupivacaine.

Esters:

- are the most common topical anaesthetics;
- have a shorter duration of action;
- are metabolised by tissue esterases;
- have a high incidence of allergy (including anaphylaxis);
- examples include amethocaine (tetracaine), cocaine, procaine, benzocaine.

Adverse effects

- Most of the adverse effects of local anaesthetics are due to high plasma concentrations of the drug, which mainly affect the cardiac and central nervous systems, i.e. cardiac toxicity, vasodilation, hypotension and seizures.
- The adverse effects can be due to an individual's sensitivity to local anaesthetics, the use of a high dose of local anaesthetic or (more commonly) due to an accidental injection of the local anaesthetic into the general circulation.
- To avoid adverse effects of local anaesthetics, maximum safe doses for age and weight are recommended and should be strictly followed (Bryant et al. 2002).

Dose, onset time, peak effect and half-life

Addition of vasoconstrictors (most often adrenaline) to the local anaesthetic solution prolongs the effect of the local anaesthetic by slowing the rate of absorption and thus the rate of metabolism, especially in single-shot local anaesthetic techniques, e.g. caudal and limb blocks (brachial plexus block, femoral nerve block; Bryant et al. 2002). Other drugs may be added to local anaesthetics (usually in regional anaesthesia techniques) to give an added analgesic effect: clonidine, opioids (commonly fentanyl, morphine or hydromorphone) or ketamine. Longer-acting local anaesthetics (e.g. bupivacaine, ropivacaine or levobupivacaine) provide more effective analgesia for regional techniques than short-acting local anaesthetics (e.g. lignocaine) (ANZCA 2005). (See Chapter 7 for a detailed discussion about regional anaesthesia.)

4.8.3 Topical local anaesthetics

- *Topical* local anaesthetics are extremely effective for the management of procedure-related pain in children, especially for venepuncture and insertion of intravenous cannulae (Murat et al. 2003).
- Local anaesthetic *gel or liquid* may be applied to open wounds, however this must be used with caution, as it is difficult to estimate the total dose given.
- Various local anaesthetic combinations have been developed for both topical and local application. These include mixtures of lignocaine, epinephrine (adrenaline) and tetracaine (LET) and (until recently), tetracaine (or lignocaine), adrenaline and cocaine (TAC or LAC) (Murat et al. 2003; Sinha et al. 2006; Young 2005).
- Cocaine-containing preparations are no longer recommended for use with children, as they have been associated with serious adverse events, including seizures and death (Murat et al. 2003).
- The most commonly used local anaesthetics for children are topical preparations, e.g. EMLA®, amethocaine (Ametop® or AnGel®) and 4% lignocaine (ELA-Max® or LMX$_4$®).

There is considerable difference in the pharmacology of amethocaine and EMLA® (Table 4.11). The vasodilatory effects, faster onset and prolonged duration of action make amethocaine the topical anaesthetic drug of choice, however due to the higher rates of allergic reactions, some children need to use EMLA® instead.

> A Cochrane systematic review of six RCTs ($n = 534$) found that amethocaine was more effective than EMLA® for intravenous cannulation pain. The review emphasised the importance of ensuring that the creams are left on for the correct amount of time. This is an important issue, as children with a high level of anticipatory fear may become more distressed if the cream is left on for an insufficient time and they experience pain despite expecting (and being promised) anaesthesia (Lander et al. 2006).

Table 4.11   A comparison of the properties of amethocaine and EMLA®

	Amethocaine (Ametop®, AnGel®)	EMLA® (Eutectic Mixture of Local Anaesthetics)
Drug	4% tetracaine (amethocaine)	2.5% lignocaine + 2.5% prilocaine
Route	Topical	Topical
Onset of action	*Quick acting:* Venepuncture: 30 min IV cannulation: 45 min	*Slower acting:* Venepuncture: 60–90 min IV cannulation: 90–120 min
Contact time	Remove after 1 h	Remove after 2–4 h
Duration of action after removal	*Long acting:* 4–6 h	*Short acting:* 1–2 h
Adverse effects	Vasodilation Skin erythema (redness), itching, oedema Blistering if left in situ for too long	Vasoconstriction Skin blanching
Age	Licensed from 1 month of age	Licensed from 6 months of age

Source: Harvey and Morton (2007)

4.8.4 Ketamine

Overview
Ketamine:

- is an anaesthetic agent that has powerful analgesic properties, even at very low (sub-anaesthetic) doses;
- currently has three main paediatric applications: anaesthesia, procedural sedation and analgesia;
- is a very useful method of pain control as a low-dose infusion and has increasing applications for managing complex acute and cancer pain in both adults and children;
- has significant opioid-sparing effects, reducing opioid consumption by up to 30% (ANZCA 2005).

Little paediatric data exists despite its growing use among paediatric pain management clinicians, however Anderson and Palmer (2006) suggests it can be used as a sole agent or a co-analgesic.

Action
- Ketamine is a N-methyl-D-aspartate (NMDA) receptor antagonist, therefore it blocks pain wind-up (see Chapter 2 for details of wind-up and hyperalgesia).
- Ketamine's main role is to reduce opioid-induced tolerance and hyperalgesia, thus it is probably most efficacious for escalating pain or as a rescue analgesic drug for pain that is poorly responsive to opioid analgesics (ANZCA 2005).
- Single doses of ketamine are less effective than an infusion (in combination with opioid infusion/PCA or alone) as it has a very short half-life (Lin and Durieux 2005).

Metabolism/elimination
- Ketamine is metabolised in the liver with minimal drug remaining for renal excretion, thus it is useful to use for patients with renal or hepatic dysfunction.

Adverse effects
- The main side effect of ketamine is dysphoria, especially vivid dreams and hallucinations. This occurs in 10% of patients and may be similar to the rates of dysphoric effects of opioids (Anderson and Palmer 2006).
- In contrast to opioid analgesics, respiratory depression and cardiovascular changes are minimal.
- When used at higher doses for procedural sedation, increased salivation, agitation and emergence reactions have been reported.
- At the low doses used for acute pain management (e.g. 50–200 microgram/kg/h) adverse effects are minimal apart from dysphoria, and are often well tolerated if patients are warned what to expect and know that the effects are limited to the duration of the infusion.

Dose, onset time, peak effect and half-life
Routes of ketamine administration include intravenous, oral, intrathecal, epidural, and subcutaneous (Table 4.12).

Table 4.12 Ketamine doses

Drug	Route	Dose	Onset/Peak/Duration
Ketamine *(analgesia infusion)*	IV	IV infusion: 0.05–0.2 mg/kg/hr (as co-analgesic or sole agent)	Onset time: < 1 min
Ketamine *(procedural pain)*	Oral	5 mg/kg	Onset time: 10–20 min Peak effect: 20–30 min
Ketamine *(procedural pain)*	IV	IV bolus: 1–2 mg/kg	Onset time: < 1 min Peak effect: 5–10 min t1/2: 2–3 h

When used for procedural pain ketamine should be administered by a suitably trained clinician with advanced airway management skills. (See Chapter 10 for further discussion)
Source: Lin and Durieux (2005); Brislin and Rose (2005); Anderson and Palmer (2006); Rose (2007); Morton (2008)

4.8.5 Nitrous oxide

Overview
Nitrous oxide:

- is an anaesthetic gas;
- has analgesic effects and sedative and amnesic properties;
- has a very low solubility in blood, thus it reaches the brain very quickly. This results in its rapid onset and offset.

> In children nitrous oxide is primarily used for anaesthesia and procedural pain management. For discussion about the use of nitrous oxide for procedural pain management see Chapter 10.

4.8.6 Other adjuvant analgesic drugs

Little paediatric data exists about the use of other adjuvant analgesic drugs, with the majority of publications being case studies with small patient numbers. However, these drugs offer alternatives to traditional analgesic drugs with growing evidence in the adult research literature of their efficacy. As paediatric analgesic drug research increases, these adjuvant analgesic drugs are likely to be used more commonly for children, thus a brief overview is included. Unless otherwise stated the following information refers to adult studies.

Anticonvulsants
(e.g. gabapentin, pregabalin, carbamazepine, valproate, topiramate)

- Anticonvulsants work by reducing neuronal excitability (Knotkova and Pappagallo 2007).
- The physiology of pain (see Chapter 2) and of epilepsy are similar, which is why anticonvulsants are efficacious as analgesics.
- They are effective in treatment of chronic neuropathic pain and may be efficacious for acute neuropathic pain (ANZCA 2005).
- They are used for treatment of chronic pain in children, although they are not licensed for this indication (see Chapter 8).
- Carbamazepine has more adverse effects than other anticonvulsants and is used less frequently since gabapentin became available (Serpell 2005).
- Gabapentin is effective in reducing postoperative pain and anxiety in adults (ANZCA 2005).

- Topiramate has recently been approved for migraine prophylaxis in adults (Golden et al. 2006).

Tricyclic antidepressants
(e.g. amitriptyline, nortriptyline, imipramine, desipramine)

- Tricyclic antidepressants (TCAs) work by blocking the re-uptake of serotonin and noradrenaline at the nerve synapse (Serpell 2005).
- TCAs have rapid onset of analgesic effects in addition to their antidepressant effects.
- Their additional effects of improved sleep and mood elevation may also improve pain.
- TCAs are effective for chronic neuropathic pain (ANZCA 2005).
- TCAs are more effective than selective serotonin reuptake inhibitors (SSRIs) for neuropathic pain (Serpell 2005).

Selective serotonin reuptake inhibitors
(e.g. fluoxetine, sertraline, citalopram, duloxetine)

- There is no evidence that SSRIs are better than a placebo for treating pain (Serpell 2005; ANZCA 2005).

Other antidepressants
(e.g. venlafaxine)

- Works by blocking inhibiting serotonin and noradrenaline with less sedation and fewer adverse effects than TCAs (Serpell 2005).
- Effective for treating established neuropathic pain, however they are less effective than TCAs (Knotkova and Pappagallo 2007).

Alpha-2 agonists
(e.g. clonidine, dexmedetomidine)

- Alpha-2 agonists work by reducing central sympathetic output and increasing firing of inhibitory neurones on descending pain pathways (see Chapter 2) (Buck 2006).
- The alpha-2 agonists clonidine and dexmedetomidine produce sedation and analgesia without impairing respiration (Hall et al. 2001).
- Clonidine can be used as an anxiolytic and analgesic and is also useful to control the symptoms of opioid and benzodiazepine withdrawal (Brislin and Rose 2005).
- Clonidine improves postoperative analgesia, however it causes sedation and hypotension at higher doses (ANZCA 2005).
- Clonidine can be used orally, intravenously and via epidural (Kokinsky and Thornberg 2003).
- Dexmedetomidine reduced opioid use by 50% when used as a sedative agent in the ICU setting (ANZCA 2005).
- Dexmedetomidine is being used as an alternative to benzodiazepines for sedation in the paediatric ICU setting and as a sedative for procedural sedation in children (Buck 2006).

Topical drugs
(e.g. capsaicin, topical NSAIDs, topical local anaesthetic)

- A number of medications have an analgesic effect when applied topically to the skin (McCleane 2007).
- They have fewer adverse effects as they are not taken systemically (Serpell 2005).
- Capsaicin is extracted from chilli peppers and is effective for the treatment of diabetic neuropathies, polyneuropathy and other neuropathic pains. It works by inactivating

C-fibres and depleting nerve endings of substance P (see Chapter 2) (Serpell 2005; McCleane 2007).

- Clonidine can have both a central and peripheral action when administered topically. It reduces hyperalgesia in sympathetically maintained pain (see Chapter 8) (McCleane 2007).
- Topical lignocaine can decrease the pain of herpetic neuralgia (Serpell 2005).

Antispasticity drugs
(e.g. baclofen)

- Baclofen is an effective antispasmodic agent, which acts on GABA receptors at the spinal cord level (see Chapter 2).
- In children it is administered orally or intrathecally for the treatment of severe spasticity and dystonia associated with conditions such as cerebral palsy (Albright and Ferson 2006).

Benzodiazepines
(e.g. midazolam, diazepam, lorazepam, clonazepam)

- Benzodiazepines relieve skeletal muscle spasms and reduce muscle tone, thus reducing pain, particularly following orthopaedic surgery (Brislin and Rose 2005).
- Benzodiazepines may be used as adjunct analgesic drugs to systemic or regional analgesics (Brislin and Rose 2005).

The use of antiemetics and laxatives is discussed in Chapter 7.

Summary

- Many analgesic drugs have not been tested in children or are administered *off-label*.
- Misconceptions about analgesic drugs, particularly opioids, contribute to the under-treatment of pain in children.
- Confusion about opioid terminology leads to anxiety in families and healthcare professionals and suboptimal pain management practice.
- Combining analgesic drugs with non-drug strategies ensures better pain management outcomes.
- Nurses need to be aware of the hepatic and renal function of their patients and the need for reduced doses of analgesic drugs if these are impaired.
- The route of drug administration affects the onset and efficacy of a drug. There are a range of advantages and disadvantages for children with different administration routes, which should be considered prior to analgesic selection.
- Analgesic drugs should be selected using a stepwise approach based on the type and severity of pain, onset and peak effect of the drug, benefits, risks and adverse effects.
- The main analgesic drugs fall into three categories: non-opioids, opioids and adjuvant analgesic drugs.
- Improved knowledge about pharmacology should enable nurses to make better decisions about appropriate selection of analgesic drugs, increase awareness of the impact and management of adverse effects, and improve individual nurses' ability to advocate for better analgesic prescribing.

Useful web resources

Australian and New Zealand College of Anaesthetists, Faculty of Pain Medicine: www.fpm.anzca.edu.au

Department of Pain Medicine and Palliative Care, Beth Israel Medical Center, New York: www.stop-pain.org

Free Nurses Continuing Education (CE) activities on Medscape: www.medscape.com/nurses

International Association for the Study of Pain: www.iasp-pain.org

Medline Plus information about pain management: www.nim.nih.gov/medlineplus/pain.html

Prescription drug information: www.drugs.com

References

Albright, A.L. and Ferson, S.S. (2006) Intrathecal baclofen therapy in children, *Neurosurgical Focus*, 21(2): E3, 1–6.

Anderson, B.J. and Palmer G.M. (2006) Recent developments in the pharmacological management of pain in children, *Current Opinion in Anaesthesiology*, 19: 285–292.

Australian and New Zealand College of Anaesthetists and Faculty of Pain Medicine [ANZCA] (2005) *Acute Pain Management: Scientific Evidence*, 2nd edition, Australian and New Zealand College of Anaesthetists, Melbourne.

Ballantyne, J.C. and LaForge, K.S. (2007) Opioid dependence and addiction during opioid treatment of chronic pain, *Pain*, 129: 235–255.

Begg, E.J. (2003) *Instant Clinical Pharmacology*, Blackwell Publishing, Oxford.

Berde, C.B. and Sethna, N.F. (2002) Analgesics for the treatment of pain in children, *New England Journal of Medicine*, 347(14): 1094–1103.

Bozkurt, P. (2005) Use of tramadol in children. *Pediatric Anesthesia*, 15: 1041–1047.

Brislin, R.P. and Rose, J.B. (2005) Pediatric acute pain management, *Anesthesiology Clinics of North America*, 23: 789–814.

Brown, T.C.K. and Fisk, G.C. (1992) Paediatric anaesthetic pharmacology. In Brown, T.C.K. and Fisk, G.C. (eds.) *Anaesthesia for Children* (2nd edition), Blackwell Scientific Publications, Oxford, pp. 25–52.

Bryant, B., Knights, K. and Salerno, E. (2003) *Pharmacology for Health Professionals*, Elsevier (Australia) Pty Ltd.

Buck, M.L. (2006) Dexmedetomidine for sedation in the pediatric intensive care setting, *Pediatric Pharmacotherapy*, 12(1): 1–4.

Chandrasekharan, N.V., Dai, H., Roos. K.L., Evanson, N.K., Tomsik, J., Elton, T.S. and Simmons, D.L. (2002) COX-3, a cyclooxygenase-1 variant inhibited by acetaminophen and other analgesic/antipyretic drugs: cloning, structure, and expression, *Proceedings of the National Academy of Sciences of the USA*, 99(21): 13926–13931.

Charlton, J.E. (ed). (2005) *Core Curriculum for Professional Education in Pain* (3rd edition), IASP Task Force on Professional Education, IASP Publications, Seattle.

Eisenberg, E., Marinangeli, F., Birkhahn, J., Paladini, A. and Varrassi, G. (2005) Time to modify the WHO analgesia ladder? *Pain, Clinical Updates*, XIII(5): 1–4.

Golden, A.S., Haut, S.R. and Moshe, S.L. (2006) Nonepileptic uses of antiepileptic drugs in children and adolescents, *Journal of Pediatric Neurology*, 34(6): 421–432.

Greco, C. and Berde, C. (2005) Pain management for the hospitalised pediatric patient, *Pediatric Clinics of North America*, 52: 995–1027.

Hall, J.E., Uhrich, T.D. and Ebert, T.J. (2001) Sedative, analgesic and cognitive effects of clonidine infusions in humans, *British Journal of Anaesthesia*, 86(1): 5–11.

Harrop, J.E. (2007) Management of pain in children, *Archives of Disease in Childhood, Education and Practice Edition*, 92: ep101-ep108.

Harvey, A.J. and Morton, N.J. (2007) Management of procedural pain in children, *Archives of Disease in Childhood, Education and Practice Edition*, 92: ep2–ep26.

Henneberg, S.W. and Nilsson, L.B. (2007) Acute paediatric pain: review, *Current Anaesthesia and Critical Care*, 18(3): 126–134.

Jovey, R.D., Ennis, J. Gardner-Nix, J., Goldman, B., Hays, H., Lynch, M and Moulin, D. (2003) Use of opioid analgesics for the treatment of chronic non-cancer pain: a consensus statement and guidelines from the Canadian Pain Society, 2002, *Pain Research and Management*, 8(Suppl A): 3A–14A.

Kanneh, A. (2002a) Paediatric pharmacological principles: an update Part 1: Drug development and pharmacodynamics, *Paediatric Nursing*, 14(8): 36–42.

Kanneh, A. (2002b) Paediatric pharmacological principles: an update Part 2: Pharmacokinetics: absorption and distribution, *Paediatric Nursing*, 14(9): 39–43.

Knotkova, H. and Pappagallo, M. (2007) Adjuvant analgesics, *Medical Clinics of North America*, 91: 113–124.

Kokki, H. (2003) Nonsteroidal anti-inflammatory drugs for postoperative pain: a focus on children, *Pediatric Drugs*, 5(2): 103–123.

Kokinsky, E. and Thornberg, E. (2003) Postoperative pain control in children: a guide to drug choice, *Pediatric Drugs*, 5(11): 751–762.

Lander, J.A., Weltman, B.J. and So, S.S. (2006) EMLA and amethocaine for reduction of children's pain associated with needle insertion. *Cochrane Database of Systematic Reviews*, (3): CD004236.

Lin, C. and Durieux, M.E. (2005) Ketamine and kids: an update, *Pediatric Anesthesia*, 15: 91–97.

Lönnqvist, P.-A. and Morton, N.S. (2005) Postoperative analgesia in infants and children, *British Journal of Anaesthesia*, 95(1): 59–68.

McCleane, G. (2007) Topical analgesics, *Medical Clinics of North America*, 91: 125–139.

Morton, N.S. (2007) Management of postoperative pain in children, *Archives of Disease in Childhood, Education in Practice Edition*, 92: ep14-ep19.

Morton, N.S. (2008) Ketamine for procedural sedation and analgesia in pediatric emergency medicine: a UK perspective, *Pediatric Anesthesia*, 18: 25–29.

Murat, I., Gall, O. and Tourniaire, B. (2003) Procedural pain in children, evidence-based best practice and guidelines, *Regional Anesthesia and Pain Medicine*, 28: 561–572.

Neal, M.J. (2002) *Medical Pharmacology at a Glance* (4th edition), Blackwell Science, Oxford.

Rang, H.P., Dale, M.M., Ritter, J.M. and Moore, P.K. (2003) *Pharmacology* (5th edition), Churchill Livingstone, London.

Remy, C., Marret, E. and Bonnet, F. (2006) State of the art of paracetamol in acute pain therapy, *Current Opinion in Anesthesiology*, 19: 562–565.

Rose, M. (2007) Systemic analgesics for children, *Anaesthesia and Intensive Care Medicine*, 8(5): 184–188.

Serpell, M. (2001) Pharmacological treatment of chronic pain, *Anaesthesia and Intensive Care*, 6(2): 39–42.

Sinha, M., Christopher, N.C., Fenn, R. and Reeves, L. (2006) Evaluation of nonpharmacologic methods of pain and anxiety management for laceration repair in the pediatric emergency department, *Pediatrics*, 117: 1162–1168.

Williams, D.G., Patel, A. and Howard, R.F. (2002) Pharmacogenetics of codeine metabolism in an urban population of children and its implications for analgesic reliability, *British Journal of Anaesthesia*, 89: 839–845.

World Health Organization (1996) *Cancer Pain Relief*, 2nd edition, World Health Organization, Geneva.

World Health Organization (1998) *Cancer Pain Relief and Palliative Care in Children*, World Health Organization, Geneva.

World Health Organization (2007) *Promoting Safety of Medicines for Children*, World Health Organization, Geneva.

Yaster, M., Karolinski, K. and Maxwell, L. (1997) Opioid agonists and antagonists. In Yaster, M., Krane, E. J., Kaplan, R. F., Cote, C. J. and Lappe D. G. (eds.) *Pediatric Pain Management and Sedation Handbook*, Mosby, St. Louis, pp. 29–50.

Young, K.D. (2005) Pediatric procedural pain, *Annals of Emergency Medicine*, 45: 160–171.

CHAPTER 5
Non-Drug Methods of Pain Relief
Alison Twycross

Introduction

This chapter will provide an overview of some of the most commonly used non-drug methods available to aid the relief of pain in children. Within this chapter each non-drug method will be discussed in turn, the relevant research summarised, and the implications for practice identified. Non-drug interventions can be classified into three groups: *sensory, cognitive-behavioural and cognitive interventions* (Figure 5.1). Psychological preparation and play are discussed in Chapter 10. The non-drug methods will be discussed in alphabetical order. Non-drug methods that can be used to relieve pain in infants are also discussed. (The use of aromatherapy, herbs, naturopathy, homeopathy and the manipulative techniques – chiropractic and osteopathy – are not within the remit of this chapter.)

5.1 Acupuncture

What is acupuncture?

- Acupuncture is a system of ancient medicine, healing and Eastern philosophy originating in China.
- Acupuncture is based on the theory that energy (Chi) flows through the body along channels known as *meridians,* which are connected by acupuncture points.
- If the flow of energy is obstructed, pain results (Rusy and Weisman 2000; Kemper and Gardiner 2003).
- The energy flow is restored by inserting needles at acupuncture points along the meridians involved, which eliminates or reduces pain (Rusy and Weisman 2000; Kemper and Gardiner 2003).

5.1.1 Using acupuncture to relieve children's pain: research evidence

There is little research about the use of acupuncture in children. This is attributed in part to the view that children dislike needles (Kemper et al. 2000).

- The effectiveness of using acupuncture to treat migraine in children ($n = 22$) was tested by Pintov et al. (1997) using a randomised controlled trial. Acupuncture was found to reduce the frequency and severity of migraines.

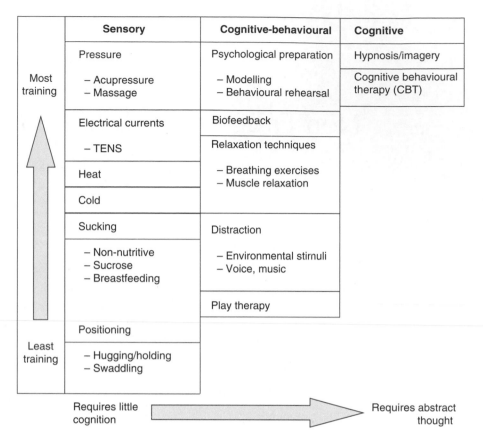

Figure 5.1   Non-drug interventions of pain relief (adapted from Vessey and Carlson 1996).

- Sixty-seven percent of children ($n = 47$) (and 60% of their parents) referred to an acupuncturist for chronic pain problems thought that acupuncture was a positive experience, with 70% of children and 59% of parents reporting definite pain relief (Kemper et al. 2000).
- In Lin et al.'s (2002) study, children ($n = 243$) with chronic pain were treated with acupuncture. Children received an average of 8.4 sessions of acupuncture therapy over a six-week period. Pain intensity scores decreased significantly. The children experienced *overall improvement of well-being* and also reported increased attendance at school, improved sleep patterns, and the ability to take part in more extracurricular activities. No side effects or complications were reported.
- A combined acupuncture and hypnotherapy package was used by Zeltzer et al. (2002) for children ($n = 31$) with chronic pain. Ninety percent of patients completed the six-week course. No adverse effects were reported and both children and parents reported significant improvements in children's pain and functioning.

A review of the use of acupuncture as a pain relieving intervention for children has been undertaken by Kundu and Berman (2007).

Most children find acupuncture an acceptable treatment for chronic pain.
  The research evidence available suggests that acupuncture is an effective treatment for chronic pain.
  An alternative to traditional acupuncture using needles is *laser acupuncture* (Kundu and Berman 2007).

5.2 Biofeedback

What is biofeedback?

Biofeedback involves measuring physiological indicators such as blood pressure, heart rate, skin temperature, sweating and muscle tension and conveying such information to the person to raise awareness and conscious control of the related physiological activities.

Types of biofeedback include finger temperature, α-electroencephalography (EEG) biofeedback, muscle electromyography (EMG) and temporal pulse biofeedback (McGrath et al. 2003).

Each of these methods is used to alert the patient to muscle tension, which allows them to recognise the early signs of tension and implement relaxation techniques.

5.2.1 Using biofeedback to relieve children's pain: research evidence

Biofeedback has been shown to be particularly effective in the treatment of headaches:

- Hermann and Blanchard (2002) reviewed 15 studies that used *thermal biofeedback* alone or with other treatments and found that two-thirds of paediatric migraine sufferers had a 50% reduction in symptoms.
- Scharff et al. (2002) compared *thermal biofeedback* to an attention placebo (hand cooling) and a waiting list group. Children ($n = 36$) with migraine, and their parents, were randomly assigned to the three groups. Children in the hand-warming group were more likely to achieve clinical improvement in migraine. These differences were still evident six months after the study.
- Arndorfer and Allen (2001) explored the efficacy of a *thermal biofeedback* treatment package as an intervention with children ($n = 5$), aged 8–14 years, with tension headache. All participants demonstrated clinically significant reduction in one or more headache parameter (frequency, duration, intensity) following treatment. At six-month follow up, four of the five participants were headache free.
- Hermann and Blanchard (2002) also reviewed three studies that used *electromyography biofeedback* to treat children with tension headaches; there was an 80–90% success rate in these studies.

Biofeedback has also been used with children with other types of pain:

- The use of biofeedback to manage pain associated with juvenile rheumatoid arthritis was explored by Lavigne et al. (1992). Children ($n = 8$) who received progressive muscle relaxation, electromyography biofeedback and thermal biofeedback experienced a reduction in their pain.
- Significant reductions in pain were also noted by children ($n = 8$) with sickle cell disease, who participated in biofeedback-assisted relaxation sessions including electromyography biofeedback and thermal biofeedback (Cozzi et al. 1987).

Further research is needed but biofeedback appears to reduce the pain associated with headache, and may have a place in the treatment of other types of chronic pain in children.

5.3 Cognitive Behavioural Therapy

What is cognitive behavioural therapy?

Cognitive behavioural therapy (CBT) aims to improve the way that an individual manages and copes with their pain. The child is taught to use techniques such as distraction, relaxation and biofeedback to help them manage their pain.

BOX 5.1

Focus of cognitive behavioural therapy

Poltorak and Benore (2006) provide an overview of the use of cognitive behavioral therapy for pain management. They state that the focus is multifaceted and includes:

1. Alteration of maladaptive behaviours
2. Alteration of self-statements, images and feelings that interfere with adaptive functioning
3. Alteration of assumptions and beliefs that contribute to the habitual perceptions and reactions
4. Training in new behaviours and ways of thinking that promote healthier functioning

---

Box 5.1 provides a summary of the focus of cognitive behavioural therapy. Strategies that are used include *cognitive restructuring, cognitive distraction* and *activity-rest cycling* (Poltorak and Benore 2006).

5.3.1 Using cognitive behavioural therapy to relieve children's pain: research evidence

Several studies have explored the effectiveness of cognitive behavioural therapy (CBT) in the management of children's pain:

- Jay et al. (1987) compared the efficacy of CBT, oral valium or a minimal treatment-attention (control group) in reducing children's distress during bone marrow aspirations. Children ($n = 56$), aged 3–14 years, with leukaemia took part in the study. Children receiving CBT had significantly lower behavioural distress, lower pain ratings, and lower pulse rates than the control group. Children in the valium group exhibited no significant differences from the control group except that they had lower diastolic blood pressure.
- In Dahlquist et al.'s (1985) study children ($n = 3$), aged 11–14, undergoing cancer chemotherapy were coached in cue-controlled muscle relaxation, controlled breathing, pleasant imagery and positive self-talk during chemotherapy venepuncture. There was a 46–68% reduction from baseline levels of observed behavioural distress during the intervention. Medical personnel's and child's self-report ratings of the children's distress during venepuncture also decreased during intervention.
- Jay et al. (1991) investigated whether the combination of oral valium and CBT would result in increased efficacy of the CBT. Children ($n = 83$) were randomly assigned to receive CBT or CBT plus valium while undergoing either a bone marrow aspiration or a lumbar puncture. No significant differences were found between the two groups.
- Surjala et al. (1995) compared the effectiveness of CBT and relaxation and massage for the management of oral mucositis pain associated with cancer treatment. Children ($n = 94$) took part in this randomised control trial. CBT was found to be as effective as a combination of relaxation and imagery.
- Liossi and Hatira (1999) compared the use of hypnosis and CBT with children ($n = 30$), aged 5–15 years, undergoing bone marrow aspirations. The children were randomised to one of three groups: hypnosis; a package of cognitive behavioural skills; and no intervention (control group). Children receiving either hypnosis or CBT reported less pain and pain related anxiety than the control group. Children in the hypnosis group exhibited less anxiety or behavioural distress than those in the CBT group.
- In Eccleston et al.'s (2003) study adolescents ($n = 57$) with chronic pain and an accompanying adult ($n = 57$) completed a three-week residential programme of group CBT. Post-treatment adolescents reported significant improvements in relation to disability and physical function. Three months post-treatment adolescents maintained physical improvements and reduced anxiety, disability and somatic awareness. At three months 64% of participants had improved school attendance with 40% having returned to full-time education.

A Cochrane review exploring the effectiveness of pyschological interventions for the management of sickle cell disease pain included three studies. Some evidence for the effectiveness of cognitive behavioural therapy was found. Further research is needed (Anie and Green 2000).

> Cognitive behavioural therapy appears to be a useful pain-relieving strategy, particularly for children with chronic pain or experiencing repeated painful procedures. More research is needed in this area.

5.4 Distraction

> ### What is distraction?
> Distraction involves *distracting* the child from their pain.
>   The effectiveness of distraction can be explained by the *gate control theory* (see Chapter 2). The use of distraction techniques closes the *gate* because pain is put at the periphery of awareness with attention being focused on the distraction device rather than on the pain.

5.4.1 Using distraction to relieve children's pain: research evidence

The effectiveness of distraction as a pain relieving intervention has been explored in more research studies than other non-drug methods. This is perhaps because it is relatively easy for the nurse, and other healthcare professionals, to use distraction methods to help children cope with pain. The results of key studies are summarised below:

- Vessey et al. (1994) used a kaleidoscope to distract children ($n = 100$: randomly assigned to either group) during blood-taking while children in the control group were comforted by the nursing staff. The children using the kaleidoscope were significantly ($p < 0.001$) calmer and experienced less pain.
- However, in another randomised controlled study by Carlson et al. (2000) that explored the effectiveness of distraction using the *illusion kaleidoscope,* no difference was found between the groups ($n = 384$), aged 4–18 years, undergoing venepuncture or the insertion of an intravenous cannula.
- The use of distraction techniques with preschoolers ($n = 31$) having intramuscular injections and subcutaneous port access was explored by Dahlquist et al. (2002a). They found that developmentally appropriate distraction techniques reduced children's observed anxiety levels.
- Distraction using a developmentally appropriate electronic toy was also found to be effective for children ($n = 6$), aged 2–9 years, undergoing repeated needle sticks (Dahlquist et al. 2002b).
- Distraction techniques were found to be a useful addition to analgesic drugs for children ($n = 24$) with musclo-skeletal pain in the accident and emergency department (Tanabe et al. 2002).
- Cassidy et al. (2002) found that watching cartoons on TV did not distract children while having routine vaccinations nor did it reduce their pain (control group: $n = 29$; experimental group: $n = 33$).
- Similar findings have been found among children ($n = 13$) with burns (Landolt et al. 2002).
- However, Bellini et al. (2006) found that for children ($n = 69$: randomly assigned to experimental or control group) watching TV was a more effective distraction technique than mothers engaged in active distraction.

- Sinha et al. (2006) found that the use of distraction techniques reduced the sensory and affective components of pain among children (n = 240), aged 6–18 years, undergoing laceration repair in the accident and emergency department.

A Cochrane review of both cognitive-behavioural and cognitive interventions for the management of needle-related pain found *distraction* to be particularly effective (Uman et al. 2006).

> Distraction appears to be useful tool for reducing children's pain. However, the effectiveness of distraction as a non-drug method of pain relief is influenced by the method used. Perhaps unsurprisingly, active methods of distraction appear to be more helpful than passive methods.

5.4.2 Using distraction techniques in practice

To determine an effective distraction strategy the nurse should involve the child and parents in identifying what is particularly interesting to the child. The characteristics of an effective distraction technique for brief episodes of pain are outlined in Box 5.2. Box 5.3 suggests examples of distraction with children.

BOX 5.2

Characteristics of effective distraction strategies for brief episodes of pain

The distraction technique must be:

1 Interesting to the child
2 Consistent with the child's energy level and ability to concentrate
3 Stimulating to the major senses:
   - hearing
   - vision
   - touch
   - movement
4 Capable of providing a change in stimuli when the pain changes, e.g., increasing stimuli as pain increases

Source: Adapted from McCaffery and Beebe (1989)

BOX 5.3

Examples of distraction strategies for use with children

Singing
Games and puzzles
Blowing bubbles or windmill toys
Blowing an imaginary feather off the doctor's nose
Reading pop up books
Playing with a kaleidoscope
Breathing out/controlled breathing
Looking in a mirror to see the view through a nearby window
Watching television or a video; playing interactive computer games
Listening through headphones to stories or music

5.4.3 Using virtual reality as a distraction technique

In the last decade several studies describe using virtual reality as a distraction technique, which involves using a computer and a visual simulation game:

- Virtual reality distraction has been shown to be effective in distracting children ($n = 11$) receiving intravenous chemotherapy (Schneider and Workman 2000).
- Virtual reality distraction was also shown to reduce children's distress during (central venous) port access procedures for children ($n = 20$), aged 7–14 years, with oncology conditions (Wolitzky et al. 2005).
- A virtual reality game combined with analgesic drugs was found to be more effective at reducing a children's ($n = 9$) pain during burn dressings than analgesic drugs alone (Das et al. 2005).
- Virtual reality was found to be effective in distracting children ($n = 20$) while having an intravenous cannula sited (Gold et al. 2006).
- Distraction using virtual reality techniques to manage pain associated with (central venous) port access and venepuncture was found to be more effective than self-selected distracters for children with cancer ($n = 50$) (Wolitzky et al. 2005).

> Virtual reality appears to be a useful method for distracting children from their pain.

5.4.4 Involving parents in distraction techniques

Parents can assist with a number of distraction activities but may need guidance from healthcare professionals as to how they can best help their child. Children describe parental presence as being an excellent distracter from *things which hurt* (Woodgate and Kristjanson 1996; Polkki et al. 2003). The results of several studies indicate that when parents are taught how to distract their child during a painful procedure, children experience less anxiety and pain (Greenberg et al. 1999; Manimala et al. 2000; Kleiber et al. 2001; Walker et al. 2006). Teaching parents distraction techniques for their child has a twofold effect: it reduces parental feelings of helplessness and benefits the child by reducing their distress. Parents need to be helped to select a distraction technique that is appropriate for their child (Boxes 5.2, 5.3).

5.5 Heat and Cold

> Topical sources of heat and cold can be applied to a painful area and are useful for pain relief or comfort (McCaffery and Pasero 1999).
> The underlying mechanisms of pain relief from heating and cooling are uncertain (McCaffery and Pasero 1999).

5.5.1 Using heat and cold to relieve children's pain: research evidence

Only one study has explored the use of cold as a pain-relieving intervention for children:

- Ebner (1996) explored whether cold therapy decreased the perceived pain associated with intramuscular injections in children. Children ($n = 40$), aged 10–18 years, were randomly assigned to the control or experimental group. The experimental group had an ice pack placed on the injection site for 15 minutes prior to injection, whereas the control group received injections according to hospital protocol. Ice was not shown to be significant in reducing procedural pain.

Anecdotal evidence suggests that the use of heat and cold are useful. Indeed, several authors cite them as useful non-drug methods of pain relief:

- McCarthy et al. (2003) state that the application of superficial cold or heat is used as part of physiotherapy when pain is present. Cold is recommended within the first 24–48 hours of the injury to prevent swelling while heat is usually used after the first 24–48 hours.
- Dampier and Shapiro (2003) also state that heat packs and hot baths are helpful for sickle cell disease pain but that cold usually makes the pain associated with sickle cell disease worse.
- A Cochrane review, included nine studies, and found that heat wraps can reduce back pain in adults, but that the evidence for cold treatment is sparse. There is moderate evidence that heat provides a short-term reduction in pain, but there are no good data showing whether or not cold therapy has any effect (French et al. 2006).

For further information about using topical heating and cooling for pain relief see Chapter 9 of McCaffery and Pasero (1999).

> The use of heat and cold as pain relieving interventions need further research.

5.6 Hypnosis

Within this section the term *hypnosis* will be used to encompass both hypnosis and guided imagery. (The terms hypnosis and guided imagery are often used inter-changeably but the methods used within research papers are not always comparable. The reader is advised to check the original papers for the actual method used.)

> ### What is hypnosis?
>
> Hypnosis is an altered state of consciousness using intensified attention within a relaxed physical state to allow a trance state that is different from both the normal waking state and any of the stages of sleep (Kuttner and Solomon 2003).
>
> Hypnosis involves helping children to focus their attention away from the feared components of a procedure and to focus on an imaginative experience that is viewed as comforting, safe, fun or intriguing (Zeltzer et al. 1997).

5.6.1 Using hypnosis to relieve children's pain: research evidence

- Hypnosis was found to be significantly better at reducing pain associated with bone marrow aspirations and lumbar punctures in children with cancer than non-hypnotic techniques ($p < 0.05$) (Zeltzer and LeBaron 1982).
- The use of hypnosis with children ($n = 24$), aged 9–17 years, undergoing cardiac catheterisation was investigated by Pederson (1995). Hypnosis did not reduce children's pain during catheterisation but did reduce the distress behaviours demonstrated during the procedure.
- Children ($n = 52$) admitted for elective surgery were assigned to an experimental or control group in Lambert's (1996) study. The experimental group were taught hypnosis by

the researcher; each child was asked to select an enjoyable image, which was incorporated into an individually tailored relaxation exercise. The children in the experimental group had significantly less postoperative pain ($p < 0.01$) and shorter hospital stays than children in the control group.

- In Huth et al.'s (2004) study children, aged 7–12 years, admitted for tonsillectomy and/or adenoidectomy were randomly assigned to two groups. Children ($n = 36$) in the experimental group watched a videotape on the use of imagery and then listened to a 30-min audio-tape about imagery a week before surgery. Children ($n = 37$) in the attention-control group received an equal amount of preoperative time from the investigator and drew on art paper after preoperative data was collected while the investigator talked with the mother and/or child. The children who received the hypnosis training had significantly lower pain scores ($p = 0.04$) in the first four hours postoperatively.
- Children ($n = 10$) with recurrent abdominal pain were trained in relaxation and hypnosis. Pain diaries were completed at 0, 1 and 2 months and demonstrated a significant (67%) decrease in pain during the therapy (Ball et al. 2003).
- Similar findings were obtained in a study by Weydert et al. (2006) with children ($n = 22$), aged 5–18 years, with recurrent abdominal pain.
- Liossi et al. (2006) compared the effectiveness of a local anaesthetic cream (EMLA) and self-hypnosis with the use of EMLA alone or the use of EMLA with attention (from the researcher in the form of nonmedical play, and nonmedical verbal interactions). Children ($n = 45$), aged 6–16 years, were randomised into the three groups. Children in the group receiving EMLA cream and hypnosis demonstrated less anticipatory anxiety ($p < 0.001$) and less procedural pain and anxiety ($p < 0.001$).

A systematic review of eight studies ($n = 313$) by Richardson et al. (2006) compared hypnosis with other cognitive and cognitive behavioural interventions for the management of procedural pain in children with cancer. There was some evidence of effectiveness.

A systematic review carried out by Uman et al. (2006) examining psychological interventions for the management of needle-related pain in children found hypnosis to be an effective method.

> Hypnosis (or guided imagery) appears to be an effective way of reducing recurrent abdominal pain in children. There is also evidence that hypnosis can help children cope with painful procedures and postoperative pain.

5.7 Massage

What is massage?

Massage therapy involves manipulation of the body by combining tactile and kinaesthetic stimulation performed in purposeful sequential application (Tsao et al. 2006).
   The precise mechanism of action is not known (Ireland and Olson 2000).

5.7.1 Using massage to relieve children's pain: research evidence

There is very little research about massage as a pain-relieving intervention. The two studies summarised below were carried out by the same research team:

- Children ($n = 20$), aged 5–14 years, with juvenile rheumatoid arthritis had a 15-minute session with their parents every day for a month. Children received either a massage session or a relaxation session. At followup both children and parents in the massage group reported less pain than those in the relaxation group (Field et al. 1997).

- In Hernandez-Reif et al.'s (2001) study, children (n = 24) with severe burns were assigned to either a massage therapy group or an attention-control group. Children were either massaged for 15 minutes prior to a dressing change or engaged in 15 minutes of informal conversation. Children in the massage group demonstrated minimal behavioural indicators of distress while children in the control group demonstrated multiple indicators of distress.

An overview about the use of massage therapy in children can be found in Beider et al. (2007).

> Massage appears to help children cope with chronic pain and with the pain associated with burns dressings.

5.8 Relaxation

> ### What is relaxation?
>
> Relaxation involves helping a child to *relax*.
>   The effectiveness of relaxation can also be explained by the *gate control theory* (see Chapter 2). By relaxing, the *gate* is closed.
>   For the young child relaxation may simply consist of being held in a comfortable well-supported position or being rocked in a wide rhythmical arc.
>   With older children relaxation involves teaching the children to engage in progressive relaxation of the muscle groups (Chen et al. 2000; McGrath et al. 2003).

5.8.1 Using relaxation to relieve children's pain: research evidence

Several review papers have examined studies exploring the use of relaxation techniques to relieve children's pain:

- Holden et al. (1999) undertook a review of empirical treatment studies and concluded that relaxation was an effective treatment for recurrent migraine and tension headaches in children and adolescents.
- Following a review of 13 studies in the area, muscle relaxation was found to be an effective pain-relieving intervention for procedural pain by Powers (1999).
- The results of seven randomised controlled trials conducted with adolescents (n = 288) over a 20-year period were examined by Larsson et al. (2005). Therapist-assisted relaxation was found to be an effective treatment for adolescents suffering from recurrent tension headaches or migraine.
- A Cochrane review that included 18 studies about the use of psychological treatments for chronic pain in children found relaxation was effective in reducing the severity and frequency of chronic headaches in children and adolescents (Eccleston et al. 2006).

> Relaxation appears to be an effective pain-relieving intervention for recurrent migraine and tension headaches. The effectiveness of relaxation for relieving other types of pain needs further research.

Further information about using relaxation techniques in practice can be found in Chapter 9 of McCaffery and Beebe (1989) or in Rickard (1994).

5.9 Transcutaneous Electric Nerve Stimulation

> **What is TENS?**
>
> TENS is a method for stimulating nerves through electrodes applied to the skin; it is effective for the symptomatic treatment of both acute and chronic pain (Smith and Madsen 2003).
>
> TENS is a safe, non-invasive pain-relieving strategy for partially or completely blocking the pain sensation (McCarthy et al. 2003).
>
> The analgesic effect of the TENS has been explained by the gate control theory, which suggests that stimulation of the large-diameter afferent nerve fibres can close the gate (McCarthy et al. 2003). (See Chapter 2 for more information about the gate control theory.)

5.9.1 Using TENS to relieve children's pain: research evidence

Only one study has examined the use of TENS to relieve children's pain:

- TENS was found to be effective for venepuncture pain in a blinded placebo-controlled trial of school children (*n* = 514) aged 5–17 years (Lander and Fowler-Kerry 1993).

Further information about using TENS in practice can be found in Chapter 5 of McCaffery and Beebe (1989) and Lin (2003).

> TENS is used fairly widely to manage children's pain. Further research is needed about its effectiveness.

5.10 Non-drug Methods for Infants

There are several non-drug methods that can be used specifically for infants. These are described in this section, in alphabetical order. Many of these methods need further research to prove their effectiveness in reliving pain (Cignacco et al. 2007).

5.10.1 Administration of sucrose

The administration of a sucrose solution to infants as a strategy for managing procedural pain has been examined in several studies:

- Several studies have also demonstrated the analgesic effects of non-nutritive sucking using sweet-tasting solutions in full and pre-term infants (Bucher et al. 1995; Haourari et al. 1995; Johnston et al. 1999).
- In a randomised controlled trial (*n* = 201), *sucrose* was more effective than *EMLA* for the reduction of pain and distress behaviours during venepuncture (Gradin et al. 2002).
- A systematic review of the efficacy of sucrose suggests that it is a safe and effective method of reducing procedural pain from one off events (Stevens et al. 1998).
- Information about the optimum dose of sucrose remains inconclusive (Stevens et al. 1998).

> The administration of sucrose appears to be an effective method for managing procedural pain in infants. Further research is needed about the optimum dose.

5.10.2 Breastfeeding

A systematic review of the effectiveness of breastfeeding or supplemental breast milk in relieving procedural pain in neonates was carried out by Shah et al. (2006):

- Breastfeeding or supplemental breast milk (i.e. given via a bottle or nasogastric tube) reduces pain and distress behaviour
- Breastfeeding is more effective than *swaddling* or the use of a dummy (pacifier), and has a similar efficacy to the administration of sucrose.

Other studies reported in 2007 support these conclusions:

- Efe and Ozer (2007) found that breastfeeding was an effective way of relieving pain during neonatal immunisations.
- Efe and Savaser (2007) found no difference in the analgesic effect of breastfeeding and the administration of sucrose during venepuncture.

> More research is needed but it appears that breastfeeding can be used to relieve procedural pain in neonates.

5.10.3 Facilitated tucking (or containment)

> **What is facilitated tucking?**
>
> Facilitated tucking involves placing a cloth or blanket over a neonate and holding them so that their limbs are in close proximity to their trunk.
>   This differs from swaddling because the neonate is not completely wrapped in the blanket and is being held in position.

The use of facilitated tucking has been tested in three studies with randomised samples of 30–40 neonates. Cignacco et al. (2007) reviewed these studies and concluded that facilitated tucking appeared to be effective in reducing procedural pain in neonates.

5.10.4 Kangaroo care (or skin-to-skin contact)

> **What is kangaroo care?**
>
> Kangaroo care involves the neonate being taken out of the incubator or cot and laid on the bare skin of their mother or father (Cignacco et al. 2007).

- A study carried out with preterm neonates ($n = 74$), over the age of 32 weeks gestation, demonstrated that kangaroo care produces a reduction in the pain response (Johnston et al. 2003). There was a significant reduction in pain response following a painful procedure compared to neonates in a control group at 30, 60 and 90 seconds post-procedure.

> Kangaroo care appears to be a useful strategy for managing pain in neonates.

5.10.5 Environment

- Managing environmental factors such as bright lights and reducing the volume of monitor alarms are effective ways of reducing and/or preventing pain in the infant (Stevens 1999; Franck and Lawhon 2000).
- Maintaining a normal sleep/wake cycle within the intensive care unit by dimming lights at night has also been shown to promote well-being in the infant (Franck and Lawhon 2000).

5.10.6 Non-nutritive sucking (NNS)

> **What is non-nutritive sucking?**
>
> Non-nutritive sucking refers to the use of a dummy (or pacifier) with an infant to promote sucking without breast or formula milk (Cignacco et al. 2007).

- There is an increasing body of research that demonstrates the calming effect of a dummy (pacifier) during painful procedures (Stevens 1999; Gibbins et al. 2002).
- In one study, infants ($n = 150$) were randomised to six groups. Infants in the dummy (pacifier) group recorded lower pain scores than all the infants except those in the sucrose plus dummy (pacifier) group (Carbajal et al. 1999).

5.10.7 Positioning

- Anatomically neutral positioning affects an infant's physiological and behavioural responses (Stevens 1999).
- However, prone positioning was not effective in reducing pain during single heel lances in preterm infants (Stevens et al. 1999).
- Care should be taken to position an infant as normally as possible despite the need to attach monitors, probes, etc.

5.10.8 Rocking

- Rocking a child is an appropriate and effective method of pain relief for younger children (Korner 1988; Stevens et al. 1999).
- In one studys rocking was found to be as effective as non-nutritive sucking in reducing crying (Campos 1994).

5.10.9 Swaddling

> **What is swaddling?**
>
> Swaddling involves wrapping the infant in a cloth or blanket to make them feel secure.

- Fearon et al. (1997) found that, with preterm infants ($n = 15$) aged above 31 weeks of gestation, swaddling after a painful procedure resulted in a reduced pulse rate. Inconclusive results were obtained among infants aged less than 31 weeks of gestation.

- However, Balantyne et al. (1999) and Huang et al. (2004) found that swaddling helped reduce infants' responses to procedural pain even with infants aged less that 31 weeks of gestation.
- Further, in a meta-analysis of 108 term and preterm neonates, Prasopkittikun and Tilskulchai (2003) concluded that positive effects from swaddling were present in all the neonates but lasted for a significantly shorter time in younger neonates.

> Swaddling has been shown to be effective in reducing procedural pain in neonates, but further research is needed (Cignacco et al. 2007).

5.10.10 Using non-drug methods in practice

Many of the non-drug methods described in this chapter can be used by nurses, and other healthcare professionals, with very little training. Other techniques such as hypnosis require healthcare professionals to obtain a recognised qualification. When implementing the non-drug methods described in this chapter the skills of the whole multidisciplinary team are important; play therapists and clinical psychologists play a vital role. However, despite what is known about the usefulness of non-drug methods as pain relieving strategies, several studies have found evidence that nurses do not use them in practice (Pederson and Harbaugh 1995; Polkki et al. 2001; Twycross 2007).

Summary

- There are a number of non-drug methods that can be used to relieve children's pain.
- There are non-drug methods that can be used specifically to relieve infants' pain.
- Several of the non-drug methods can be used relatively easily in practice; others require special training.
- Many of the studies exploring the effectiveness of these non-drug methods have small samples and in some cases the results are inconsistent. Further research is needed.
- Nurses, and other healthcare professionals, need to evaluate their pain management practices as several studies have suggested non-drug methods are not routinely used.

> **Useful web resources**
>
> Pain Clinical Update on Psychological Interventions of the Acute and Chronic Pain in Children: Available from: http://www.iasppain.org/AM/AMTemplate.cfm?Section=Home&TEMPLATE=/CM/ContentDisplay.cfm&CONTENTID=2271

> **Other useful resources**
>
> Tsao, J.C.I., Meldrum, M. and Zeltzer, L.K. (2005) Complementary and alternative medicine approaches for pediatric pain. In Finley, G.A., McGrath, P.J. and Chamber, C.T. (eds.) *Bringing Pain Relief to Children: Treatment Approaches*, Humana Press, Totowa, pp. 131–158.

References

Anie, K.A. and Green, J. (2000) Psychological therapies for sickle cell disease and pain. *Cochrane Database of Systematic Reviews*, Issue 3. Art. No.: CD001916.
Arndorfer, R.E. and Allen, K.D. (2001) Extending the efficacy of a thermal biofeedback treatment package to the management of tension-type headaches in children, *Headache*, 41: 183–192.

Ball, T.M., Shapiro, D.E., Monhelm, C.J. and Weydert, J.A. (2003) A pilot study of the use of guided imagery for the treatment of recurrent abdominal pain in children, *Clinical Pediatrics*, 42(6): 527–532.

Ballantyne, M., Stevens, B., McAllister, M., Dionne, K. and Jack, A. (1999) Validation of the premature infant pain profile in the clinical setting, *Clinical Journal of Pain*, 15: 297–303.

Beider, S., Mahrer, N.E. and Gold, J.I. (2006) Pediatric massage therapy: AN overview for clinicians, *Pediatric Clinics of North America*, 54: 1025–1041.

Bellini, C.V., Cordelli, D.M., Raffaelli, M., Ricci, B., Margese, G. and Buonocore, G. (2006) Analgesic effect of watching TV during venipuncture, *Archives of Disease in Childhood*, 91: 1015–1017.

Bucher, H.U., Moser, T., von Siebenthal, K., Keel, M., Wolf, M. and Duc, G. (1995) Sucrose reduces pain reaction to heel lancing in pre-term infants: A placebo-controlled randomised and masked study, *Pediatric Research*, 38(3):332–335.

Campos, R.G. (1994) Rocking and pacifiers: two comforting interventions for heelstick pain, *Research in Nursing and Health*, 17(5):321–31.

Carbajal, R., Chauvet, X., Couderc, S. and Olivier-Martin, M. (1999) Randomised trial of analgesic effects of sucrose, glucose, and pacifiers in term neonates, *British Medical Journal*, 319(7222):1393–1397.

Carlson, K.L., Broome, M. and Vessey, J.A. (2000) Using distraction to reduce reported pain, fear and behavioural distress in children and adolescents: a multisite study, *Journal of the Society of Pediatric Nursing*, 5(2): 75–86.

Cassidy, K-L., Reid, G.J., MGrath, P.J., Finley, G.A., Smith, D.J., Szudek, E.A. and Morton, B. (2002) Watch needle, watch TV: audiovisual distraction in preschool immunization, *Pain Medicine*, 3(2): 108–118.

Chen, E., Joseph, M. and Zeltzer, L.K. (2000) Behavioral and cognitive interventions in the treatment of pain in children, *Pediatric Clinics of North America*, 47(3): 513–525.

Cignacco, E., Hamers, J.p.H., Stoffel, L., van Lingen, R.A., Gessler, P., McDougall, J. and Nelle, M. (2007) The efficacy of non-pharmacological interventions in the management of procedural pain in pre-term and term neonates: a systematic literature review, *European Journal of Pain*, 11: 139–152.

Cozzi, L., Tryon, W.W. and Sedlacek, K. (1987) The effectiveness of biofeedback-assisted relaxation in modifying sickle cell crisis, *Biofeedback Self Regulation*, 12: 51–61.

Dahlquist, L.M., Gil, K.M., Armstrong, F.D., Ginsberg, A. and Jones, B. (1985) Behavioral management of children's distress during chemotherapy, *Journal of Behavior Therapy and Experimental Psychiatry*, 16(4): 325–329.

Dahlquist, L.M., Pendley, J.S., Landthrip, D.S., Jones, C.L. and Streber, C.P. (2002a) Distraction intervention for preschoolers undergoing intramuscular injections and subcutaneous port access, *Health Psychology*, 21(1): 94–99.

Dahlquist, L.M., Busby, S.M., Slifer, K.J., Tucker, C.L., Eischen, S., Hilley, L. and Sulc, W. (2002b) Distraction for children of different ages who undergo repeated needle sticks, *Journal of Pediatric Oncology Nursing*, 19(1): 22–34.

Dampier, C. and Shapiro, B.S. (2003) Management of pain in sickle cell disease. In Schechter, N.L., Berde, C.B. and Yaster, M. (eds.) *Pain in Infants, Children and Adolescents*, 2nd edition, Lippincott, Williams & Wilkins, Baltimore, pp. 489–516.

Das, D.A., Grimmer, K.A., Sparnon, A.L., McRae, S.E. and Thomas, B.H. (2005) The efficacy of playing a virtual reality game in modulating pain for children with acute burn injuries: a randomised control trial, *BMC Pediatrics*, 5(1): 1–10.

Ebner, C.A. (1996) Cold therapy and its effect on procedural pain in children, *Issues in Comprehensive Pediatric Nursing*, 19(3): 197–208.

Eccleston, C., Malleson, P.N., Clinch, J., Connell, H. and Sourbut, C. (2003) Chronic pain in adolescents: evaluation of a programme of interdisciplinary cognitive behaviour therapy, *Archives of Disease in Childhood*, 88(10): 881–885.

Eccleston, C., Yorke, L., Morely, S., Williams, A.C. and Mastroyannopoulou, K. (2006) Psychological therapies for the management of chronic and recurrent pain in children and adolescents, *The Cochrane Library*, 4 (CD003968).

Efe, E. and Ozer, Z.C. (2007) The use of breastfeeding for pain relief during neonatal immunization injections, *Applied Nursing Research*, 20: 10–16.

Efe, E. and Savaser, S. (2007) The effect of two different methods used during peripheral venous blood collection on pain reduction in neonates, *Ağrı Ağrı Dergisi*, 19(2): 49–56.

Fearon, I., Kisilevsky, B.S., Hains, S.M., Muir, D.W. and Tranmer, J. (1997) Swaddling after heel lance: age-specific effects on behavioral recovery in preterm infants, *Journal of Developmental & Behavioral Pediatrics*, 18(4): 222–232.

Field, T., Hernandez-Reif, M., Seligman, S., Krusnegor, J., Sunshine, W., Rivas-Chacon, R., Schanberg, S. and Kuhn, C. (1997) Juvenile rheumatoid arthritis: BENEFITS from massage therapy, *Journal of Pediatric Psychology*, 22(5): 607–617.

Franck, L. and Lawhon, G. (2000) Environmental and behavioural strategies to prevent and manage neonatal pain. In Anand, K.J.S., Stevens, B.J. and McGrath, P.J. (eds.) *Pain in Neonates*, 2nd edition, Elsevier, Amsterdam, pp. 203–216.

French, S.D., Cameron, M., Walker, B.F., Reggars, J.W, and Esterman, A.J. (2006) Superficial heat or cold for low back pain. *Cochrane Database of Systematic Reviews*, Issue 1. Art. No.: CD004750.

Gibbins, S., Stevens, B., Hodnett, E., Pinelli, J., Ohlsson, A. and Darlington, G. (2002) Efficacy and safety of sucrose for procedural pain relief in preterm and term neonates, *Nursing Research*, 51(6): 375–382.

Gold, J.I., Kim, S.H., Kant, A.J., Rizzo, M.H. and Skip, A. (2006) Effectiveness of virtual reality for pediatric pain distraction during IV placement, *Cyberpsychology and Behavior*, 9(2): 207–212.

Gradin, M., Eriksson, M., Holmqvist, G., Holstein, Á. and Schollin, J. (2002) Pain reduction at venipuncture in newborns: oral glucose compared with local anesthetic cream, *Pediatrics*, 110(6):1053–1057.

Greenberg, R.S., Billett, C., Zahurak, M. and Yaster, M. (1999) Videotapes increase parental knowledge about pediatric pain, *Pediatric Anaesthesia*, 89: 899–903.

Haouari, N., Wood, C., Griffiths, G. and Levene, M. (1995) The analgesic effect of sucrose in full term infants: a randomised controlled trial, *British Medical Journal*, 310: 1498–1500.

Hermann, C. and Blanchard, E.B. (2002) Biofeedback in the treatment of headache and other childhood pain, *Applied Psychophysiology & Biofeedback*, 27(2): 143–62.

Hernandez-Reif, M., Field, T., Largie, S., Hart, S., Redzepi, M., Nierenberg, B. and Peck, T.M. (2001) Children's distress during burn treatment is reduced by massage therapy, *Journal of Burn Care and Rehabilitation*, 22(2): 191–195.

Holden, E.W., Deichmann. M.M. and Levy, J.D. (1999) Empirically supported treatments in pediatric psychology: recurrent pediatric headache, *Journal of Pediatric Psychology*, 24: 91–109.

Huang, C.M., Tung, W.S., Kuo, L.L. and Chang, Y.J. (2004) Comparison of pain responses of premature infants to heelstick between containment and swaddling, *Nursing Research*, 12: 31–40.

Huth, M.M., Broome, M.E. and Good, M. (2004) Imagery reduces children's post-operative pain, *Pain*, 110: 439–448.

Ireland, M. and Olson, M. (2000) Massage therapy and therapeutic touch in children: state of the science, *Alternative Therapies in Health and Medicine*, 6(5): 54–63.

Jay, S.M., Elliott, C.H., Katz, E. and Siegel, S.E. (1987) Cognitive-behavioral and pharmacologic interventions for children's distress during painful medical procedures, *Journal of Consulting and Clinical Psychology*, 55(6): 860–865.

Jay, S.M., Elliott, C.H., Woody, P.D. and Siegel, S. (1991) An investigation of cognitive-behavior therapy combined with oral valium for children undergoing painful medical procedures, *Health Psychology*, 10(5): 317–22.

Johnston, C.C., Stevens, B.J., Franck, L.S., Jack, A., Stremler, R. and Platt, R. (1999) Factors explaining lack of response to heel stick in preterm infants, *Journal of Obstetric, Gynecologic and Neonatal Nursing*, 28(6): 587–594.

Johnston, C.C., Stevens, B., Pinelli, J., Gibbins, S., Filion, F., Jack, A., Steele, S., Boyer, K. and Veilleux, A. (2003) Kangaroo care is effective in diminishing pain response in preterm neonates, *Archives of Pediatrics & Adolescent Medicine*, 157(11): 1084–1088.

Kemper, K.J. and Gardiner, P. (2003) Complementary and alternative medical therapies in pediatric pain treatment. In Schechter, N.L., Berde, C.B. and Yaster, M. (eds.) *Pain in Infants, Children and Adolescents*, 2nd edition, Lippincott, Williams & Wilkins, Baltimore, pp. 449–461.

Kemper, K.J., Sarah, R., Silver-Highfield, E., Xiarhos, E., Barnes, L. and Berde, C. (2000) On pins and needles? pediatric patients' experiences with acupuncture, *Pediatrics*, 105: 941–947.

Kleiber, C., Croft-Rosenberg, M. and Harper, D.C. (2001) Parents as distraction coaches during IV insertion: a randomised study, *Journal of Pain and Symptom Management*, 22(4): 851–861.

Korner, A.F. (1988) Early intervention with preterm infants. In Hibbs, E.D. (ed.) *Children and Families: Studies in Prevention and Intervention*, International Universities Press, Madison, pp. 53–62.

Kundu, A. and Berman, B. (2007) Acupuncture for pediatric pain and symptom management, *Pediatric Clinics of North America*, 54: 885–899.

Kuttner, L. and Solomon, R. (2003) Hypnotherapy and imagery for managing children's pain. In Schechter, N.L., Berde, C.B. and Yaster, M. (eds.) *Pain in Infants, Children and Adolescents*, 2nd edition, Lippincott, Williams & Wilkins, Baltimore, pp. 317–328.

Lambert, S.A. (1996) The effects of hypnosis/guided imagery on the postoperative course of children, *Developmental and Behavioral Pediatrics*, 17(5): 307–310.

Lander, J. and Fowler-Kerry, S. (1993) TENS for children's procedural pain, *Pain*, 52:209–216.

Landolt, M.A., Marti, D., Widmer, J., and Meuli, M. (2002) Does cartoon movie distraction decrease burned children's pain behaviour? *Journal of Burn Care and Rehabilitation*, 23(1): 61–65.

Larsson, B., Carlsson, J., Fichtel, A. and Melin, L. (2005) Relaxation treatment of adolescent headache sufferers: results from a school-based replication series, *Headache*, 45: 692–704.

Lavigne, J.V., Ross, C.K., Berry, S.L., Hayford, J.R. and Pachman, L.M. (1992) Evaluation of a psychological package for treating pain in juvenile rheumatoid arthritis, *Arthritis Care and Research*, 5: 101–110.

Lin, Y-C. (2003) Acupuncture. In Schechter, N.L., Berde, C.B. and Yaster, M. (eds.) *Pain in Infants, Children and Adolescents*, 2nd edition, Lippincott, Williams & Wilkins, Baltimore, pp. 462–470.

Lin, Y., Bioteau. A. and Lee, A. (2002) Acupuncture for the treatment of pediatric pain: a pilot study, *Medical Acupuncture*, 14(1): 45–46.

Liossi, C. and Hatira, P. (1999) Clinical hypnosis versus cognitive behavioral training for pain management with pediatric cancer patients undergoing bone marrow aspirations, *International Journal of Clinical & Experimental Hypnosis*, 47(2): 104–116.

Liossi, C., White, P. and Hatira, P. (2006) Randomized clinical trial of local anesthetic versus a combination of local anesthetic with self-hypnosis in the management of pediatric procedure-related pain. *Health Psychology*, 25(3): 307–315.

Manimala M.R., Blount R.L. and Cohen L.L. (2000) The effects of parental reassurance versus distraction on child distress and coping during immunizations, *Children's Healthcare*, 29(3): 161–177.

McCaffery, M. and Beebe, A.B. (1989) *Pain: Clinical Manual for Nursing Practice*, C V Mosby, St Louis.

McCaffery, M. and Pasero, C. (1999) Practical nondrug approaches to pain. In McCaffery, M. and Pasero, C. (eds.) *Pain: Clinical Manual*, 2nd edition, Mosby, St Louis, pp. 399–427.

McCarthy, C.F., Shea, A.M. and Sullivan, P. (2003) Physical therapy management of pain in children. In Schechter, N.L., Berde, C.B. and Yaster, M. (eds.) *Pain in Infants, Children and Adolescents*, 2nd edition, Lippincott, Williams & Wilkins, Baltimore, pp. 434–448.

McGrath, P.J., Dick, B. and Unruh, A.M. (2003) Psychologic and behavioural treatments of pain in children and adolescents. In Schechter, N.L., Berde, C.B. and Yaster, M. (eds.) *Pain in Infants, Children and Adolescents*, 2nd edition, Lippincott, Williams & Wilkins, Baltimore, pp. 303–316.

Pederson, C. (1995) Effect of imagery on children's pain and anxiety during cardiac catheterization, *Journal of Pediatric Nursing*, 10(6): 365–374.

Pederson, C. and Harbaugh, B.L. (1995) Nurses' use of nonpharmacologic techniques with hospitalised children, *Issues in Comprehensive Pediatric Nursing*, 18: 91–109.

Pintov, S., Lahat, E., Alstein, M., Vogel, Z. and Barg, J. (1997) Acupuncture and the opioid system: implications in the management of migraine, *Pediatric Neurology*, 17: 129–133.

Polkki, T., Vehvilamen-Julkunen, K. and Pietila, A-M. (2001) Nonpharmacological methods in relieving children's postoperative pain: a survey on hospital nurses in Finland, *Journal of Advanced Nursing*, 34(4): 483–492.

Polkki, T., Pietila, A-M. and Vehvilamen-Julkunen, K. (2003) Hospitalized children's descriptions of their experiences with postsurgical pain-relieving methods, *International Journal of Nursing Studies*, 40: 33–44.

Poltorak, D.Y. and Benore, E. (2006) Cognitive-behavioral interventions for physical symptom management in pediatric palliative medicine, *Child and Adolescent Psychiatric Clinics of North America*, 15: 683–691.

Powers, S.W. (1999) Empirically supported treatments in pediatric psychology: procedure-related pain, *Journal of Pediatric Psychology*, 24: 131–145.

Prasopkittikun, T. and Tilkskulchai, F. (2003) Management of pain from heel stick in neonates: an analysis of research conducted in Thailand, *Journal of Perinatal and Neonatal Nursing*, 7: 304–312.

Richardson, J., Smith, J.E., McCall, G. and Pilkington, K. (2006) Hypnosis for procedure-related pain and distress in pediatric cancer patients: a systematic review of effectiveness and methodology related to hypnosis interventions, *Journal of Pain and Symptom Management*, 31(1): 70–84.

Rickard, J. (1994) *Relaxation for Children*, 2nd edition, Australian Council for Educational Research, Melbourne, Victoria.

Rusy, L.M. and Weisman, S.J. (2000) Complementary therapies for acute pediatric pain management, *Pediatric Clinics of North America*, 47(3): 589–599.

Scharff, L., Marcus, D.A. and Masek, B.J. (2002) A controlled study of minimal-contact thermal biofeedback treatment in children with migraine, *Journal of Pediatric Psychology*, 27(2): 109–119.

Schneider, S.M. and Workman, M.L. (2000) Virtual reality as a distraction intervention for older children receiving chemotherapy, *Pediatric Nursing*, 26(6): 593–597.

Shah, P.S., Aliwalas, L.L. and Shah, V. (2006) Breastfeeding or breast milk for procedural pain in neonates. *Cochrane Database of Systematic Reviews*, 3: CD004950.

Sinha, M., Christopher, N.C., Fenn, R. and Reeves, L. (2006) Evaluation of nonpharmacologic methods of pain and anxiety management for laceration repair in the pediatric emergency department, *Pediatrics*, 117(4): 1162–1168.

Smith, J.L. and Madsen, J.R. (2003) Neurosurgical procedures for the treatment of pediatric pain. In Schechter, N.L., Berde, C.B. and Yaster, M. (eds.) *Pain in Infants, Children and Adolescents*, 2nd edition, Lippincott, Williams & Wilkins, Baltimore, pp. 329–338.

Stevens, B. (1999) Pain in infants. In McCaffery, M. and Pasero, C. (eds.) *Pain: Clinical Manual*, 2nd edition, Mosby, St Louis, pp. 626–673.

Stevens, B., Johnston, C., Franck, L., Petryshen, P., Jack, A. and Foster, G. (1999) The efficacy of developmentally sensitive interventions and sucrose for relieving procedural pain in very low birth weight neonates, *Nursing Research*, 48(1): 35–43.

Stevens, B., Yamada, J. and Ohlsson, A. (1998) Sucrose for analgesia in newborn infants undergoing painful procedures, *Cochrane Database of Systematic Reviews*, Issue 2. Art. No. CD001069.

Surjala, K.L., Donaldson, G.W., Davis, M.W., Kippes, M.E. and Carr, J.E. (1995) Relaxation imagery and cognitive-behavioral training reduce pain during cancer treatment: a controlled clinical trial, *Pain*, 63: 189–198.

Tanabe, P., Ferket, K., Thomas, R., Paice, J. and Marcantonio, R. (2002) The effect of standard care, ibuprofen, and distraction on pain relief and patient satisfaction in children with musculoskeletal trauma, *Journal of Emergency Medicine*, 28(2): 118–125.

Tsao, J.C.I., Meldrum, M. And Zeltzer, L.K. (2006) Efficacy of complementary and alternative medicine approaches for pediatric pain: state of the science. In Finley, G.A., McGrath, P.J. and Chamber, C.T. (eds.) *Bringing Pain Relief to Children: Treatment Approaches*, Humana Press, Totowa, pp. 131–158.

Twycross, A. (2007) Children's nurses' post-operative pain management practices: an observational study, *International Journal of Nursing Studies*, 44(6): 869–881.

Uman, L.S., Chambers, C.T., McGrath, P.J. and Kisely, S. (2006) Psychological interventions for needle-related procedural pain and distress in children and adolescents, *Cochrane Reviews* 18(4): CD005179.

Vessey, J.A. and Carlson, K.L. (1996) Nonpharmacological interventions to use with children in pain. *Issues in Comprehensive Pediatric Nursing*, 19:169–182.

Vessey, J.A., Carlson, K.L. and McGill, J. (1994) Use of distraction with children during a painful procedure, *Nursing Research*, 43(6): 369–372.

Walker, L.S., Williams, S.E., Smith, C.A., Garber, J., Van Slyke, D.A. and Lipani, T.A. (2006) Parent attention versus distraction: impact on symptom complaints by children with and without chronic functional abdominal pain, *Pain*, 122: 43–52.

Weydert, J.A., Shapiro, D.E., Acra, S.A., Monheim, C.J., Chambers, A.S. and Ball, T.M. (2006) Evaluation of guided imagery as treatment for recurrent abdominal pain in children: a randomised control trial, *BMC Pediatrics*, 6:29, 1–10.

Wolitzky, K., Fivush, R., Zimand, E., Hodges, L. and Rothbaum, B.O. (2005) Effectiveness of virtual reality distraction during a painful medical procedure in pediatric oncology patients, *Psychology and Health*, 20(6): 817–824.

Woodgate, R. and Kristjanson L. (1996) A young child's pain: how parents and nurses 'take care', *International Journal of Nursing Studies*, 33(3): 271–284.

Zeltzer, L. and LeBaron, S. (1982) Hypnosis and nonhypnotic techniques for reduction of pain and anxiety during painful procedures in children and adolescents with cancer, *Journal of Pediatrics*, 101(6): 1032–1035.

Zeltzer, L.K., Bush, J.P., Chen, E. and Riveral, A. (1997) A psychobiologic approach to pediatric pain: Part 1. History, physiology, and assessment strategies, *Current Problems in Pediatrics*, 27(6): 225–253.

Zeltzer, L.K., Tsao, J.C.I., Stelling, C., Powers, M., Levy, S. and Waterhouse, M (2002) A phase 1 study on the feasibility of an acupuncture/hypnotherapy intervention for chronic pediatric pain, *Journal of Pain and Symptom Management*, 24: 437–446.

CHAPTER 6
Pain Assessment
Jennifer Stinson

Introduction

This chapter will provide an overview of the assessment of pain in children from neonates to adolescents. The difference between pain assessment and measurement will be highlighted, the key steps in pain assessment identified and the need to take a pain history discussed. Self-report and behavioural and physiological indicators of pain in children will be reviewed. The need for clear documentation about pain assessment and how regularly pain assessment should be undertaken are also discussed. Information about commonly used pain tools will be provided and the factors that need to be considered when choosing a pain assessment tool will be outlined. Research relating to nurses' pain assessment practices is discussed in Chapter 11.

6.1 Nurses' Role in Pain Assessment

Many healthcare professionals are involved, either directly or indirectly, in the assessment of children's pain. However, nurses have the most contact with children receiving healthcare. This places them in a unique position to identify children who are experiencing pain; to appropriately assess the pain and its impact on the child and family; to relieve pain using available resources; and to evaluate the effectiveness of those actions. This chapter will provide the theoretical knowledge required by nurses to enable them to successfully assess pain in children.

6.2 Pain Measurement and Pain Assessment

Pain measurement generally describes the quantification of pain intensity. For example, we commonly ask 'How much does it hurt?' The emphasis is on the quantity, extent or degree of pain (Johnston 1998).

Pain assessment is a broader concept than measurement and involves clinical judgment based on observation of the nature, significance and context of the child's pain experience (Johnston 1998).

The majority of pain assessment tools focus on *measuring* pain intensity. However, a wider *assessment* provides information such as where the pain is and what it is like. This helps the nurse to make decisions regarding the most likely cause of the pain and to choose the most appropriate intervention.

Pain assessment includes measurement (e.g. pain intensity) but the emphasis is on the multidimensional nature of pain.

Pain assessment involves exploring the:

- intensity of the pain;
- location of the pain;
- duration of the pain;
- sensory qualities of the pain (e.g. word descriptors);
- cognitive aspects of the pain (e.g. perceived impact on aspects of everyday life);
- affective aspects of the pain experience (e.g. pain unpleasantness);
- contextual and situational factors that may influence the child's perception of pain (see Chapter 3).

6.2.1 Assessing pain in children

Pain assessment is the first step in the management of pain. To treat pain effectively, ongoing assessment of the presence and severity of pain and the child's response to treatment is essential (American Academy of Pediatrics and American Pain Society 2001). Pain assessment poses many challenges in infants and children because of:

- the subjective and complex nature of pain;
- developmental and language limitations that preclude comprehension and self-report;
- dependence on others to infer pain from behavioural and physiological indicators.

(McCaffery and Pasero 1999)

When assessing pain in children there are three key steps (Box 6.1).

BOX 6.1

Key steps: pain assessment

Step 1: Record a pain history
Step 2: Assess the child's pain using a developmentally appropriate pain assessment tool
Step 3: Reassess pain having allowed time for pain relieving interventions to work

---

Parents and significant family members know their child best and can recognise subtle changes in manner or behaviour. They have a particularly important role in pain assessment and should be involved at all three steps.

Step 1: Recording a pain history

Recording a thorough history of the child's prior pain experiences and current pain complaints is the first step in pain assessment. Standardised pain history forms (Hester and Barcus 1986; Acute Pain Management Guideline Panel 1992; Ball and Binder 1995; Hester et al. 1998) have been developed for talking with children and parents about the pain. For the child in acute pain, the questions outlined in Table 6.1 usually provide sufficient information and can be included within the nursing admission process.

For a child with chronic pain a more detailed pain history needs to be taken. This includes information about:

- the description of the pain;
- associated symptoms;
- temporal or seasonal variations;
- impact on daily living (e.g. school, sport, play and self-care);
- pain relief measures used.

Table 6.1 Pain history for children with acute pain

Child's questions	Parent's questions
Tell me what pain is	What word(s) does your child use in regard to pain?
Tell me about the hurt you have had before	Describe the pain experiences your child has had before
Do you tell others when you hurt? If yes, who?	Does your child tell you or others when he or she is hurting?
What do you want to do for yourself when you are hurting?	How do you know when your child is in pain?
What do you want others to do for you when you are hurt?	How does your child usually react to pain?
What don't you want others to do for you when you hurt?	What do you do for your child when he or she is hurting?
What helps the most to take your hurt away?	What does your child do for him- or herself when he or she is hurting?
Is there anything special that you want me to know about when you hurt? (If yes, have child describe)	What works best to decrease or take away your child's pain?
	Is there anything special that you would like me to know about your child and pain? (If yes, describe)

Source: Hester and Barcus (1986); Hester et al. (1998)

Further detail about questions to ask children and parents about chronic pain can be seen in Box 6.2.

BOX 6.2

Pain history questions for children with chronic pain and their parents/carers

Description of pain

Type of pain – *Is the pain acute* (e.g. medical procedures, postoperative pain, accidental injury), *recurrent* (e.g. headaches) *or chronic* (e.g. juvenile idiopathic arthritis)?
Onset of pain – *When did the pain begin? What were you doing before the pain began? Was there any initiating injury, trauma or stressors?*
Duration – *How long has the pain been present?* (e.g. hours/days/weeks/months)
Frequency – *How often is pain present? Is the pain always there or is it intermittent? Does it come and go?*
Location
Where is the pain located? Can you point to the part of the body that hurts? (Body outlines can be used to help children indicate where they hurt)
   Children aged three to four years or older can mark an X to indicate painful areas, shade in with crayons areas of pain or choose different colours to represent varying degrees of pain intensity.
Does the pain go anywhere else? (e.g. radiates up or down from the site that hurts) Pain radiation can also be indicated on body diagrams.
Intensity
What is your pain intensity at rest? What is your pain intensity with activity? (Use an appropriate pain assessment tool)

BOX 6.2 Continued

Over the past week what is the least pain you have had? What is the worst pain you have had? What is your usual level of pain?

Quality of pain

School-age children can communicate about pain in more abstract terms.

Describe the quality of your pain? (e.g. word descriptors such as sharp, dull, achy, stabbing, burning, shooting or throbbing)

Word descriptors can provide information on whether the pain is nociceptive or neuropathic in nature or a combination.

Associated symptoms

Are there any other symptoms that go along with or occur just before or immediately after the pain? (e.g. nausea, vomiting, light-headedness, tiredness, diarrhoea, or difficulty walking)

Are there any changes in the colour or temperature of the affected extremity or painful area? (These changes most often occur in children with conditions such as complex regional pain syndromes)

Temporal or seasonal variations

Is the pain affected by changes in seasons or weather?

Does the pain occur at certain times of the day? (e.g. after eating or going to the toilet)

Impact on daily living

Has the pain led to changes in daily activities and/or behaviours? (e.g. sleep disturbances, change in appetite, decreased physical activity, change in mood, or a decrease in social interactions or school attendance)

What level would the pain need to be so that you could do all your normal activities? (e.g. tolerability) *What level would the pain need to be so that you won't be bothered by it?* (rated on similar scale as pain intensity)

What brings on the pain or makes the pain worse? (e.g. movement, deep breathing and coughing, stress, etc.)

Pain relief measures

What has helped to make the pain better?

What medication have you taken to relieve your pain? If so, what was the medication and did it help? Were there any side effects?

It is important to also ask about the use of physical, psychological and complementary and alternative treatments tried and how effective these methods were in relieving pain (see Chapter 5).

The degree of pain relief or intensity of pain after a pain-relieving treatment/intervention should be determined.

Other factors that affect an individual child's perception of pain should also be considered. These are discussed in Chapter 3.

Step 2: Assessing the child's pain using a developmentally appropriate pain assessment tool

The three approaches to measuring pain are:

- self-report (that is, what the child says);
- behavioural (that is, how the child behaves);
- physiological indicators (that is, how the child's body reacts).

These measures are used separately or in combination in a range of pain assessment tools that are available to use in practice. Self-report measures are considered the *gold standard* and should be used with children who are:

- old enough to understand and use self-report scale (e.g. three years of age and older);
- not overtly distressed.

(Stinson et al. 2006)

With infants, toddlers, preverbal, cognitively impaired and sedated children behavioural pain assessment tools should be used (Von Baeyer and Spagrud 2007). If the child is overtly distressed (e.g. due to pain, anxiety or some other stressor), no meaningful self-report can be obtained at that point in time. The child's pain can be estimated using behavioural pain assessment tools until such time as the child is less distressed (e.g. following the administration of analgesic drugs).

6.3 Self-Report Tools

Several self-report pain assessment tools have been designed for use with school-aged children.

6.3.1 Verbal rating scales

- Verbal rating scales (VRS) consist of a list of simple word descriptors or phases to denote varying degrees or intensities of pain.
- Each word or phrase has an associated number.
- Children are asked to select a single word or phrase that best represents their level of pain intensity and the score is the number associated with the chosen word.
- One example of a VRS is using word descriptors of *not at all* = 0, *a little bit* = 1, *quite a lot* = 2 and *most hurt possible* = 3 (Goodenough et al. 1997).

6.3.2 Faces pain scales

- Faces pain scales present the child with drawings or photographs of facial expressions representing increasing levels of pain intensity (Figs 6.1 to 6.3).
- The child is asked to select the picture of a face that best represents their pain intensity and their score is the number (rank order) of the expression chosen.
- Faces scales have been well validated for use in children aged 5–12 years (Champion et al. 1998; Stinson et al. 2006).
- There are two types of faces scales – line drawings (e.g. Faces pain scale – revised, Figure 6.1) and photographs (e.g. Oucher, Figure 6.3).
- Faces pain scales with a happy and smiling *no pain* face or faces with tears for *the most pain possible* have been found to affect the pain scores recorded. For example, the smiling lower anchor of the Wong-Baker FACES Pain Scale (Figure 6.2) has been found to produce higher pain ratings than those with neutral faced anchors (Chambers and Craig 1998). Therefore, faces pain scales with neutral expressions for *no pain* such as that developed by Hicks et al. (2001) (Figure 6.1) are generally recommended.
- Some of the more commonly used and well-validated faces pain scales are outlined in Table 6.2.

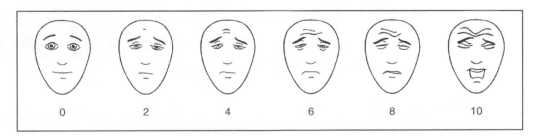

Figure 6.1 Faces Pain Scale – Revised (FPS-R; Hicks et al. 2001). From Pain, 2001; 93: 173–183. Used with permission from IASP. Numbers are for reference and are not shown to children. Scale and instructions in many languages are available online for clinical and research use at www.painsourcebook.ca.

Table 6.2   Validated faces pain tools

Measure	Characteristics	Considerations
Faces Pain Scale-Revised (FPS-R) (Hicks et al. 2001)	The Faces Pain Scale-Revised (FPS-R) was altered so that the Faces Pain Scale (FPS) was compatible in scoring with other self-rating and observational scales. Six gender-neutral faces (Figure 6.1). Faces ranged from *no pain* to *as much pain as is possible*. Scored 0–10	Intended for use in children 5–12 years of age but has been used in children 4–18 years of age. Well-established evidence of reliability, validity and ability to detect change (Stinson et al. 2006). High clinical utility (quick and easy to use). Translated into more than 30 languages. Disadvantages include limited evidence regarding interpretability of scores and mixed evidence about the acceptability of the scale with children
Oucher–photographic scale (Beyer 1984)	Six photographs of culturally specific faces presented vertically alongside Oucher numerical rating scale (Figure 6.3). Scored 0–10. Caucasian, Hispanic, Afro-American and Asian scales	Intended for use in children 3–7 years of age but has been used in children 3–18 years of age. Well-established evidence of reliability, validity and ability to detect change. Its use in younger children (3–4 year olds) requires further testing (Stinson et al. 2006). Moderate clinical utility. Mixed acceptability compared to other faces scales. Disadvantages: Photos are not gender or ethnically neutral and are of children with acute rather than chronic pain, limiting the range of clinical contexts it can be used in. Practical issues: cost to purchase scales and need to disinfect between patients
Wong-Baker FACES Pain Scale (Wong and Baker 1988)	Six hand-drawn faces ranging from smiling to crying (Figure 6.2). Face 1 = 'no hurt', face 2 = 'hurts a little bit', face 3 = 'hurts little more', face 4 = 'hurts whole lot', face 5 = 'hurts worst'. Scored 0–5 or 0–10	Intended for use in children 3–18 years. Well-established evidence of reliability, validity and ability to detect change (Stinson et al. 2006). High clinical utility (quick and simple to use, requires minimal instruction). High acceptability (well liked by children and healthcare professionals). Translated into 10 languages. Readily available (can be obtained free of charge) and easily reproduced by photocopying. Wearable pins are available for purchase. Disadvantages include: smiling *no pain* face results in higher reported pain scores compared to neutral face (Chambers and Craig 1998; Chambers et al. 2005), worst pain face has tears and not all children cry when in pain

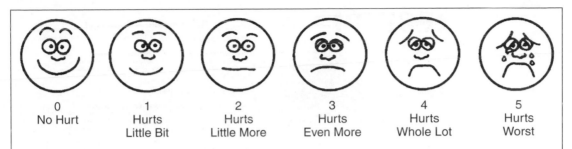

0
No Hurt

1
Hurts
Little Bit

2
Hurts
Little More

3
Hurts
Even More

4
Hurts
Whole Lot

5
Hurts
Worst

Original instructions:

Explain to the person that each face is for a person who feels happy because he has no pain (hurt) or sad because he has some or a lot of pain. Face 0 is very happy because he doesn't hurt at all. Face 1 hurts just a little bit. Face 2 hurts a little more. Face 3 hurts even more. Face 4 hurts a whole lot. Face 5 hurts as much as you can imagine, although you don't have to be crying to feel this bed. Ask the person to choose the face that best describes how he is feeling.

Rating scale is recommended for person's age 3 years and older.

Brief word instructions: Point to each face using the words to describe the pain intensity. Ask the child to choose face that best describes own pain and record the appropriate number.

Figure 6.2 Wong Baker FACES Pain Scale. Reproduced with permission from Hockenberry, M.J., Wilson, D., Winkelstein ML: Wong's Essentials of Pediatric Nursing, ed. 7, St. Louis, 2005, p. 1259. Used with permission, Mosby. Can be downloaded for clinical use from: http://www.mosbysdrugconsult.com/WOW/facesReproductions. html#DownloadFACES

6.3.3 Numerical pain scales

- A numerical rating scale (NRS) consists of a range of numbers (e.g. 0–10 or 0–100) that can be represented in verbal or graphical format (Figure 6.4).
- Children are told that the lowest number represents *no pain* and the highest number represents *the most pain possible*. The child is instructed to circle, record or state the number that best represents their level of pain intensity.
- Verbal NRS tend to be the most frequently used pain intensity measure with children over eight years of age in clinical practice.
- They have the advantage that they can be verbally administered without a print copy and are easy to score. They do require numeracy skills and, therefore, should be used in older school-aged children and adolescents.
- While there is evidence of their reliability and validity in adults, verbal NRS have undergone very little testing in children.
- An example of a well-validated scale incorporating a graphic NRS is the Oucher (Beyer 1984; Figure 6.3). The Oucher comprises two separate scales: the photographic faces scale and a 0–10 vertical NRS. Older school-aged children and adolescents are meant to use the NRS.

6.3.4 Graphic rating scales

- The most commonly used graphic rating scale is the Pieces of Hurt Tool (Hester 1979).
- This tool consists of four red poker chips, representing *a little hurt* to *the most hurt you could ever have*.
- The child is asked to select the chip that represents his/her pain intensity and the tool is scored from 0 to 4.
- The Pieces of Hurt Tool has been well validated for acute procedural and hospital-based pains and is recommended for use in young pre-school children (Stinson et al. 2006).

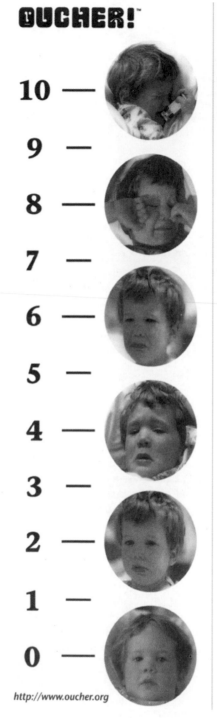

OUCHER!™

10 —
9 —
8 —
7 —
6 —
5 —
4 —
3 —
2 —
1 —
0 —

http://www.oucher.org

THE OUCHER: A SUMMARY

What is the OUCHER?

The OUCHER is a poster developed for children to help them communicate how much pain or hurt they feel. There are two scales on the OUCHER: A number scale for older children and a picture scale for younger children.

Which scale should be used?

Children who are able to count to 100 by ones or tens and who understand, for example, that 71 is greater than 43, can use the numerical scale. Children who do not understand numbers should use the picture scale. Some children who are able to use the number scale might prefer to use the picture scale. Ask the child which scale he or she would prefer.

How do I use the OUCHER?

Picture scale: The following is an example of how to explain the picture scale to a younger child. The words can be changed when using the picture scale with an older child.

This is a poster called the OUCHER. It helps children tell others how much hurt they have. (For younger children, it might be useful to ask: Do you know what I mean by hurt? If the child is not sure, then an explanation should be provided.) Here's how this works. This picture shows not hurt (point to the bottom picture), this picture shows just a little bit of hurt (point to the 2nd picture), this picture shows a little more hurt (point to the 3rd picture), this picture shows even more hurt (point to the 4th picture), this picture shows a lot of hurt (point to the 5th picture), and this picture shows the biggest hurt you could ever have (point to the 6th picture). Can you point to the picture that shows how much hurt you are having right now?

Once a children selects a picture, their picture selection is changed to a number score from 0-10.

    10 – Picture at the top of the scale
    8 – Second picture from the top
    6 – Third picture from the top
    4 – Fourth picture from the top
    2 – Fifth picture from the top
    0 – Picture at the bottom of the scale

Number scale: The following is an example of how to explain the number scale.

This is a poster called the OUCHER. It helps children tell others how much hurt they have. Here's how it works. 0 means no hurt. Here (point to the lower third of the scale, about 1 to 3), this means you have little hurts; here (point to the middle third of the scale, about 3 to 6) it means you have middle hurts. If your hurt is about here (point to the upper third of the scale, about 6 to 9), it means you have big hurts. But if you point to 10, it means you have the biggest hurt you could ever have. Can you point to the number (or tell me which number) that is like the hurt you are having right now?

The pain score for the number scale is the exact number from 0 to 10 that the child gives you.

What does the score mean? How should it be used?

The person who has pain is the expert or the one who knows best how the pain feels. The OUCHER score gives parents, teachers, nurses, and doctors some idea of how much pain the child is feeling. OUCHER scores can be used as a means to see if certain actions used to relieve pain, such as rest, applying heat or cold, eating or drinking, and medicine make a difference in how much pain the child feels. OUCHER scores can be recorded over a period of hours or days and would be useful information to share with nurses and doctors.

Remember, OUCHER scores only communicate how much pain the child is feeling. Other observations, such as changes in activity, location of the pain, what it feels like, and how long it lasts, are important. If you, as a parent or teacher, are concerned about the child's pain, you should contact your health care provider.

For information about the Oucher, write to: Dr. Judith E. Beyer, P.O. Box 411714, Kansas City, MO 64141 or go to the www.OUCHER.com website.

http://www.oucher.org

Figure 6.3   Oucher. The Caucasian version of the Oucher was developed and copyrighted in 1983 by Judith E. Beyer, Ph.D., RN (University of Missouri-Kansas City School of Nursing, USA). Reproduced with permission from Dr Judith Beyer. Available from: http://www.oucher.org/the_scales.html.

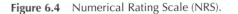

Figure 6.4 Numerical Rating Scale (NRS).

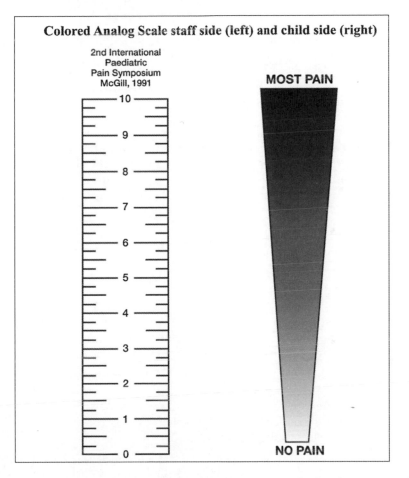

Figure 6.5 Colour Analogue Scale. From Pain, 1996; 64: 435–443. Used with permission from IASP ©1996. International Association for the Study of Pain.

- The Pieces of Hurt Tool is easy to use and score and the instructions have been translated into several languages including Arabic, Thai and Spanish.
- Drawbacks to its use include cleaning the chips between patient use and the potential for losing chips.

6.3.5 Visual analogue scales

- Visual analogue scales (VAS) require the child to select a point on a vertical or horizontal line where the ends of the line are defined as the extreme limits of pain intensity.
- The child is asked to make a mark along the line to indicate the intensity of their pain. There are many versions of VAS for use with children.
- In addition, creative strategies have been employed to improve the reliability and validity of VAS for use in children by using graphic or other methods to enhance the child's understanding of the measure (e.g. colour analogue scale; McGrath et al. 1996, Figure 6.5).

- VAS have been extensively researched and have been recommended for most children aged eight years and older (Stinson et al. 2006).
- While VAS are easy to reproduce, photocopying may alter the length of the line, and may require the extra step of measuring the line, which increases the burden and likelihood for errors.

6.3.6 Multidimensional pain tools

Although pain intensity is the most commonly recorded measure of a painful episode, a more comprehensive pain assessment is often necessary, for example, for children with chronic pain. In this situation it is necessary to assess factors such as pain triggers, the types of sensations that are experienced and how the pain interferes with aspects of everyday life. Table 6.3 outlines three self-report pain tools that have been shown to be reliable and valid multidimensional pain measures.

Pain diaries are another way to track pain in children with recurrent or chronic pain. While paper-based diaries have been used in clinical and research practice for decades, they are prone to recall biases and poor compliance. More recently, real-time data collection methods using electronic hand-held diaries have been developed for children with recurrent and chronic pain (Palermo et al. 2004; Stinson et al. 2006, 2008).

> For further information about self-report tools see Stinson et al. (2006).

6.4 Behavioural Tools

The tools developed to assess pain in infants and young children generally use behavioural indicators of pain. A wide range of specific expressive behaviours have been identified in infants and young children that are indicative of pain:

- individual behaviours (e.g. crying and facial expression);
- large movements (e.g. withdrawal of the affected limb, touching the affected area, and the movement or tensing of limbs and torso);
- changes in social behaviour or appetite;
- changes in sleep/wake state or cognitive functions.

A variety of observational or behavioural pain measures have been developed and validated for use in infants and children (Tables 6.4, 6.5).

> **Observational tools** are indicated for children who are:
>
> - Too young to understand and use self-report scales (e.g. less than four years old)
> - Too distressed to use self-report scales
> - Impaired in their cognitive or communicative abilities
> - Very restricted by bandages, surgical tape, mechanical ventilation or paralysing drugs
> - Whose self-report ratings are considered to be exaggerated, minimised or unrealistic due to cognitive, emotional or situational factors
>
> *Source:* von Baeyer and Spagrud (2007)

Table 6.3   Validated multidimensional self-report pain tools

Measure	Components	Considerations
Adolescent Pediatric Pain Tool (APPT) (Savedra et al. 1989) (Figure 6.6)	Pain intensity measured using: • a 0–100 mm word graphic rating scale • body outline to describe location of pain • word descriptors	Originally developed for children and adolescents with postoperative pain; has been used in children with acute and chronic disease-related pain (e.g. cancer, sickle cell disease, arthritis) Intended for use in children 5–16 years of age; used in children from 4–18 years Well established evidence of reliability, validity and ability to detect change Advantages: easy to use, well-liked, requires minimal training and takes 3–6 minutes to complete
Pediatric Pain Assessment Tool (PPAT) (Abu-Saad 1990)	Pain intensity measured using: • 0–10 cm VAS • body outline (number of body areas marked) • 32 word descriptors	Initially developed for acute medical and postoperative pain; has also been used with recurrent pain (headaches) and chronic pain (arthritis) Intended for use in children 5–16 years of age; used in children up to 17 years Well-established evidence of reliability and validity and some evidence of ability to detect change Child, parent and healthcare professional forms Easy to use and little time to complete
Pediatric Pain Questionnaire (PPQ) (Varni et al. 1987)	Pain intensity measured using: • 0–10 cm VAS anchored with happy and sad faces for present and worst pain • gender neutral body outline to describe location of pain (number of body areas marked) • pain intensity (choosing four of eight coloured crayons to represent various levels of pain intensity from none, mild, moderate and severe) • 46 word descriptors to assess the sensory, affective and evaluative qualities of pain	Originally developed for children and adolescents with recurrent and chronic pain (e.g. juvenile arthritis) Intended for use in children 5–16 years of age; used in children 4–18 years Child, adolescent and parent versions Well-established evidence of reliability and validity and some evidence of ability to detect change Advantages: minimal training and takes 10–15 minutes to complete Children younger than 7 years will usually need to be read the instructions to complete the VAS and body outline Free for unfunded research Website: www.pedsgl.org

Assessing pain in ventilated infants and children remains a special challenge for nurses (Ramelet et al. 2004; Boyle et al. 2006). Ventilated children may not be able to express their pain because:

• they are intubated;
• they are sedated (with or without pharmacological paralysis);
• they have neurological impairment.

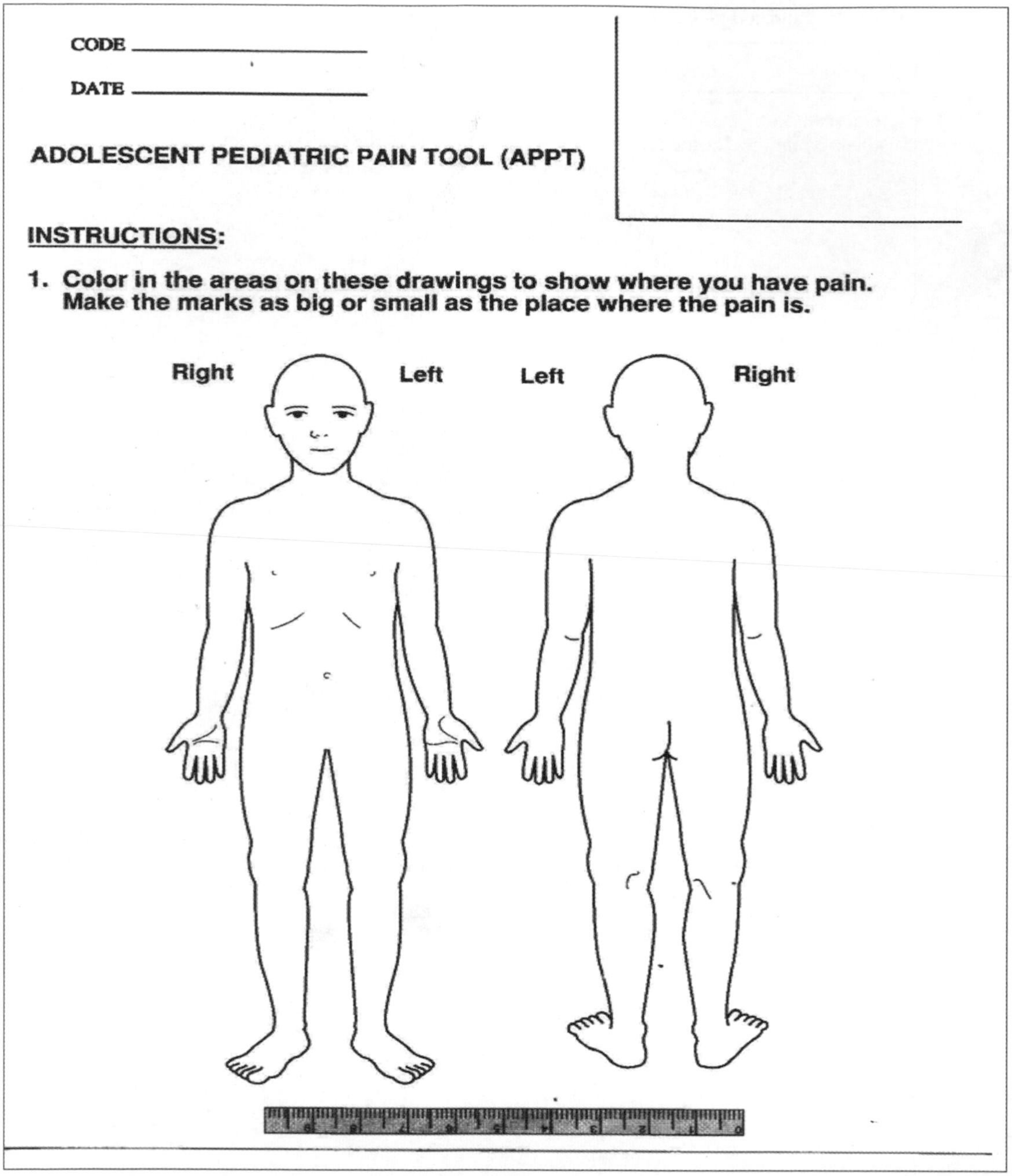

CODE _____

DATE _____

ADOLESCENT PEDIATRIC PAIN TOOL (APPT)

INSTRUCTIONS:

1. **Color in the areas on these drawings to show where you have pain. Make the marks as big or small as the place where the pain is.**

Right   Left   Left   Right

Figure 6.6   Body outline from Adolescent Pediatric Pain Tool (APPT). Permission to reproduce from M.C. Savedra, M.D. Tesler, W.L. Holzemer and J.A. Ward, University of California, San Francisco, School of Nursing, San Francisco, CA. Copyright © 1989, 1992.

Table 6.4 Validated behavioural tools

Measure	Indicators	Considerations
Children's Hospital of Eastern Ontario Pain Scale (CHEOPS) (McGrath et al. 1985)	Crying, facial expression, verbalisations, torso activity, whether and how child touches wound, leg position	Intended for use in children 1–7 years of age but has been used in children 4 months to 17 years Procedural and postoperative pain Indicators are scored on a four-point scale (0,1,2,3) Range of total scores is 4–13, but no indication of what mild, moderate or severe pain score ranges would be Well-established evidence of reliability, validity and ability to detect change (von Baeyer and Spagrud 2007) Length of tool and confusing scoring system makes it complicated to use in everyday clinical practice (low/medium clinical utility) Cannot be used in intubated or paralysed patients
COMFORT Scale (Ambuel et al. 1992)	Alertness, calmness or agitation, respiratory response, blood pressure, heart rate, muscle tone, physical movement, facial tension. Recently modified to include crying for non-ventilated infants (van Dijk et al. 2000)	Intended for use in children 0 to 17 years of age but has been used in children 0 to 18 years On ventilator or in critical care (only validated tool for this purpose) Well-established evidence of reliability and validity; however inconsistent ability to detect change (von Baeyer and Spagrud 2007) Score 8 items from 1–5 with total score ranging from 8 to 40 Administration time is about 3 minutes 2 hours for training to use tool (low/medium clinical utility)
FLACC (Merkel et al. 1997) (Table 6.5)	Facial expression, leg movement, activity, cry and consolability	Intended for use in children 2 months to 8 years of age but has been used in children 0–18 years Procedural and postoperative pain Each category is scored on a 0–2 scale, which results in a total score between 0 and 10 Well-established evidence of reliability and validity; however inconsistent ability to detect change (von Baeyer and Spagrud 2007) Simple to use, score and interpret (high clinical utility) Cannot be used in intubated or paralysed patients Important to note that consolability requires (a) an attempt to console, and (b) a subjective rating of response to that intervention, which complicates the scoring Limited use in disabled children with altered limb/leg movement

Table 6.5   FLACC behavioural scale

Categories	Scoring		
	0	**1**	**2**
Face	No particular expression or smile	Occasional grimace or frown, withdrawn, disinterested	Frequent to constant frown, clenched jaw, quivering chin
Legs	Normal position or relaxed	Uneasy, restless, tense	Kicking, or legs drawn up
Activity	Lying quietly, normal position, moves easily	Squirming, shifting back and forth, tense	Arched, rigid, or jerking
Cry	No cry (awake or asleep)	Moans or whimpers, occasional complaint	Crying steadily, screams or sobs, frequent complaints
Consolability	Content, relaxed	Reassured by occasional touching, hugging, or being talked to, distractible	Difficult to console or comfort

Each of the five categories (F) Face; (L) Legs; (A) Activity; (C) Cry; (C) Consolability is scored from 0–2, which results in a total score between 0 and 10.
Reproduced with permission. FLACC Behavioral Scale © 2002. The Regents of the University of Michigan. All Rights Reserved.

Other factors that add to the complexity of assessing pain in ventilated children include:

- difficulty differentiating pain from distress, anxiety and agitation;
- the child's age (e.g. limited range of behaviours in young infants; older children may be able to self-report);
- the severity of the child's illness may alter the physiological and behavioural responses that would normally be seen in healthy children.

The COMFORT scale is the only measure that has been validated for this purpose (see Table 6.4). However the major limitation of this tool is that it does not differentiate between pain and sedation (Ramelet et al. 2004).

For further information about behavioural tools see von Baeyer and Spagrud (2007).

6.5 Physiological Indicators

Neonates and children clearly display metabolic, hormonal and physiological responses to pain. These physiological reactions all indicate the activation of the sympathetic nervous system, which is part of the autonomic nervous system, and is responsible for the *fight or flight* response associated with stress (Sweet and McGrath 1998). These physiological changes should be recognised as:

- usually reflecting stress reactions;
- being only loosely correlated with self-report of pain;
- occurring in response to other states such as exertion, fever and anxiety (von Baeyer and Spagrud 2007).

Table 6.6 Physiological signs used to assess pain (adapted from Sweet and McGrath 1998)

Observation	Change indicating pain
Heart rate	Increases when in pain (after an initial decrease)
Respiratory rate and pattern.	There is conflicting evidence about whether this increases or decreases, but there is a significant shift from baseline. Breathing may become rapid and/or shallow.
Blood pressure	Increases when a child is in acute pain
Oxygen saturation	Decreases when a child is in acute pain

> On their own, physiological indicators do not constitute a valid clinical pain measure for children. A multidimensional or composite measure that incorporates physiological and behavioural indicators, as well as self-report is, therefore, preferred whenever possible (Franck et al. 2000; von Baeyer and Spagrud 2007).

Physiological parameters that can indicate that a child is in pain are outlined in Table 6.6. Other physiological indicators of pain include sweating and dilated pupils.

6.6 Pain Assessment Tools for Neonates

There are several pain assessment tools that combine behavioural and physiological indicators as well as contextual factors (e.g. gestational age, sleep/wake state) for assessing pain in neonates. These measures have varying degrees of established reliability and validity (Table 6.7). The Premature Infant Pain Profile (PIPP) (Stevens et al. 1996) has been the most rigorously validated of these measures (Figure 6.7).

Facial activity has been the most comprehensively studied behavioural pain assessment measure in neonates. It is the most reliable and consistent indicator of pain across populations and types of pain (Craig 1998). The facial actions associated with acute pain in neonates are identified in Box 6.3 and are portrayed in Figure 6.8.

BOX 6.3

Facial actions associated with acute pain in neonates

- Bulging brow
- Eyes squeezed tightly shut
- Deepening of nasolabial furrow
- Open lips
- Mouth stretched vertically and horizontally
- Taut tongue

Source: Craig (1998)

6.7 Pain Assessment in Cognitively Impaired Children

Infants and children with cognitive impairment or developmental delay who are unable to report pain may be at greater risk for undertreatment of pain (Box 6.4). These include children with cerebral palsy, neurodevelopmental disorders, severe developmental delay and children with pervasive developmental disorders. Pain experienced by these children is particularly difficult to assess accurately.

Infant ID Number: _____

Date:/Time: _____

Event: _____

PROCESS	INDICATOR	0	1	2	3	SCORE
Chart	Gestational age (at time of observation	36 weeks and more	32 weeks to 35 weeks, 6 days	28 weeks to 35 weeks, 6 days	Less than 28 weeks	
Observe infant 15 seconds before procedure Heart rate ___ Oxygen saturation ___	Behavioural state	Active/awake Eyes open Facial movements Crying (with eyes open or closed)	Quiet/awake Eyes open No facial movements	Active/sleep Eyes closed Facial movements	Quiet/sleep Eyes closed No facial movements	
Observe infant 30 seconds after procedure	Heart rate Max. ___	0 to 4 beats/minute increase	5 to 14 beats/minute increase	15 to 24 beats/minute increase	25 beats/minute or more increase	
	Oxygen saturation Min. ___	< 2% decrease	2% to 4% decrease	5% to 7% decrease	<7% or more decrease	
	Brow bulge	None	Minimum	Moderate	Maximum	
	Eye squeeze	None	Minimum	Moderate	Maximum	
	Nasolabial furrow	None	Minimum	Moderate	Maximum	
				Total score		

Figure 6.7   Premature Infant Pain Profile (PIPP). ©1996 Clinical Journal of Pain. Reproduced with permission.

Table 6.7   Some validated pain assessment tools for neonates

Measure	Indicators included	Considerations
CRIES (Crying, Requires O2 for saturation above 95, increased vital signs, expression, and sleeplessness) (Krechel and Bilder 1995)	Cry, oxygen saturation, heart rate/blood pressure, expression and sleeplessness	Full-term neonates (32–60 weeks gestational age) Postoperative pain measure Each indicator is rated on a three point scale (0,1,2) that results in a total score ranging from 0–10 Evidence of reliability and validity (Duhn and Medves 2004) and some evidence of ability to detect change Easy to remember and use (*high clinical utility*) Uses oxygenation as a measure, which can be affected by many other factors BP measurements may upset neonates
Neonatal Infant Pain Scale (NIPS) (Lawrence et al. 1993)	Facial expression, cry, breathing patterns, arms, legs, state of arousal	Preterm and term infants Procedural pain measure Operational definitions for indicators are provided Each indicator is scored on a two-point (0,1) or three-point (0,1,2) scale at 1-minute intervals, before, during, and following a procedure Evidence of reliability and validity (Duhn and Medves 2004) Hard to remember (*limited clinical utility*) Cannot be used in intubated or paralysed patients
Premature Infant Pain Profile (PIPP) (Stevens et al. 1996) (Figure 6.8)	Gestational age, behavioural state, heart rate and oxygen saturation, brow bulge, eye squeeze, and nasolabial furrow	Preterm and term infants (e.g. 28–40 weeks gestation) Initially developed for procedural pain, requires further evaluation with very low birth weight neonates and with non-acute and post-surgical pain populations Includes contextual indicators (e.g. gestational age and behavioural state) Each indicator is evaluated on a four-point scale (0,1,2,3) for a possible total score of 18–21 based on the gestational age of the infant Total score of 6 or less generally indicates minimal or no pain, while scores greater than 12 indicate moderate to severe pain Most rigorously evaluated tool; evidence of reliability, validity and ability to detect change Pain assessments take 1 minute (*high clinical utility*)

PIPP Training CD-ROM (approximately 20 minutes for training) available from: Dr. Sharyn Gibbins at sharyn.gibbons@sunnybrook.ca (Gibbins et al. 2007)

BOX 6.4

Reasons for increased risk of undertreatment of pain in cognitively impaired children

- Multiple medical problems may cause or be a source of pain
- Undergo multiple procedures that are often painful
- Idiosyncratic behaviours, such as moaning or laughing, may mask expression of pain
- Many pain behaviours, such as changes in facial expression and patterns of sleep or play, are already inconsistent and difficult to interpret because of physical problems
- Comfort of these children may be valued less by society

Source: McGrath (1998)

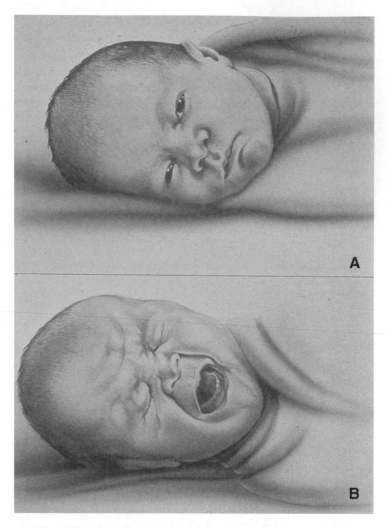

Figure 6.8   Neonatal pain facial expression. Facial behaviour in infant in quiet wake state prior to heel rub and the reaction to heel-lance. From Pain, 1987; 28: 395–410. Used with permission from IASP ©1987. International Association for the Study of Pain.

While these children are generally unable to report pain, credible assessment can usually be obtained from the parent or another person who knows the child well (Breau et al. 2002; Hunt et al. 2004, 2007). However, proxy judgements have been shown to underestimate the pain experience of others (Chambers and Craig 1998; St. Laurent-Gagnon et al. 1999; Kelly et al. 2002).

Factors to consider in the assessment of pain in children with a significant cognitive impairment include:

- underlying neurological condition/process;
- developmental level (e.g. cognition, communication, motor function);
- usual behaviour and health condition (e.g. baseline condition);
- usual means of communication (e.g. verbal, non-verbal);
- caregiver's views;
- impact of concurrent illnesses;
- differential diagnosis (e.g. consider all sources of distress and pain) (Oberlander et al. 1999).

Behavioural cues used to identify pain in cognitively impaired children

- Facial expression
- Vocalizations (e.g. moaning)
- Changes in posture and movements
- Physiological changes (such as, sweating, pallor or flushing)
- Alterations in sleeping and eating
- Change in mood and sociability

Source: McGrath et al. (1998); Fanurik et al. (1999)

Parents and caregivers tend to report a diversity of behavioural responses to pain but the categories outlined above are common to almost all children and provide cues to caregivers that their child might be experiencing pain. This underlines the importance of obtaining a thorough baseline history from caregivers of children with cognitive impairments.

While there are several pain assessment tools for this population, the most well-validated measure is the Non-Communicating Children's Pain Checklist – Revised (NCCPC-R) (Breau et al. 2002, Figure 6.9). The Paediatric Pain Profile has also been developed for use with this group of children (Hunt et al. 2004, 2007) (see http://www.ppprofile.org.uk/).

For further information about the assessment of pain in cognitively impaired children see Oberlander and Symons (2006).

6.8 Choosing the Right Pain Assessment Measure

There is an abundance of reliable, valid and clinically useful pain assessment tools for assessing pain in neonates, infants, children and adolescents (Duhn and Medves 2004; Stinson et al. 2006; von Baeyer and Spragrud 2007). However, no easily administered, widely accepted, uniform technique exists for assessing pain for **all** children (Franck et al. 2000; Stinson et al. 2006; Von Baeyer and Spagrud, 2007). Box 6.5 identifies some of the factors that need considering when selecting a pain tool for use in everyday practice.

Within the hospital setting it will probably be necessary to have more than one pain assessment tool to cater for all patient groups.

Each pain assessment tool should, whenever possible, use a **common metric** – e.g. all rate pain from 0–10 or 0–5.

This means that a pain score of 5 will mean the same whichever pain assessment tool you are using and will thus aid effective communication about each child's pain.

For more information about why a common metric is important see Hicks et al. (2001).

The key points to consider when choosing a pain assessment tool are outlined in Box 6.6.

0 = NOT AT ALL	1 = JUSTA LITTLE	2 = FAIRLYOFTEN	3 = VERYOFTEN		NA = NOT APPLICABLE

I. Vocal

v1. Moaning, whining, whimpering (fairly soft)...	0	1	2	3	NA
2. Crying (moderately loud)..	0	1	2	3	NA
3. Screaming/yelling (very loud)...	0	1	2	3	NA
4. Aspecific sound or word for pain (e.g. a word, cry or type of laugh)....................	0	1	2	3	NA

II. Social

5. Not cooperating, cranky, irritable, unhappy..	0	1	2	3	NA
6. Less interaction with others, withdrawn...	0	1	2	3	NA
7. Seeking comfort or physical closeness	0	1	2	3	NA
8. Being difficult to distract, not able to satisfy or pacify...........................	0	1	2	3	NA

III. Facial

9.　Afurrowed brow..	0	1	2	3	NA
10. A change in eyes, including: squinching of eyes, eyes opened wide, eyes frowning	0	1	2	3	NA
11. Turning down of mouth, not smiling	0	1	2	3	NA
12. Lips puckering up, tight, pouting, or quivering....................................	0	1	2	3	NA
13. Clenching or grinding teeth, chewing or thrusting tongue out	0	1	2	3	NA

IV. Activity

14. Not moving, less active, quiet...	0	1	2	3	NA
15. Jumping around, agitated, fidgety..	0	1	2	3	NA

V. Body and Limbs

16. Floppy	0	1	2	3	NA
17. Stiff, spastic, tense, rigid	0	1	2	3	NA
18. Gesturing to or touching part of the body that hurts	0	1	2	3	NA
19. Protecting, favoring or guarding part of the body that hurts	0	1	2	3	NA
20. Flinching or moving the body part away, being sensitive to touch...................	0	1	2	3	NA
21. Moving the body in a specific way to show pain (e.g. head back, arms down, curls up, etc.)	0	1	2	3	NA

VI. Physiological

22. Shivering	0	1	2	3	NA
23. Change in color, pallor	0	1	2	3	NA
24. Sweating, perspiring	0	1	2	3	NA
25. Tears...	0	1	2	3	NA
26. Sharp intake of breath, gasping..	0	1	2	3	NA
27. Breath holding..	0	1	2	3	NA

VII. Eating/Sleeping

28. Eating less, not interested in food...	0	1	2	3	NA
29. Increase in sleep...	0	1	2	3	NA
30. Decrease in sleep..	0	1	2	3	NA

SCORE SUMMARY:

Category:	I	II	III	IV	V	VI	VII	TOTAL
Score:								

Figure 6.9　Non-Communicating Children's Pain Checklist – Revised (NCCPC-R). Reproduced with permission from Dr Lynn Breau. Version 01.2004 © 2004 Lynn Breau, Patrick McGrath, Allen Finley, Carol Camfield.

6.9 How Often Should Pain be Assessed?

Effective pain management depends on regular assessment of the presence and severity of pain and the patient's response to pain management interventions. Every patient should have their pain assessed:

- on admission to hospital;
- when they visit an emergency department or an ambulatory clinic;

> **BOX 6.5**
>
> **Choosing a pain assessment tool for everyday use**
>
> The tool needs to be:
>
> - *reliable* (e.g. consistent and trustworthy ratings regardless of time, setting or who is administering measure);
> - *valid* (e.g. unequivocally measures a specific dimension of pain);
> - *responsive* (e.g. able to detect change in pain due to treatment);
> - *feasible* to use (e.g. simple to use and not long, short training time, easy to administer and score);
> - *practical* (e.g. for assessing different types of pain).
>
> The tool should also be:
>
> - developmentally and culturally appropriate for the client group;
> - easily and quickly understood by patients;
> - well liked by patients, clinicians and researchers;
> - inexpensive and easy to obtain, reproduce, distribute and disinfect;
> - available in various languages or easily translatable.
>
> *Source:* Hester et al. (1998); McCaffery and Pasero (1999); Twycross and Shields (2005); Von Baeyer (2006); McGrath (2007)

- at least once per shift (if they are an inpatient);
- before, during and after an invasive procedure.

Pain should be assessed very regularly following surgery and/or if the patient has a known painful medical condition. Pain should be assessed hourly for the first six hours. After this, if the pain is well controlled, it can be assessed less frequently (e.g. every four hours). If the pain is fluctuating, regular assessment should continue for 48–72 hours; after this the pain intensity will normally have peaked and be starting to subside. (The management of acute pain is discussed in more detail in Chapter 7.)

6.9.1 Documentation

Regular assessment and documentation facilitates effective treatment and communication among members of the healthcare team, patient and family. Pain is considered to be the *fifth vital sign* and, therefore, should be assessed and documented along with the other vital signs. Putting mechanisms in place that make documentation of pain easy for clinicians helps ensure consistent documentation. Standardised forms/tools for the

> **BOX 6.6**
>
> **Key points to consider when choosing a pain assessment tool**
>
> - Selection of the right instrument will depend on the child's condition, age, ethnic background, and the child's cognitive/developmental level
> - Careful explanation and appropriate timing of administration are necessary
> - It is helpful for children to have an opportunity to practise using the tool before pain is expected, e.g. in a surgical pre-admission programme
> - Offer the child a chance to practise using the scale by having them rate hypothetical situations that would produce low (e.g. paper cut) and high levels of pain (e.g. stepping on a nail)
>
> *Source:* McCaffery and Pasero (1999); Von Baeyer (2006)

documentation of pain allow for the initial assessment and ongoing re-assessment (e.g. admission assessment forms, vital signs chart). They can also be used for the documentation of the efficacy of pain-relieving interventions. Including pain intensity as part of the vital signs record allows for pain to be assessed, documented and taken as seriously as other vital signs.

Summary

- Pain assessment is vital for effective pain management.
- The first step in assessing pain is recording a pain history.
- The second step in pain assessment is assessing the child's pain using a developmentally appropriate pain assessment tool.
- The third step is evaluating the effectiveness of the pain-relieving interventions implemented.
- Validated and reliable pain assessment tools are available for children of all ages.
- The child's self-report of pain is considered the *gold standard*.
- Physiological, behavioural and self-report indicators can all be used to assess children's pain.
- Pain should be assessed regularly to detect for the presence of pain and to evaluate the effectiveness of treatments.
- Documentation of pain facilitates regular reassessment of pain and follow-up.

Useful web resources

Great Ormond Street Hospital for Children NHS Trust (GOSH) and UCL Institute of Child Health (ICH): http://www.ich.ucl.ac.uk/gosh/clinicalservices/Pain_control_service/Custom%20Menu_02 (Provides information on RCN pain assessment guidelines and recommended pain assessment tools in children.)

Partners Against Pain: http://www.partnersagainstpain.com/index-mp.aspx?sid=3 (Provides printable PDFs of commonly used paediatric pain scales.)

Ped-IMMPACT: http://www.immpact.org/meetings.html (Recommendations for the design, execution and interpretation of paediatric pain clinical trials including PDFs of systematic reviews of self-report and observational pain tools for 3–18 years.)

References

Abu-Saad, H.H., Kroonen, E. and Halfens, R. (1990) On the development of a multidimensional Dutch pain assessment tool for children, *Pain*, 43(2): 249–256.

Acute Pain Management Guideline Panel (1992) *Acute pain management in infants, children, and adolescents: operative and medical procedures. Quick reference guide for clinicians*, AHCPR, Pub. No. 92-0020, Rockville, Md., Agency for Health Care Policy and Research, Public Health Service, U.S. Dept. of Health and Human Services.

Ambuel, B., Hamlett, K.W., Marx, C.M. and Blumer, J.L. (1992) Assessing distress in pediatric intensive care environments: the COMFORT scale, *Journal of Pediatric Psychology*, 17: 95–109.

American Academy of Pediatrics and American Pain Society (2001) The assessment and management of acute pain in infants, children and adolescents, *Pediatrics*, 108(3): 793–797.

Ball, J. and Bindler, R. (1995) Pain assessment and management. In Ball, J. and Bindler, R. (eds.) *Pediatric Nursing: Caring for Children*, Appleton & Lange, Connecticut, p. 183.

Beyer, J.E. (1984) *The Oucher: A User's Manual and Technical Report*, Hospital Play Equipment, Evanston, Illinois.

Boyle, E.M., Freer, Y., Wong, C.M., McIntosh, N. and Anand, K.J.S. (2006) Assessment of persistent pain or distress and adequacy of analgesia in preterm ventilated infants, *Pain*, 124: 87–91.

Breau, L.M., McGrath, P.J., Camfield, C. and Finley, G.A. (2002) Psychometric properties of the Non-communicating Children's Pain Checklist – Revised, *Pain*, 99: 349–357.

Chambers, C.T. and Craig, K.D. (1998) An intrusive impact of anchors in children's faces pain scales, *Pain*, 78(1): 27–37.

Chambers, C., Hardial, J., Craig, K., Court, C. and Montgomery, C. (2005) Faces scales for the measurement of postoperative pain intensity in children following minor surgery, *Clinical Journal of Pain*, 21(3): 277–285.

Champion, G.D., Goodenough, B., von Baeyer, C.L. and Thomas, W. (1998) Measurement of pain by self-report. In Finley, G.A. and McGrath, P.J. (eds.) *Measurement of Pain in Infants and Children: Progress in Pain Research and Management*, Vol. 10, IASP Press, Seattle, pp. 123–160.

Craig, K.D. (1998) The facial display of pain in infants and children. In Finley, GA, McGrath, PJ (eds.) *Measurement of Pain in Infants and Children: Progress in Pain Research and Management*, Vol. 10, IASP Press, Seattle, pp. 103–121.

Duhn, L.J. and Medves, J.M. (2004) A systematic integrative review of infant pain assessment tools, *Advances in Neonatal care*, 4(3): 126–140.

Fanurik, D., Koh, J.L., Schmitz, M.L., Harrison, R.D. and Conrad, T.M. (1999) Children with cognitive impairment: parent report of pain and coping, *Developmental and Behavioral Pediatrics*, 20(4): 228–234.

Franck, L.S., Greenberg, C.S. and Stevens, B. (2000) Pain assessment in infants and children, *Pediatric Clinics of North America*, 47(3): 487–512.

Gibbins S., Maddalena P., Yamada, J. and Stevens, B. (2007) Testing the satisfaction and feasibility of a computer-based teaching module in the neonatal intensive care unit, *Advanced Neonatal Care*, 7(1): 43–49.

Goodenough, B., Thomas, W., Champion, G., McInerney, M., Young, B., Juniper K. and Ziegler, J.B. (1997) Pain in 4 to 6 year-old children receiving intramuscular injections: a comparison of the faces pain scale with Oucher self-report and behavioural measures, *Clinical Journal of Pain*, 13(1): 60–73.

Hester, N. (1979) The preoperational child's reaction to immunization, *Nursing Research*, 28(4): 250–255.

Hester, N.O. and Barcus, C.S. (1986) Assessment and management of pain in children, Pediatrics, *Nursing Update*, 1(14): 1–8.

Hester, N.O., Foster, R.L., Jordan-Marsh, M. Ely, E., Vojir, C.P. and Miller, K.L. (1998) Putting pain measurement into clinical practice. In Finley, G.A. and McGrath, P.J. (eds.) *Measurement of Pain in Infants and Children: Progress in Pain Research and Management*, Vol. 10, IASP Press, Seattle, pp. 179–198.

Hicks, C.L., von Baeyer, C.L., Spafford, P.A., van Korlaar, I. and Goodenough B. (2001) The Faces Pain Scale – Revised: toward a common metric in pediatric pain measurement, *Pain*, 93: 173–183.

Hunt, A., Goldman, A., Seers, K., Crichton, N., Mastroyannopoulou, K., Moffat, V., Oulton, K. and Brady, M. (2004) Clinical validation of the paediatric pain profile, *Developmental Medicine and Child Neurology*, 46(1): 9–18.

Hunt, A., Wisbeach, A., Seers, K., Goldman, A., Crichton, N., Perry, L. and Mastroyannopoulou, K. (2007) Development of the paediatric pain profile: role of video analysis and saliva cortisol in validating a tool to assess pain in children with severe neurological disability, *Journal of Pain and Symptom Management*, 33(3): 276–289.

Johnston, C. (1998) Psychometric issues in the measurement of pain. In Finley, G.A. and McGrath, P.J. (eds.) *Measurement of Pain in Infants and Children: Progress in Pain Research Management*, Vol. 10, IASP Press, Seattle, pp. 5–20.

Kelly, A.M., Powell, C.V. and Williams, A. (2002) Parent visual analogue scale ratings of children's pain do not reliably reflect pain reported by child, *Pediatric Emergency Care*, 18(3): 159–162.

Krechel, S.W. and Bildner, J. (1995) CRIES: a new neonatal postoperative pain measurement score. Initial testing of validity and reliability, *Pediatric Anesthesia*, 5: 53–61.

Lawrence, J., Alcock, D., McGrath, P., Kay, J., MacMurray, S.B. and Dulberg, C. (1993) The development of a tool to assess neonatal pain, *Neonatal Network*, 12: 59–66.

McCaffery, M. and Pasero, C. (1999) *Pain: Clinical Manual*, 2nd edition, Mosby, St Louis.

McGrath, P.A. (2007) Pain assessment in children. In R.F. Schmidt and W.D. Willis (eds.) *Encyclopedia of Pain*, pp. 1645–1648. Springer-Verlag, Berlin, Heidelberg, New York.

McGrath, P.A., Seifert, C., Speechley, K., Booth, J., Stitt, L. and Gibson, M. (1996) A new analogue scale for assessing children's pain: an initial validation study, *Pain*, 64: 435–443.

McGrath, P.J. (1998) Behavioral measures of pain. In Finley, G.A. and McGrath, P.J. (eds.) *Measurement of Pain in Infants and Children: Progress in Pain Research Management*, Vol. 10, IASP Press, Seattle, 83 –102.

McGrath, P.J., Johnson, G., Goodman, J.T., Schillinger, J., Dunn, J. and Chapman, J. (1985) CHEOPS: a behavioral scale for rating postoperative pain in children. In Fields, H.L., Dubner, R. and Cervero. F. (eds.) *Proceedings of the Fourth World Congress on Pain: Advances in Pain Research and Therapy*, Vol. 9, Raven Press, New York, pp. 395–401.

McGrath, P.J., Rosmus, C., Campbell, M.A. and Hennigar, A. (1998) Behaviours caregivers use to determine pain in non-verbal, cognitively impaired individuals, *Developmental Medicine and Child Neurology*, 40: 340–343.

Merkel, S.I., Voepel-Lewis, T., Shayevitz, J.R. and Malviya, S. (1997) The FLACC: a behavioral scale for scoring postoperative pain in young children, *Pediatric Nursing*, 23(3): 292–297.

Oberlander, T.F., and Symons, F. (2006) *Pain in Children and Adults with Developmental Disabilities*, Paul H. Brookes Publishing Company, Baltimore.

Oberlander, T.F, O'Donnell, M.E. and Montgomery, C.J. (1999) Pain in children with significant neuro-logical impairment, *Developmental and Behavioral Pediatrics*, 20(4): 235–243.

Palermo, T., Valenzuela, D. and Stork, P. (2004) A randomized trial of electronic versus paper pain dia-ries in children: impact on compliance, accuracy, and acceptability, *Pain*, 107: 213–219.

Ramelet, A, Abu-Saad, H.H., Rees, N. and McDonald, S. (2004) The challenges of pain measurement in critically ill young children: a comprehensive review, *Australian Critical Care*, 17(1): 33–45.

Savedra, M.C., Tesler, M.D., Holzemer, W.L. and Ward, J.A. (1989) *Adolescent Pediatric Pain Tool (APPT): Preliminary User's Manual*, University of California, San Francisco, School of Nursing, San Francisco, CA.

Stevens, B., Johnston, C., Petryshen, P. and Taddio, A. (1996) Premature Infant Pain Profile: develop-ment and initial validation, *Clinical Journal of Pain*, 12: 13–22.

Stinson, J., Yamada, J., Kavanagh, T., Gill, N. and Stevens, B. (2006) Systematic review of the psy-chometric properties and feasibility of self-report pain measures for use in clinical trials in children and adolescents, *Pain*, 125(1–2): 143–157.

Stinson, J., Stevens, J., Feldman, B., Streiner, D., McGrath, P., Dupuis, A., Gill, N. and Petroz, G. (2008) Construct validity of a multidimensional electronic pain diary for adolescents with arthritis. *Pain*, 136(3): 281–292.

St. Laurent-Gagnon, T., Bernard-Bonnin, A.C. and Villeneuve, E. (1999) Pain evaluation in preschool children and by their parents, *Acta Paediatrica*, 88(4): 422–427.

Sweet, S.D. and McGrath, P.J. (1998) Physiological measures of pain. In G.A. Finley and P.J. McGrath (eds.) *Measurement of Pain in Infants and Children: Progress in Pain Research Management*, Vol. 10, IASP Press, Seattle, pp. 59–81.

Twycross, A. and Shields, L. (2005) Reliability and validity in practice: assessment tools, *Paediatric Nursing*, 17(9): 43.

van Dijk, N., de Boer, J.B., Koot, H.M., Tibboel, D., Passchier, J. and Duivenvoorden, H.J. (2000) The reliability and validity of the COMFORT scale as a postoperative pain instrument in 0 to 3-year-old infants, *Pain*, 84: 367–377.

Varni, J.W., Thompson, K.L. and Hanson, V. (1987) The Varni/Thompson Pediatric Pain Questionnaire: I. Chronic musculoskeletal pain in juvenile rheumatoid arthritis, *Pain*, 28: 27–38.

von Baeyer, C.L. (2006) Children's self-reports of pain intensity: scale selection, limitations and interpre-tation, *Pain Research and Management*, 11(3): 157–162.

von Baeyer, C.L. and Spagrud, L.J. (2007) Systematic review of observational (behavioural) measures for children and adolescents aged 3 to 18 years, *Pain*, 127: 140–150.

Wong, D.L. and Baker, C.M. (1988) Pain in children: comparison of assessment scales, *Pediatric Nursing*, 14(1): 9–17.

CHAPTER 7

Managing Acute Pain in Children

Stephanie J. Dowden

Introduction

Children continue to experience moderate to severe unrelieved pain postoperatively (Polkki et al. 2003; Vincent and Denyes 2004; Johnston et al. 2005) despite the evidence to guide practice being readily available. This chapter will discuss the causes and experience of acute pain in childhood. Pharmacological and non-drug strategies for managing acute pain in both hospital and community settings will be reviewed. The management of procedural pain is discussed in Chapter 10. Details about the pharmacology and doses of analgesic drugs are discussed in Chapter 4. However, some specific modalities used in hospital settings (e.g. intravenous opioid infusions and regional anaesthesia techniques) will be discussed in detail in this chapter. Information about dosing regimes and guidance about best-practice clinical management will also be provided.

7.1 What is Acute Pain?

Acute pain by definition is short-lived, lasting hours, days or weeks. It is usually of recent onset and has a defined course with a direct causal relationship to a disease, injury or medical procedure (Ready and Edwards 1992). Acute pain usually resolves completely as healing takes place. Pain lasting over three months is classified as chronic or persistent; however, it is likely that acute pain and chronic pain are on a continuum, rather than being separate entities (Australian and New Zealand College of Anaesthetists and Faculty of Pain Medicine [ANZCA] 2005). (See Chapter 2 for further information about the mechanism of pain and Chapter 8 for a detailed discussion about chronic pain.)

7.2 Causes of Acute Pain in Childhood

There are a number of causes of acute pain in childhood, ranging from common to rare. The most common acute pain is the day-to-day pain caused by minor trauma – scrapes, bruises and grazes that occur during normal play and activity. The majority of these pains require little more than a band-aid, an ice pack, a hug and reassurance. For moderate acute pain episodes, children may require interventions from their family doctor, school nurse or community healthcare professional. These pains are generally easily managed with simple analgesic drugs and non-drug interventions. Severe acute pain episodes are likely to require treatment in the hospital setting and need stronger analgesic drugs and non-drug interventions to achieve pain control. (See Chapter 4 for further information on

Table 7.1   Causes of acute pain

Cause	Examples
Childhood illnesses (see also Chapter 8)	Earache (otalgia), pharyngitis, headache, abdominal pain, musculoskeletal pain, dental caries
Trauma	Soft tissue injuries, lacerations, fractures, burns
Surgery	Postoperative pain and complications of surgery
Medical conditions	Sickle-cell disease, haemophilia, renal colic, pancreatitis, Crohn's disease, ulcerative colitis, osteogenesis imperfecta
Cancer (see also Chapters 8 & 9)	Disease process, cancer treatment, mucositis, bone pain, neuropathies
Medical procedures (see also Chapter 10)	Blood tests, insertion of intravenous cannulae, wound dressings, immunisations, lumbar puncture, bone marrow aspiration
Acute exacerbation of chronic pain (see also Chapters 8 and 9)	Migraine, arthritis, oesophagitis, gastritis

Source: Schechter (2006)

the pharmacology of analgesic drugs and Chapter 5 for a review of the non-drug methods.) Causes of acute pain are identified in Table 7.1 and will be discussed further below.

7.2.1 Childhood illnesses and minor trauma

The commonest reasons for children presenting to family doctors with acute pain are otalgia (from otitis media), pharyngitis and minor trauma (Schechter 2006). Presentations for acute pain to school nurses are primarily for adolescent-specific conditions (e.g. menstrual pain, minor musculoskeletal trauma, headaches and abdominal pain). More serious causes of acute pain may initially present to family doctors or school nurses, prior to referral to hospital for further management or may be followed up in the community following discharge from hospital.

7.2.2 Medical conditions

Sickle cell disease (SCD) is a significant medical cause of acute pain in childhood. A UK cohort study ($n = 253$) found sickle cell crisis was the commonest clinical event with SCD, reaching a peak incidence in early adolescence (Telfer et al. 2007). In between these acutely painful episodes (unlike with many other medical conditions) the majority of patients are well with minimal pain. Most other medical causes of acute pain in childhood (e.g. arthritis, systemic lupus erythematosus, haemophilia, inflammatory bowel disease or epidermolysis bullosa) have combined acute and chronic pain components, which consist of acute pain episodes on a background of chronic pain (McClain 2006).

Children with cancer experience significant acute pain. Acute cancer pain may be caused by the disease process, medical and surgical treatment or medical procedures undertaken for investigations (WHO 1998). Like other medical causes of acute pain there can be combined chronic and acute pain components.

Children with developmental disabilities (such as Down syndrome, cerebral palsy and autism) are a particular group with very high prevalence rates (75–85%) of pain (Oberlander and Symons 2006). They experience acute pain from multiple sources (Table 7.2) as well as chronic pain due to their underlying condition, which is compounded further by their cognitive impairment and communication difficulties (Oberlander and Symons 2006). This group of children often have their pain unrecognised and consequentially undertreated.

Table 7.2 Pain in children with developmental disabilities

Cause	Example
Assistive devices	Pressure areas or rubbing from orthotics, splints, prostheses
Surgery	Scoliosis surgery, femoral osteotomy, tendon transfers, release of muscle contractures
Oral health	Periodontal disease, dental caries, temporomandibular pain
Drug toxicity	Adverse effects of medications, especially anticonvulsants, e.g. pancreatitis, mucositis, neuropathies
Gastrointestinal disorders	Gastro-oesphageal reflux, gastritis, oesophagitis, mucositis, constipation, gastric feeding tube problems
Musculoskeletal	Hip dislocation, spasticity, muscle spasm, positioning difficulties, immobility, joint problems
Childhood illnesses	Late recognition/presentation of childhood illnesses with consequential increased pain, illness severity and complications

Source: Oberlander and Symons (2006)

7.2.3 Trauma

Trauma is the most common cause of acute pain in school-aged children. It is primarily dealt with by emergency medical responders and in hospitals, although some children may initially be managed by family doctors and school nurses.

7.2.4 Surgery/medical investigations

Surgical procedures and medical investigations are the most common reasons for hospitalised children to experience acute pain.

7.3 Pain Assessment

Pain assessment is discussed in detail in Chapter 6. However, it is important to emphasise that for the child in acute pain a thorough assessment is essential to determine the most appropriate intervention. Acute medical pain is perhaps the most difficult to assess as it can present in a range of ways and is often the result of a significant exacerbation of a chronic health condition (e.g. acute abdominal pain with Crohn's disease or a joint bleed with haemophilia). The acute pain associated with these conditions can cause considerable suffering and distress; added to this is the complexity of assessing acute pain episodes in children and adolescents with underlying chronic pain. If the child also has a developmental disability this adds to the difficulty of pain assessment.

Acute pain following trauma and/or surgery is primarily due to tissue damage. However, several other factors may contribute, particularly in the immediate postoperative or postinjury phase. All possible sources of pain and discomfort should be considered including haemorrhage and haematoma, compartment syndrome, pain from blocked catheters or drains, bladder spasms, intravenous cannulae, muscle spasms, nausea and itching. Each of these requires different interventions.

7.4 Non-drug Methods of Pain Relief

Non-drug methods of pain relief are discussed in detail in Chapter 5. Methods that have been shown to be most effective to manage acute pain in children are outlined in Figure 7.1.

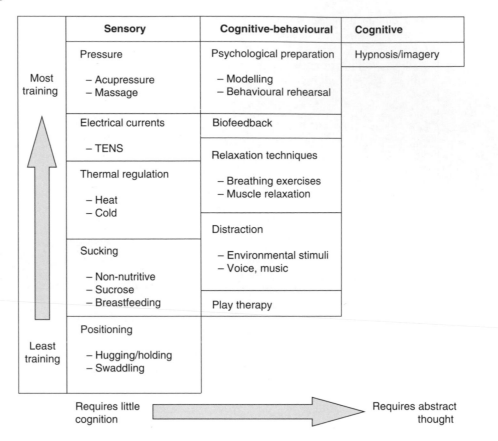

Figure 7.1   Non-drug methods of pain relief for acute pain management (adapted from Vessey and Carlson 1996).

7.5 Analgesic Drug Interventions

7.5.1 WHO analgesic ladder

The World Health Organization (WHO) analgesic ladder (WHO 1996), discussed in Chapter 4, offers a stepwise approach to pain management (Box 7.1) that suggests as pain increases or decreases the analgesic drugs being administered should be adjusted

---

BOX 7.1

Stepwise approach to pain management

Step 1 (mild pain)

• Administer a non-opioid, e.g. paracetamol and/or NSAID (e.g. ibuprofen or diclofenac).

Step 2 (moderate pain)

• Continue step 1 medications and add a simple opioid (e.g. codeine or dihydrocodeine).

Step 3 (severe pain)

• Continue step 1 and 2 medications and add strong opioid (e.g. morphine or fentanyl or hydromorphone or oxycodone or diamorphine).
• Consider the addition of regional anaesthesia (e.g. epidural or nerve block).

Adjuvant analgesics may be added at any step according to the type and quality of the pain.

accordingly. As acute pain is short-lived, once the initial acute pain is controlled, a step-down, rather than a step-up approach should be used, as the pain should diminish over several hours or days. If the pain does not lessen as expected this may indicate possible complications or an alternative diagnosis that needs to be investigated. Pain problem-solving will be discussed later in this chapter.

7.5.2 Pain management in the community setting

Most minor pains of childhood are managed by parents in the home, using non-drug methods or over-the-counter analgesic drugs (step 1 medications). Moderate pain that might necessitate a visit to the family doctor or school nurse can be well controlled with step 1 or step 2 medications and/or the use of local anaesthetics in the majority of situations.

7.5.3 Pain management in the hospital setting

Within the hospital, pain may be minor, moderate or severe and all steps of the analgesia ladder may be required to manage the pain.

7.5.4 Research evidence for analgesics in acute pain

Despite the small number of medications licensed for use in children (see Chapter 4) there is a good research base demonstrating the efficacy and acceptability for their use in the treatment of acute pain in children.

Non-opioids

Paracetamol and non-steroidal anti-inflammatory drugs (NSAIDs) provide effective analgesia for minor childhood conditions and after minor surgery, have an opioid-sparing effect after major surgery, and cause less nausea and vomiting than opioids:

- In a randomised controlled trial comparing 8-hourly doses of ibuprofen or paracetamol or placebo to treat children ($n = 219$) with otitis media pain, ibuprofen was more effective than paracetamol and significantly more effective than placebo (Bertin et al. 1996).
- In a recent study with children ($n = 201$), ibuprofen and paracetamol or ibuprofen alone was more effective than paracetamol alone for pain immediately following dental surgery (Gazal and Mackie 2007).
- In a study involving children ($n = 120$), intra-operative ketorolac was as effective as morphine, but produced less postoperative vomiting following dental surgery (Purday et al. 1996).
- In a study including children ($n = 50$), rectal diclofenac was as effective as morphine, but caused significantly less nausea and vomiting following squint surgery (Wennström and Reinsfelt 2002).
- The use of simple analgesics has also been shown to reduce the need for opioids following tonsillectomy (Oztekin et al. 2002; Pickering et al. 2002), minor orthopaedic surgery (Hiller et al. 2006) and thoracic surgery (Aydin et al. 2007).
- When used in combination with other analgesic drugs (multimodal analgesia) NSAIDs decrease opioid consumption by 30–40% (Morton and O'Brien 1999; Pickering et al. 2002; Viitanen et al. 2003) and improve analgesia quality (Morton and O'Brien 1999).

Local anaesthetics

Local anaesthetics can be administered as single doses topically or infiltrated into the area of surgery or injury:

- In a study of children ($n = 54$) with otitis media who had received paracetamol a topical otic (ear) preparation containing antipryine, benzocaine and glycerin (Auralgan®) was found to be more effective than olive oil drops (a common home remedy) in reducing otalgia 30 minutes following installation in the ear canal (Hoberman et al. 1997).

- A Cochrane review of 33 studies which included children ($n = 1984$) found dorsal penile nerve block to be the most effective intervention for neonatal circumcision. EMLA® was also effective, but not as effective as the nerve block (Brady-Fryer et al. 2004).
- Local anaesthetic infiltration prior to tonsillectomy was found to reduce pain and analgesic requirement postoperatively in children ($n = 90$) (Naja et al. 2005).
- The topical preparations EMLA® and amethocaine (tetracaine) 4% gel or cream are comparable in efficacy for procedural pain management in children, but EMLA® requires a longer application time (Murat et al. 2003).

Local anaesthetics for regional anaesthesia   Local anaesthetics, with or without opioids or other adjuvant analgesics (such as clonidine and ketamine), can also be administered via caudal epidural, epidural or peripheral nerve blocks during and following surgery:

- In a study involving children ($n = 99$) having sub-umbilical surgery, intra-operative caudal levobupivacaine, bupivacaine and ropivacaine provided similar analgesic efficacy, but bupivacaine produced a longer motor block and longer analgesic action postoperatively (Locatelli et al. 2005).
- A systematic review of 17 randomised controlled trials (RCTs) found clonidine caused consistent prolonging of analgesia when added to caudal local anaesthetic blocks (Ansermino et al. 2003).
- Addition of clonidine or ketamine to caudal local anaesthetic infusions improved analgesia compared to local anaesthetic alone for children ($n = 60$) (De Negri et al. 2001).
- The addition of opioids to epidurals has been challenged, as the increased risk of opioid-related adverse effects combined with an insignificant increase in analgesia compared to local anaesthetic alone suggests alternate analgesics (such as clonidine or ketamine) may offer better outcomes (Lönnqvist et al. 2002).

Opioids
- Borland et al. (2007) in a RCT compared the efficacy of intranasal fentanyl with intravenous morphine for children ($n = 67$) with long-bone fractures. There were no serious adverse events and both drugs provided comparable analgesia.
- Kokki et al. (2006) compared buccal (into the cheek) versus sublingual administration of oxycodone in children ($n = 30$) undergoing surgery and found absorption was similar for either route of instillation.
- Neonates and infants are more sensitive to morphine than older children; however, individual variation is significant, which means doses should be calculated by age, weight and clinical status, then titrated to effect (Bouwmeester et al. 2003).

Tramadol
- Tramadol was more effective than paracetamol alone (Pendeville et al. 2000) and equally as effective as morphine (Engelhardt et al. 2002) following minor surgery.

7.6 Pain Management Guidelines

A detailed list of pain management guidelines are provided in Chapter 1. Several guidelines specific to acute pain management are outlined in Box 7.2.

BOX 7.2

Guidelines relating to acute pain management

Australian and New Zealand College of Anaesthetists and Faculty of Pain Medicine (2007) *Acute Pain Management: Scientific Evidence*, Updated 2nd edition, Australian and New Zealand College of Anaesthetists, Melbourne. Available from: http://www.anzca.edu.au/resources/books-and-publications/acutepain_update.pdf

Australian and New Zealand College of Anaesthetists and Faculty of Pain Medicine (2005) *Acute Pain Management: Scientific Evidence*, 2nd edition, Australian and New Zealand College of Anaesthetists, Melbourne. (Pain in children addressed in Chapter 10 Section 1). Available from: http://www.anzca.edu.au/resources/books-and-publications/acutepain.pdf

Howard, R., Carter, B., Curry, J., Morbon, N., Rivett, K., Rose, M., Tyrrell, J., Walker, S. and Williams, G. (2008) Good Practice in Postoperative and Procedural Pain Management, *Pediatric Anesthesia*, 18: 1–81. http://www.blackwell-synergy.com/toc/pan/18/S1

Scottish Intercollegiate Guidelines Network (SIGN) (2004) *Safe Sedation of Children Undergoing Diagnostic and Therapeutic Procedures: A National Clinical Guideline*. Available from: http://www.apagbi.org.uk/docs/sign58.pdf

---

7.6.1 Optimising the safety of analgesic drugs

Optimising the safety of analgesic drugs requires appropriate education of all involved (healthcare professionals, families and patients) and careful attention to the organisational aspects of analgesic drug administration (ANZCA 2005). Strategies for optimising the safe administration of the analgesic drugs are outlined in Box 7.3.

BOX 7.3

Optimising the safe administration of analgesic drugs

- Appropriate patient selection: suitable for the patient's medical condition, developmental age, surgery/procedure, emotional state, concurrent medication and pre-existing conditions.
- Staff adequately trained and supported, with sufficient staff numbers to safely monitor patients.
- Education about all aspects of analgesia to medical and nursing staff, children and families.
- Clearly identified and readily accessible protocols and guidelines to aid/guide practice.
- Equipment designed to minimise risk: labels, specific pumps, charts, documentation, etc.
- Regular monitoring for efficacy and side effects of analgesia.
- Reportable safety limits individualised to each patient or age groups.
- Emergency management protocols, e.g. sedation/respiratory depression, hypotension management.
- Acute pain service or pain link nurses to guide/direct staff.
- Regular audit.

Source: Ragg (1997b); Macintyre (2001); ANZCA (2005)

7.6.2 Aims for the management of acute pain

The aims of managing acute pain in children are:

- rapid identification of pain;
- adequate analgesia adjusted to the individual's needs and medical condition;
- prevention of pain;

- reduced surgical stress response;
- decreased adverse effects;
- adequate analgesics for exacerbations of pain;
- use of combinations of analgesic drugs;
- pain control after discharge from hospital
                    (Kokinsky and Thornberg 2003; Lönnqvist and Morton 2005;
                                               Pyati and Gan 2007).

Consequences of poorly managed postoperative pain

The consequences of unrelieved pain are identified in Chapter 1. It is important to remember that unrelieved postoperative pain may result in:

- increased morbidity (due to respiratory complications related to hypoventilation);
- increased hospital stay;
- slowed recovery time;
- slowed return to normal life activities;
- decreased patient and family satisfaction;
- increased risk of chronic pain.

7.6.3 Suggested pain management regimes for acute pain

Children have widely variable analgesia requirements, thus any analgesic regime needs to take this into consideration. Table 7.3 outlines suggested analgesia regimes for different acute pain presentations.

Practice point

Multimodal analgesia is where several different types of analgesic drugs with different mechanisms of action are used in combination to optimise the analgesic effect, which:
- allows for lower drug doses, thus minimises the adverse effects of analgesics;
- gives more balanced analgesia;
- allows analgesia to be individualised to the patient or patient group;
- targets pain at different points of pain pathway (see Chapter 2)

Source: Duedal and Hansen (2007); Pyati and Gan (2007).

7.6.4 Opioid analgesia

The administration of oral opioid analgesia for the management of severe pain using combinations of long-acting (slow release) and short-acting (normal release) opioids is discussed in Chapter 9. The use of intermittent opioid bolus, opioid infusion and PCA (patient-controlled analgesia) is considered below.

Intermittent opioid bolus
- Intramuscular injections are strongly disliked by children and are less effective for analgesia than intravenous methods of opioid delivery (ANZCA 2005).
- Intravenous opioids are safe and effective for children of all ages (ANZCA 2005).

Table 7.3 Suggested analgesia regimes for different acute pain presentations

Cause of pain	Mild pain	Moderate pain	Severe pain	Comments
Medical (e.g. sickle cell disease, inflammatory bowel disease)	Step 1 analgesic drugs and non-drug methods (e.g. heat, massage)	Add step 2 analgesic drugs	Add step 3 analgesic drugs (e.g. opioid infusion or PCA)	*Pain usually settles quickly once medical condition stabilises*
Minor surgery/Day stay surgery	Step 1 analgesic drugs plus local anaesthetic (LA) infiltration OR regional anaesthesia (RA) (e.g. caudal)	Add step 2 analgesic drugs	Add step 3 analgesic drugs (e.g. intermittent IV opioid dose)	*Discharge with regular step 1 analgesic drugs for 48 h*
Moderate surgery (Possibly fasting postoperatively)	Step 1 analgesics (via IV route if fasting) plus LA infiltration OR peripheral nerve block OR RA (e.g. caudal or epidural)	Add step 2 analgesic drugs if allowed oral intake OR if fasting add step 3 analgesics (e.g. intermittent IV opioid dose)	Add step 3 analgesic drugs (e.g. intermittent IV opioid dose OR opioid infusion /PCA)	*Discharge with regular steps 1 and 2 analgesic drugs for 2–4 days*
Major surgery (May be fasting postoperatively)	Step 1 analgesic drugs (given IV if fasting) plus LA infiltration OR peripheral nerve block OR RA (e.g. epidural)	(Not used in initial stages)	Add step 3 analgesic drugs (e.g. continuous opioid infusion or PCA plus ketamine or tramadol)	*If risk of bleeding delay NSAIDs for 24 h Continue RA for 24–48 h (72 h for orthopaedic surgery)*
				Discharge with regular steps 1 and 2 analgesic drugs for 3–5 days For major orthopaedic or thoracic surgery discharge with step 3 analgesic drugs for 2–4 weeks
Respiratory compromise (e.g. severe cerebral palsy, muscular dystrophies or chronic lung disease)	Step 1 analgesic drugs (via IV route if fasting) plus LA infiltration OR RA (e.g. caudal or epidural)	(Not used in initial stages)	Avoid opioids: consider tramadol, clonidine or ketamine as main analgesics	*Caution for drug interactions with usual medications (e.g. sedatives or anticonvulsants)*

Source: Davies and Oni (1997); Greco and Berde (2005); Kokinsky and Thornberg (2007); Morton (2007)

- Intermittent opioid boluses are used:
  - to manage short-term moderate to severe pain episodes (e.g. for dressings or fracture reduction);
  - to achieve rapid pain control prior to the commencement of a continuous analgesia technique (e.g. in the emergency department or following anaesthesia in the recovery room);
  - as a 'rescue' for pain flares (e.g. following cessation of a continuous analgesia technique or for cancer pain and palliative care; see Chapter 9).
- If more than two or three intermittent opioid bolus doses are required in a 24-hour period the analgesia should be converted to a continuous analgesia technique.
- Intermittent boluses are commonly given intravenously and can also be given intranasally.
- If the child does not have intravenous access the same intravenous dose may be given subcutaneously, preferably using a fine gauge cannula or *butterfly* infusion device that can be left in situ (if required) for subsequent doses.
- The same dose of morphine can be given via subcutaneous bolus or infusion with no difference in efficacy (Bouwmeester et al. 2001).

Tables 7.4 to 7.6 detail suggested opioid bolus dosing guidelines.

Table 7.4 Suggested child (<50 kg) **intravenous** or **subcutaneous** opioid bolus dosing guidelines

Drug	Bolus	Frequency
Morphine	50–100 microgram/kg	2–3 hourly
Fentanyl	0.5–1 microgram/kg	1–2 hourly
Hydromorphone	10–20 microgram/kg	2–4 hourly

Source: Greco and Berde (2005); Brislin and Rose (2005); Lönnqvist and Morton (2005); Rose (2007); Morton (2007)

Table 7.5 Suggested full-term neonate/infant **intravenous** morphine bolus dosing guidelines

Drug	Bolus	Frequency
Morphine	25–50 microgram/kg	3–4 hourly

Source: Brislin and Rose (2005); Rose (2007)

Table 7.6 Suggested child (over 3 years) **intranasal** opioid bolus dosing guidelines

Drug	Bolus	Frequency
Diamorphine	0.1 mg/kg	Single dose
Fentanyl	1–2 microgram/kg	Single dose

Source: Kendall et al. (2001); Borland et al. (2002); Brislin and Rose (2005); Goldman (2006); Harrop (2007)

Continuous opioid infusion or nurse controlled analgesia

Continuous opioid infusions are used for the management of moderate to severe pain that is expected to last for more than a day where PCA or oral analgesia is not suitable (due to medical condition, age, cognitive function or physical limitations). Administration via continuous infusion allows for more constant pain relief and decreases staff workload compared to administering intermittent opioid boluses.

- The opioid infusion may be administered via a PCA infusion device (but with different programming), which is referred to as nurse controlled analgesia (NCA) or administered via a standard infusion pump.
- Initial infusion rates vary according to age and should also be titrated against the individual child's response (ANZCA 2005).
- Boluses may be prescribed in addition to the continuous infusion to cover incident pain.

Pethidine is **not** routinely used for opioid infusion due to the problem of norpethidine toxicity (see Chapter 4), instead morphine, hydromorphone or fentanyl are preferable.

Tables 7.7 to 7.9 detail suggested opioid infusion dosing guidelines.

The observations that need to be recorded when an infant or child is receiving an opioid infusion or PCA are outlined in Table 7.10.

Table 7.7 Suggested child (<50 kg) **intravenous** opioid infusion dosing guidelines

Drug	Loading dose	Start rate	Infusion range	Bolus dose
Morphine	50–100 microgram/kg	20 microgram/kg/h	10–40 microgram/kg/h	10–20 microgram/kg each 10 min as required
Morphine*	50–100 microgram/kg	20 microgram/kg/h	10–30 microgram/kg/h	20 microgram/kg each 20–30 min as required
Hydromorphone	10–20 microgram/kg	3 microgram/kg/h	6 microgram/kg/h	2–4 microgram/kg each 10 min as required
Fentanyl	0.6–1 microgram/kg	0.5 microgram/kg/h	0–1.2 microgram/kg/h	0.3 microgram/kg each 5–10 min as required

*Nurse-controlled infusion.
Source: ANZCA (2005); Brislin and Rose (2005); Morton (2007); Rose (2007)

Table 7.8 Suggested **intravenous** morphine infusion dosing guidelines for infants (1–3 months)

Drug	Loading dose	Start rate	Infusion range	Bolus dose
Morphine	25–50 microgram/kg	10 microgram/kg/h	5–20 microgram/kg/h	10 microgram/kg each 30 min

Source: ANZCA 2005; Greco and Berde 2005; Rose 2007

Table 7.9   Suggested **intravenous** morphine infusion dosing guidelines for term neonates

Drug	Loading dose	Start rate	Infusion range	Bolus dose
Morphine	10–25 microgram/kg	5 microgram/kg/h	5–10 microgram/kg/h	5–10 microgram/kg each 60 min

Source: Cunliffe and Roberts (2004); Greco and Berde (2005); ANZCA (2005)

Table 7.10   Suggested observations for infants and children receiving opioid infusion or PCA

Parameter	Suggested frequency	Comments
Sedation score	1 hourly for the duration of the opioid infusion/PCA	Use a validated paediatric sedation scale (e.g. University of Michigan Sedation Scale, Box 7.5, p. 123)
Respiratory rate and heart rate	1 hourly for the duration of the opioid infusion/PCA	
Pain score	1 hourly while awake	Use a developmentally appropriate pain assessment scale (see Chapter 6)
Nausea/vomiting assessment	1 hourly for the first 12 hours, then 4-hourly as indicated	Use a validated scale
Pulse oximetry	As indicated (see Box 7.6, p. 123) or per institutional protocol	

PCA, patient-controlled analgesia

Patient-controlled analgesia

Patient-controlled analgesia (PCA) uses a programmable infusion pump to allow patients to self-administer their own intravenous analgesia.

- PCA has become the gold standard for acute pain management since its introduction into paediatric medicine in the early 1990s (McDonald and Cooper 2001; Lehmann 2005).
- The use of small, frequent boluses allows the patient to accurately titrate the analgesia to their pain thus receiving only what they need, which addresses the wide variation in individual patients' opioid requirements (McDonald and Cooper 2001; Lehmann 2005).
- PCA is used for the management of moderate to severe pain in children over five years. In some instances children as young as four years can manage PCA, but this is uncommon (McDonald and Cooper 2001).
- PCA is commonly used for postoperative pain management in children. In addition PCA may be used for trauma and burns, cancer pain, medical conditions and palliative pain (McDonald and Cooper 2001).
- PCA is safe, effective and viewed as a highly satisfactory method of analgesia delivery by staff, patient and families. Adverse effects are rare and can be reduced by the addition of opioid-sparing analgesics (e.g. paracetamol) (Ellis et al. 1999; McDonald and Cooper 2001; ANZCA 2005).

- It is important that the child's parents also understand the concept of PCA, so they can support their child in its use.
- Children who are unwilling or unable to use PCA (e.g. children under seven years or children with cognitive or physical impairment) should have an opioid infusion instead.
- Unless specifically permitted by an institutional protocol the PCA should only be used by the patient to reduce the risk of opioid-related adverse effects (particularly excess sedation and respiratory depression).
- Some institutions use a formal PCA-by-proxy protocol (allowing a parent or health-care professional as the designated proxy) for end-of-life care or for children who are opioid-tolerant. If the patient and the designated proxy are carefully chosen and educated, PCA-by-proxy is a safe and effective means of administering analgesia (American Society for Pain Management Nursing [ASPMN] 2006).

Detailed discussion and position paper about PCA-by-proxy by the American Society for Pain Management Nursing (ASPMN) can be found at:
http://www.aspmn.org/Organization/documents/PCAbyProxy-final-EW_004.pdf

---

The terminology used for PCA administration is outlined in Box 7.4.

BOX 7.4

PCA terminology

Bolus dose: When the patient presses the remote button, the PCA delivers the programmed bolus dose of analgesia.

Lockout time: This is usually set at 5–10 minutes. The PCA will not deliver a dose during lockout time, even if the button is pressed. This allows each bolus to reach peak effect before the patient has another bolus, thus reducing the risk of overdose.

Good try/Bad try: A good try is when the PCA delivers a bolus dose of analgesia. A bad try is when the patient presses the button during the lockout time and no bolus dose is delivered.

Dose duration: This ranges from 30–90 seconds, depending on the PCA infusion device used. The dose duration can be increased to prevent problems such as light-headedness or nausea associated with a rapid peak of onset of analgesia.

Background: A continuous infusion that may be added to improve analgesia. Generally a background is only required for patients with high opioid requirements. Adding a background may increase the risk of the adverse effects associated with opioids: sedation, respiratory depression, itch or nausea.

Four-hour limit: This setting is used to limit the amount of medication the patient may request in a 4-hour period (generally equivalent to 4–5 good tries/hour). There is no good evidence to show that this offers safer management. Some institutions use this setting, others not.

Source: Macintyre (2001)

To use PCA the child must:

- have the cognitive ability to associate pressing the PCA button with receiving pain relief;
- be physically able and willing to press the button to control their pain.

Table 7.11 details suggested PCA dosing guidelines.

Table 7.11   Suggested child (<50 kg) **PCA** dosing guidelines

Drug	Loading dose	Bolus dose	Lockout time	Background infusion rate	4-hour limit
Morphine	40–100 microgram/kg	20 microgram/kg	5–10 min	Nil *or* 4–10 microgram/kg/h	Nil *or* 400 microgram/kg
Hydromorphone	10 microgram/kg	2–4 microgram/kg	5–10 min	Nil *or* 0.5–2 microgram/kg/h	Nil *or* 60 microgram/kg
Fentanyl	0.5–1 microgram/kg	0.3–0.5 microgram/kg	5 min	Nil *or* 0.2–0.4 microgram/kg/h	Nil *or* 10 microgram/kg

Source: McDonald and Cooper (2001); Cunliffe and Roberts (2004); Brislin and Rose (2005); Greco and Berde (2005); ANZCA (2005); RCH (2007); Rose (2007)

The observations that need to be recorded when a child is receiving PCA are outlined in Table 7.10 (p. 120).

> ## Novel analgesic infusions
>
> There is increasing use of novel analgesics, such as tramadol or ketamine for managing acute pain in children. These are prescribed most commonly by pain management services in tertiary children's hospitals. These analgesics may be administered via PCA or a continuous intravenous infusion. At present there is limited evidence about their efficacy in children, however, the adult evidence suggests that increased use in children is likely.
>
> *Source:* Engelhardt et al. (2002); Bozkurt (2005); Lin and Durieux (2005); Anderson and Palmer (2006); Aydin et al. (2007); Dal et al. (2007)

7.6.5 Best practice management for administering intravenous opioids

Commencing the opioid infusion or PCA
- Unless the patient has received a recent dose of opioid, a loading dose should be administered when commencing an opioid infusion or PCA to ensure therapeutic plasma levels are reached quickly.
- It takes approximately four half-lives (~8 hrs for morphine/hydromorphone, ~1.5 hrs for fentanyl) for opioids to reach steady-state plasma concentration when administered as an infusion, therefore if the infusion rate is to be increased, a bolus should be given as well.

Concurrent medications
- Paracetamol, ketamine, regional anaesthesia, tramadol and NSAIDs may be administered concurrently with an opioid infusion or PCA to optimise analgesia and reduce opioid requirements and thus minimise opioid-induced adverse effects.

Precautions
- If the patient is receiving other medication that may cause sedation (e.g. antihistamines, benzodiazepines or anticonvulsants), there may be an increased risk of sedation and respiratory depression.
- Prolonged administration of opioids in the setting of impaired liver and/or renal function can alter the drug and metabolite clearance of the opioids and possibly result in accumulation and toxicity (see Chapter 4).
- Development of opioid tolerance with long-term opioid administration may require the opioid dose to be increased (see Chapter 4).

- Careful tapering of doses is important when weaning from long-term opioid administration to avoid opioid withdrawal (see Chapter 4).

The observations required for infants and children receiving opioid infusion or PCA are outlined in Table 7.10.

Practice point

- Any adverse effects relating to the analgesia should be reported urgently to the acute pain service or anaesthetist.
- The effectiveness of the analgesia should be documented in the child's healthcare record.
- For children receiving long-term opioid infusion or PCA (e.g. greater than 5 days) *less frequent* observations may be acceptable, however, this should be discussed with the acute pain service or anaesthetist.
- Any observations outside reportable limits or outside normal values for age should be reported to the acute pain service or anaesthetist.

BOX 7.5

University of Michigan Sedation Scale (UMSS)

0 – Awake and alert
1 – Minimally sedated: may appear tired/sleepy, responds to verbal conversation and/or sound
2 – Moderately sedated: somnolent/sleeping, easily aroused with light tactile stimulation or simple verbal command
3 – Deep sedation: deep sleep, arousable only with deep or significant physical simulation
4 – Unarousable
S – Patient is sleeping

Source: Malviya et al. (2002)

BOX 7.6

Indications for pulse oximetry

Pulse oximetry MUST BE used continuously in high-risk patients with:

- University of Michigan Sedation Scale (UMSS) sedation score >2
- infants under 6 months of age
- significant cardiorespiratory impairment
- sleep apnoea, snoring or airway obstruction
- spot oximetry less than 94% SaO_2

or in patients receiving:

- supplementary oxygen
- concurrent sedative agents.

Clinical indicators for 'spot' pulse oximetry are:

- tachypnoea or bradypnoea
- respiratory distress
- pallor or cyanosis or impaired oxygenation
- confusion or agitation
- hypotension
- nurse concern.

Source: Department of Anaesthesia and Pain Management, RCH, Melbourne 2007 (used with permission).

7.6.6 Management of adverse effects of opioids

Managing adverse effects of medications is an important component of successful pain management (Rusy and Weisman 2002). A variety of adverse effects occur secondary to opioid administration (see also Chapter 4). It is important to consider *all* possible causes for the adverse effects and not assume that the opioid alone is responsible. Adverse effects will be discussed in order of clinical significance.

Sedation/respiratory depression

Assessing level of sedation is the key to early identification and treatment of opioid-induced respiratory depression (Pasero and McCaffery 2002). Less opioid is required to induce sedation than respiratory depression; for this reason, monitoring of sedation is a very effective way to detect early signs of opioid toxicity.

Practice point

Respiratory depression secondary to opioid toxicity is caused by:

- decreased responses to hypercapnia and hypoxia;
- depression of the cough reflex;
- decreased minute ventilation (mainly by decreasing respiratory rate).

The best clinical indicator is increasing sedation.
Decreased rate of breathing and decreased oxygen saturation are **late** signs

Source: Pasero and McCaffery 2002

Indeed it has been suggested that due to the severe consequences of unrecognised hypoxia and its sequelae, monitoring sedation should be the sixth vital sign for patients receiving opioids. Sedation assessment should be made using a validated sedation scale to ensure consistency between healthcare professionals. If required, an opioid antagonist (most commonly, naloxone) should be carefully titrated to effect to avoid reversing all the opioid effect and inducing severe pain. All patients receiving opioids should have standing orders for naloxone administration to ensure minimal delay if naloxone administration is required. Box 7.7 suggests a protocol to manage opioid-induced respiratory depression.

Practice point

A nurse-initiated naloxone-dosing regime was introduced at Royal Children's Hospital, Melbourne, in 2006 (Box 7.7). In the first 12 months following the introduction:

- There were **no** emergency calls for opioid-induced respiratory depression.
- **No** patients needed the *resuscitation* dose of naloxone.
- **No** patients required more than 3 doses of the *excess sedation* dose.
- Nurses were able to administer naloxone using a standing order without first calling for medical advice.
- Nurses were confident drawing up naloxone using the standardised dilution protocol.

Source: Dowden, S.J. and Penrose, S. (personal communication, 15 September 2007)

BOX 7.7

Protocol to manage opioid-induced respiratory depression

If opioid-induced respiratory depression is suspected

- Stop administering the opioid
- Stimulate the patient (shake gently, call by name, ask to breathe)
- Administer oxygen
- Administer naloxone if indicated

Indications for naloxone

If patient is significantly sedated (University of Michigan Sedation Scale **3**)

- **Administer naloxone 2 microgram/kg**
- Administer bolus as an IV push and repeat every **1–2 min** until desired effect is obtained (maximum 5 doses)

If patient cannot be roused and/or is apnoeic (University of Michigan Sedation Scale **4**)

- Administer naloxone **10 microgram/kg**
- Administer bolus of naloxone as an IV push and repeat **every 1–2 min** until the desired effect is obtained (maximum 5 doses)

Suggested dilution: 0.4 mg naloxone in 20 mL normal saline = 20 microgram/mL

Continue to monitor the patient closely. Naloxone has a shorter duration of action than most opioids, thus repeated doses may be required. In some situations a naloxone infusion will be necessary.

Source: Pasero et al. (1999); Department of Anaesthesia and Pain Management, RCH, Melbourne (2007) (used with permission)

Additional sedation management options to consider:

- If receiving PCA, consider reducing or ceasing the background infusion or reducing the bolus size.
- If receiving opioid infusion, consider reducing the background infusion or reducing the bolus size.
- Optimise doses of non-opioid analgesics.
- Consider changing to a different opioid.
- Consider alternative or adjuvant analgesics.
- Review other possible contributing factors (e.g. benzodiazepines, antihistamines, prolonged anaesthesia, dose error, hypoxia, renal impairment, electrolyte imbalance).

Nausea and vomiting

- There are multiple causes for postoperative nausea and vomiting (PONV) in children (e.g. surgery, anaesthesia, prolonged fasting, opioids, antibiotics, other medications, ileus, pain, electrolyte imbalance, renal dysfunction), although opioids are commonly considered to be the primary cause.
- When deciding how best to treat PONV *all* possible causes should be considered, as this may influence antiemetic selection.

- Children have a significantly higher PONV rate than adults, which can be compounded in children with a prior history of PONV or motion sickness (Kovac 2007).
- The revised 2006 Consensus Guidelines for Managing PONV (Gan et al. 2006; Gan and Meyer 2006) suggest identifying children at high-risk for PONV, treating aggressively with prophylactic antiemetic therapy and using a combination of different antiemetic agents from different classes for best results (Table 7.12):
  - Moderate to high risk for PONV = prophylaxis with two antiemetics (different classes);
  - High risk PONV or failed prophylaxis = combination therapy with two or three antiemetics (different classes).

> Consider very low-dose opioid antagonist (e.g. naloxone infusion: 0.25–0.1 microgram/kg/h) for antiemetic-resistant PONV (Greco and Berde 2005).

Urinary retention

Urinary retention following surgery may be due to a variety of causes other than opioids, such as pain, bladder spasm, inflammation, constipation, dehydration, epidural blockade or anxiety about using a bedpan or bottle. It is not unusual for urinary retention to be multifactorial: even if one cause seems likely; others such as pre-existing neurological deficits or bladder dysfunction may have significant contributory effects (Gatti et al. 2001).

Consider:

- increasing fluid intake;
- conservative management (e.g. observation, reassurance, manual expression of bladder);
- encouragement strategies (e.g. increase privacy, commode by the bed, encourage male patients to stand up if possible, or running water).

Table 7.12   Antiemetic drugs for prevention and management of postoperative nausea and vomiting

Antiemetic class	Drug doses
$5HT_3$ antagonist	Ondansetron: 0.1–0.15 mg/kg IV/oral 8 hourly as required
	Granisetron: 40 microgram/kg IV daily as required
	Tropisetron: 0.1 mg/kg IV daily as required (maximum dose 2 mg)
Corticosteroid	Dexamethasone: single daily dose: 0.15 mg/kg IV (maximum of 3 days)
Dopamine anatagonist	Metoclopramide*: Loading dose: 0.5 mg/kg IV (maximum dose 20–30 mg); maintenance dose: 0.2 mg/kg IV/oral 6–8 hourly as required (maximum dose 20 mg)
Dopamine anatagonist	Droperidol: 10 microgram/kg IV 8-hourly as required (maximum dose 0.625 mg)
Antihistamine	Promethazine: 0.5 mg/kg IV 8-hourly as required (maximum dose 25 mg) Cyclizine: 1 mg/kg IV/oral 8-hourly as required (maximum dose 50 mg)

*In addition to being a dopamine antagonist metoclopramide has prokinetic actions on the gastrointestinal tract: enhancing gastric emptying and gut motility
$5HT_3$, histamine, dopamine and acetylcholine are all neurotransmitters involved in the process of nausea and vomiting.
Source: Gan et al. (2006); RCH (2007); Kovac (2007)

If the retention is likely to be opioid-induced, consider:

- reducing the opioid dose;
- administering very low dose of opioid antagonist (e.g. naloxone 0.5–1 microgram/kg, repeated 2–4 times as required) (Greco and Berde 2005);
- intermittent catheterisation or indwelling urinary catheter if above measures fail (use lignocaine jelly for catheterisation) (Wrede-Seaman 2005).

Pruritus (itch)

- Pruritus is commonly caused by opioid-induced histamine release and usually settles within two or three days of commencing opioids.
- Despite the tendency of clinicians to prescribe antihistamines for this problem they are not very effective and may cause sedation, constipation and urinary retention (Greco and Berde 2005).
- The use of very low dose opioid antagonist is more efficacious than antihistamine, administered as an intermittent bolus dose (e.g. naloxone 1 microgram/kg each 2–4 hours) (Greco and Berde 2005) or via infusion (e.g. naloxone 0.25–1 microgram/kg/h) (Gold et al. 2006).

Constipation

- Constipation is a common side effect of opioid administration, caused by delayed gastric emptying and decreased peristaltic activity of the bowel (Thomas 2008).
- Unlike almost all other adverse opioid effects it does not resolve after a few days (Thomas 2008).
- Preventive measures should be implemented *early* following commencement of opioid analgesics. Ideally a combination of stool softener (e.g. docusate sodium-based preparations) *and* a bowel stimulant laxative (e.g. senna-based preparations or lactulose) should be used (Thomas 2008).
- Ensuring adequate fluid intake and a high fibre dietary intake will assist in constipation management (Thomas 2008).
- Peripherally acting opioid antagonists may offer alternative management in the future, however at present these drugs are still under development (Thomas 2008).

Central nervous system effects

- The central nervous system (CNS) effects of opioids (e.g. sedation, euphoria or dysphoria) are most often short-lived in duration and resolve within several days of commencing opioids.
- The effects may be dose related, thus a reduction in the opioid dose may resolve the symptoms.
- Converting to another opioid or adding adjuvant analgesia may also help.
- If the CNS effects are severe or do not resolve with opioid dose reduction, other causes may need to be considered, such as the effect of other medications (e.g. benzodiazepines or antihistamines), hepatic or renal dysfunction, electrolyte or metabolic abnormalities, or infection (Wrede-Seaman 2005).

7.7 Regional Anaesthesia

Regional anaesthesia is the administration of local anaesthetics (LA) (often in conjunction with other drugs) into the epidural space, around a peripheral nerve plexus or into the intrathecal space to block pain transmission (see Chapters 2 and 4).

- Regional anaesthesia provides excellent pain control during and after surgery, reduces the stress response to surgery and can significantly reduce the need for opioids and other analgesic drugs postoperatively (ANZCA 2005; Lönnqvist and Morton 2005).

- The most commonly used regional anaesthesia technique in children is caudal epidural (LA injected into the caudal epidural space via the sacrococcygeal membrane), which is used for surgical procedures below the umbilical region. It is usually administered as a single dose for day-case or short-stay procedures (ANZCA 2005).
- Epidural analgesia is used in children of all ages to manage pain following major surgery to the chest, abdomen or lower limbs. It is most commonly given via a continuous infusion but can also be given via intermittent bolus or via patient controlled epidural anaesthesia (PCEA) (ANZCA 2005).
- In neonates epidurals are inserted into the caudal epidural space, then threaded to the lumbar or thoracic levels as required (ANZCA 2005).
- Other regional anaesthesia techniques may be used in children, for example, intrathecal analgesia (spinal) or peripheral nerve blocks, either as a single-dose or an infusion.
- Epidural analgesia offers superior pain relief compared to many other analgesic drug options; however, they are not without risk and need to be managed by suitably trained and experienced staff to ensure minimal complications (ANZCA 2005; Llewellyn and Moriarty 2007).

There is no consensus in paediatric pain research nor is there a clearly identified agent for preferential use in regional anaesthesia in children (Williams and Howard 2003; Brislin and Rose 2005; ANZCA 2005; Gold et al. 2006). Bupivacaine, levobupivacaine and ropivacaine are the most commonly used local anaesthetics, with or without the addition of additives (Table 7.13).

7.7.1 Best practice management for epidural infusion analgesia

The observations required for children receiving epidural infusions are outlined in Table 7.14.

Table 7.13 Local anaesthetic solutions and additives for paediatric regional anaesthesia

Local anaesthetic	Dose	Infusion rate	Neonate/Infant dose	Comments
Bupivacaine	0.0625%–0.25%	0.1–0.4 mL/kg/h	Lower concentration and infusion rate	*0.125% is the most commonly used solution*
Levobupivacaine	0.0625%–0.25%	0.1–0.4 mL/kg/h	Lower concentration and infusion rate	*0.125% is the most commonly used solution*
Ropivacaine	0.0625%–0.25%	0.1–0.4 mL/kg/h	Lower concentration and infusion rate	*0.125% is the most commonly used solution*
Additive	**Dose**		**Neonate/Infant dose**	**Comments**
Morphine	10–50 microgram/mL		Lower dose	Preservative free
Fentanyl	1–5 microgram/mL		Lower dose	
Hydromorphone	5–10 microgram/mL		Minimal data	
Clonidine	0.5–2 microgram/kg/h		May cause apnoea	
Ketamine or S-ketamine	0.5–5 mg/kg/h		Minimal data	Preservative free

Source: Cunliffe and Roberts (2004); Williams and Howard (2003); Brislin and Rose (2005); RCH (2007)

Table 7.14   Suggested observations for children receiving epidural infusion analgesia

Parameter	Suggested frequency	Comments
Sedation score	1 hourly for the duration of the epidural infusion	Use a validated paediatric sedation scale (e.g. University of Michigan Sedation Scale, see Box 7.5)
Respiratory rate and heart rate	1 hourly for the duration of the epidural infusion	
Temperature and blood pressure	1 hourly for *the first 4 hours* then 4 hourly until the epidural is ceased	
Pain score	1 hourly while awake (using developmentally appropriate pain assessment scale)	See Chapter 6 for further discussion
Vomiting score	1 hourly for the first 12 hours, then 4 hourly as indicated	Use a validated scale
Pulse oximetry	As indicated (see Box 7.6) or per institutional requirements	
Sensory and motor assessment	4 hourly	See Boxes 7.8 and 7.9

Practice point

- Any adverse effects relating to the epidural infusion should be reported urgently to the acute pain service or anaesthetist.
- Any observations outside reportable limits or outside normal values for age should be reported to the acute pain service or anaesthetist.
- The effectiveness of the analgesia should be documented in the child's healthcare record.

Assessing sensory and motor block

Assessment of sensory and motor block enables early detection of epidural complications and ensures the analgesia can be optimised. The method for assessment of sensory block is outlined in Box 7.8. Figure 7.2 demonstrates the dermatome distribution in children.

BOX 7.8

Assessment of sensory block in patients with epidural infusion

Rationale

Sensory nerve fibres respond to pain, temperature, touch and pressure. As pain and temperature nerve fibres are similarly affected by local anaesthetic drugs, changes in temperature perception indicate the area where the epidural is working.

At each vertebra, nerve roots exit from the spinal cord bilaterally. Dermatomes are areas of skin that are primarily innervated by a single spinal nerve.

It is important to assess sensory block:

- to ensure the epidural is covering the patient's pain;
- to ensure the block is not too extensive, which may increase the risk of complications.

BOX 7.8 Continued

Procedure

1 Explain procedure to patient/parent.
2 Wrap an ice cube in tissue or paper towel, leaving part exposed.
3 Place ice on an area well away from the possible dermatome cover (e.g. face or forearm) and ask the patient to tell you how cold it feels to them.
4 Apply the ice to an area likely to be numb on the same side of the body and ask the patient "Does this feel the same cold as your face/arm or different?" Patients may report the ice feeling colder, warmer or the same.
5 Apply the ice to areas above and below this point until you can determine the upper and lower margins of the block.
6 Repeat the procedure on the opposite side of the body. (Blocks may be uneven or unilateral.)
7 Document the blocked dermatomes on the observation chart. Record both the upper and lower margins of the block, e.g. T7–L1, L = R *or* R: T7–L1, L: T10–L2.
8 It is possible to assess dermatome levels on infants or non-verbal/cognitively impaired children by carefully observing flinching and facial expression in response to ice on presumed blocked and unblocked dermatomes. Another way is by observing the patient's response to movement and response to very gentle palpation of the operative site.

Source: Department of Anaesthesia and Pain Management, RCH, Melbourne 2007 (used with permission)

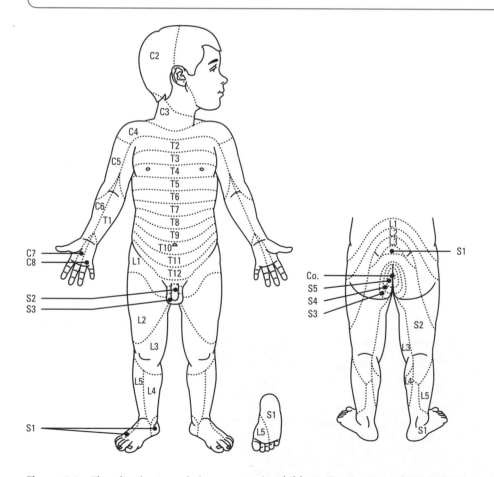

Figure 7.2 The distribution of dermatomes in children. Department of Anaesthesia and Pain Management, RCH, Melbourne, 2007 (used with permission).

Sensory block should be assessed every 4 hours and at the following times:

- in the recovery room on waking from anaesthetic;
- on return to the ward/unit from the recovery room;
- if the patient complains of pain;
- 1 hour after an epidural bolus or increase in infusion rate.

The patient should have a medical review with the acute pain service or anaesthetist if:

- sensory block is higher than T3;
- no evidence of sensory block;
- sensory block is insufficient to relieve pain.

The method for assessment of motor block is outlined in Box 7.9. Figure 7.3 demonstrates the Bromage scale to assess motor function in children.

BOX 7.9

Assessment of motor block in patients with epidural infusion

Rationale

Motor nerves (as well as sensory nerves) may be affected by local anaesthetics. It is important to assess motor block:

- to prevent pressure areas;
- to ensure the patient is safe to ambulate;
- to detect the onset of complications (e.g. epidural haematoma or abscess).

The degree of motor block on both the left and right side should be assessed using the Bromage score.

Procedure

1 Explain procedure to patient/parent.
2 Ask the patient to flex their knees and ankles. Rate their movement according to the Bromage scale. *Bromage scoring is the worldwide standard method of assessing motor function.*

Bromage score:

Bromage 0 (none)	= full flexion of knees and feet
Bromage 1 (partial)	= just able to move knees and feet
Bromage 2 (almost complete)	= able to move feet only
Bromage 3 (complete)	= unable to move feet or knees

3 Document the score on the observation chart. If motor function is different in each leg document this accordingly, e.g. Bromage L) 2, R) 0.

Source: Department of Anaesthesia and Pain Management, RCH, Melbourne 2007 (used with permission)

Motor block should be assessed every 4 hours and at the following times:

- in the recovery room on waking from anaesthetic;
- on return to the ward/unit from the recovery room;
- before the patient attempts to walk;
- 1 hour after an epidural bolus or increase in infusion rate.

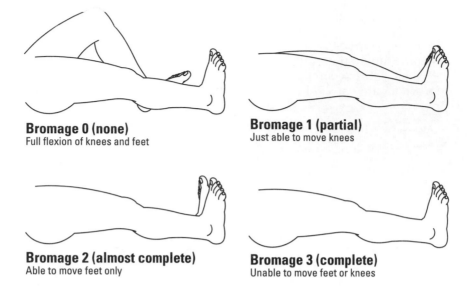

Bromage 0 (none)
Full flexion of knees and feet

Bromage 1 (partial)
Just able to move knees

Bromage 2 (almost complete)
Able to move feet only

Bromage 3 (complete)
Unable to move feet or knees

Figure 7.3 The Bromage scale to assess motor function in children. Department of Anaesthesia and Pain Management, RCH, Melbourne, 2007 (used with permission).

The patient should have a medical review with the acute pain service or anaesthetist if:

- major changes in motor function (particularly any sudden change);
- almost complete or complete motor block in legs (Bromage score 2–3);
- reduced motor function in hands or digits with thoracic epidural.

Catheter position and insertion site
- At least once during each nursing shift, the epidural insertion site should be checked for redness, tenderness, leaking and dressing integrity.
- The epidural catheter marking should be checked to ensure it has not migrated (moved).

Pressure area care
- The decreased sensation and motor blockade produced by epidural analgesia place patients at risk of developing pressure sores and nerve compression (Llewellyn and Moriarty 2007).
- Most commonly the heels, medial and lateral malleoli and sacrum are involved but *all* pressure points are at risk.
- Superficial nerves (e.g. common peroneal nerve) are vulnerable to damage from unrecognised pressure due to decreased sensation.
- The use of pressure-relief devices (e.g. air mattresses, pressure pads) and meticulous nursing care should minimise the risk (Llewellyn and Moriarty 2007).

Epidural additives
- If an *opioid* is added to the epidural solution, additional opioids or sedative agents should not be administered without prior discussion with the acute pain service or anaesthetist.

- Epidural infusions (*without* an opioid added) may be supplemented by intravenous or oral opioids to improve analgesia.
- If a patient is receiving epidural opioids and other medications that may cause sedation (e.g. antihistamines, benzodiazepines or anticonvulsants), they may be at increased risk of sedation and respiratory depression from the opioid.
- If clonidine is added to the epidural solution hypotension and sedation may result.

Anticoagulant medication

- If a patient is prescribed anticoagulant medication while receiving epidural analgesia consideration must be made to ceasing or withholding the anticoagulant medication prior to the removal of the epidural to minimise bleeding risk.

7.7.2 Minor problems and their management

Inadequate analgesia

If the patient complains of pain or appears to be in pain:

- Assess sensory block on both sides.
- Check catheter at insertion site for leaking/dislodgement.
- Check all connections for disconnection/leaking.
- Check epidural catheter position at the skin insertion site.
- Assess severity and location of pain.
- Consider surgical review if at risk of surgical complications, e.g. compartment syndrome, infection or haemorrhage.
- Manage as per institutional epidural guidelines:
  - Contact the acute pain service or anaesthetist for advice.
  - The rate may be increased or a bolus of epidural solution administered.

Leaking epidural

- If the patient is *comfortable* (suggesting the epidural is providing adequate analgesia), the dressing should be reinforced and the amount of leakage monitored. If the leaking appears excessive, discuss with the acute pain service or anaesthetist.
- If the patient is in *pain* or the epidural dressing needs changing, the acute pain service or anaesthetist should be contacted.

Occlusion

Epidural catheters are very fine and can occlude easily. If the infusion pump occludes or is not delivering the programmed rate:

- check the epidural infusion line is not occluded, trapped or kinked.
- check that taping has not caused any kinks in the catheter.
- check the infusion pump pressure.

If the cause for occlusion is not found, contact the acute pain service or anaesthetist.

Disconnection

- If the epidural becomes disconnected contact the acute pain service or anaesthetist.
  - **Do not** re-connect.
  - Wrap the two ends in a sterile towel or gauze.
  - Stop the epidural infusion.

Urinary retention

- Patients with lumbar or caudal epidural infusions are at increased risk of urinary retention. The risk is increased in patients receiving epidural opioids.
- Naloxone may be required to reverse the effect of the opioid and/or the opioid may be removed from the epidural solution.
- The patient may need to have a urinary catheter in situ.
- If a urinary catheter is required this should remain in situ until after the epidural infusion is ceased.

Complications

Contact the acute pain service or anaesthetist *urgently* if any of the following occur:

- high block >T3 (see Figure 7.2 and Table 7.15);
- back pain (see Table 7.15);
- dense motor block: Bromage score 2–3 (see Figure 7.3 and Table 7.15);
- UMSS sedation score ≥3 +/– respiratory depression (see Boxes 7.5, 7.7 and Table 7.16);
- fever >38.5°C;
- hypotension;
- signs of local anaesthetic toxicity (see Table 7.16);
- signs of local infection at the epidural entry site (e.g. erythema or discharge) (see Table 7.15);
- oedema or swelling at epidural entry site.

7.7.3 Complications of epidural analgesia and treatment guidelines

The following tables outline the different complications of epidural analgesia and treatment options. The complications are divided into epidural insertion-related problems (Table 7.15), drug-related problems (Table 7.16) and catheter-related problems (Table 7.17).

Table 7. 15 Complications related to insertion of epidural catheter

Problem	Comments	Treatment
Headache	May be due to dural tap (incidence 1–2%) May not present until patient mobilises	1 Analgesia 2 Bed rest 3 Fluids 4 Epidural blood patch if prolonged, typical postural headache
Back pain	Most commonly at insertion site Mild back pain is common and usually transient Moderate or severe back pain must be thoroughly investigated	1 Simple analgesics and reassurance for mild back pain 2 Regular review until resolved 3 If increasing pain and/or fever the patient needs urgent review
Sympathetic blockade	May cause hypotension (usually in children >8 years) The addition of clonidine to the epidural solution may increase the likelihood of hypotension	1 Posture (lie flat, *not* head down) 2 IV fluid bolus (e.g. 10mL/kg) 3 Consider removing or decreasing dose of clonidine from epidural solution
High blockade (see Figure 7.2)	Dermatome block higher than T3 Numbness or tingling in fingers or arms Horner's syndrome: miosis, ptosis, dry/warm skin on face	1 Resuscitation 2 Cease epidural infusion 3 The infusion might be recommenced at a lower rate if epidural position is confirmed

Table 7. 15   Continued

Problem	Comments	Treatment
	Respiratory distress (*intercostal block*) Bradycardia (*high thoracic block*) Unconsciousness (*total spinal block*)	
Dense motor block (see Figure 7.3)	Common immediately after surgery due to higher concentrations of solution used intra-operatively Prolonged dense motor block >6 hours after surgery must be thoroughly investigated to rule out epidural abscess or epidural haematoma	1 Regularly assess amount of motor block (using Bromage scale) 2 Report Bromage score 2–3 3 Investigate if indicated
Nerve damage	Very rare May present with weakness or numbness Usually transient	1 Neurology referral 2 Review
Epidural abscess	Very rare Presents with moderate-severe back pain, fever, sensory or motor deficits, malaise	1 Urgent investigation: full blood examination, inflammatory markers, blood culture, radiological imaging (CT/MRI) 2 Urgent neurology or neurosurgical review
Epidural haematoma	Very rare Presents with moderate to severe back pain, sensory or motor deficits	1 Urgent investigation: full blood examination, coagulation studies, radiological imaging (CT/MRI) 2 Urgent neurology or neurosurgical review

Source: Ragg (1997a) with permission; RCH (2007)

Table 7.16   Drug-related problems

Problem	Comments	Treatment
Local anaesthetic drugs		
Overdose/Toxicity	Signs of local anaesthetic toxicity may be present: dizziness, blurred vision, decreased hearing, restlessness, tremor, hypotension, bradycardia, arrythmias, seizures, sudden loss of consciousness	1 Resuscitation and management of cardiac, neurological and respiratory side effects 2 Cease epidural infusion
Allergy	Extremely rare Signs of anaphylaxis or allergic reaction may be present	1 Resuscitation, intravenous fluids, adrenaline, antihistamines and steroids 2 Cease epidural infusion
Opioids		
Respiratory depression (see Box 7.7)	Early or delayed	1 Airway management/ Resuscitation 2 Administer naloxone 3 Cease epidural infusion 4 Epidural might be recommened at a lower rate or with opioid removed from epidural solution

(Continued)

Table 7.16 Continued

Problem	Comments	Treatment
Nausea and vomiting	More common with morphine than fentanyl or hydromorphone	1 Give antiemetic(s) 2 Consider removing opioid from epidural solution
Pruritus	More common with morphine than fentanyl or hydromorphone	1 Low dose naloxone 2 Consider removing opioid from epidural solution
Urinary retention		1 Try simple measures 2 Low dose naloxone 3 Urinary catheter 4 Consider removing opioid from epidural solution
Sedation: UMSS score >3 (arousable only with deep or significant physical simulation) (see Box 7.5)		1 Cease epidural 2 Urgent assessment 3 Epidural might be recommenced at a lower rate or with opioid removed from epidural solution
Clonidine		
Sedation		1 May need clonidine dose decreased or clondine removed from epidural solution
Hypotension/ Bradycardia		1 Consider IV fluid bolus (10mL/kg) 2 Monitor urine output & BP 3 May need clonidine dose decreased or clondine removed from epidural solution

Source: Ragg (1997a) with permission; RCH (2007)

Table 7.17 Catheter-related problems

Problem	Comments	Treatment
Leakage	Common Often unrelated to effectiveness of epidural	1 Gauze pad and pressure dressing 2 Selection of occlusive dressing with high fluid permeability
Occlusion or kinking	Epidural catheters are very fine and can easily occlude or kink Kinking may be subcutaneous or on the skin where the epidural catheter or filter is secured	1 Check the catheter tubing, filter and the infusion giving set 2 Check all adhesive taping 3 Try a bolus 4 Increase the pump infusion pressure 5 Change the infusion rate
Dislodgement	Preventable with meticulous securing of epidural catheter at time of insertion and regular checks of all taping	1 Partial dislodgement may not adversely affect the block 2 Full dislodgement may mean loss of epidural blockade and require alternative analgesia
Disconnection	Preventable with meticulous connection and securing of epidural catheter and filter and regular checks of all connections	1 The commonest site for disconnection is at the filter 2 The catheter may need to be removed if disconnection occurs

Source: Ragg (1997a) with permission; RCH (2007)

7.8 Pain Problem-Solving

An important component of pain management is the ability of healthcare professionals to solve problems such as why analgesia is inadequate or why the child is not responding as expected. It is useful to think laterally, considering all possibilities. Sometimes the distress may not be due to pain; for example, infant crying can also be due to hunger, parental separation or being in an unfamiliar place. Sometimes the prescribed analgesia is inadequate for activity and the infant or child is only comfortable if they do not move.

Practice point

When assessing for efficacy of analgesia, ensure it is sufficient:

- for rest and sleep;
- for movement and turning;
- for deep breathing and coughing;
- for physiotherapy and nursing care;
- to enable mobilising;
- to allow diagnostic tests.

Source: Brislin and Rose (2005)

Asking questions such as 'If this were me or my child, what could the problem be? Would this situation be painful?' can stimulate thinking. However, it is also useful to consider that if it looks like pain and sounds like pain it probably is pain! Utilise the parent's involvement. Although they may not be able to pinpoint the cause of the pain parents can usually contribute helpful suggestions and may help identify likely causative factors.

If there is worsening pain 48 hours after surgery or at any time the pain appears *disproportional* to the surgery or underlying medical condition, the reasons for this should always be considered and thoroughly investigated *in addition* to administering analgesia. Further suggestions for problem-solving are outlined in Table 7.18.

Table 7.18   Pain problem-solving

Problem	Possible Cause/Considerations	Management
Pain escalation	What analgesia has already been given and why is it inadequate? Have simple analgesics been given regularly in addition to other analgesics?	Ensure ALL prescribed analgesics are given in a timely manner
	Has the analgesia been given as prescribed? Are the doses appropriate for the child's weight, age or condition?	Check the analgesia doses are correct If required administer additional analgesia (titrate to comfort)
	Are the infusion pumps functioning correctly? Is there a problem with drug delivery? Is the IV cannula or regional anaesthesia catheter still in situ and functioning normally?	Check the infusion delivery device(s) and ensure it is functioning correctly Check the IV cannula or regional anaesthesia catheter is still in situ and not leaking or dislodged
	Could the pain be due to a medical or surgical complication (e.g. tight plaster, compartment syndrome, haemorrhage, haematoma, blocked wound drain, ileus) that needs addressing or assessing?	Get a medical or surgical review if complications are present or could be a possible cause of the pain Address the underlying cause of the pain (e.g. split the plaster, adjust the drain(s), insert nasogastric tube)

(Continued)

Table 7.18　Continued

Problem	Possible cause/Considerations	Management
	Has a single dose regional anaesthesia block regressed, requiring initiation of alternative pain management?	Administer alternate analgesia
	Is the epidural analgesia infusion providing inadequate analgesia?	Manage as per pages 129–134
	Has the opioid infusion been appropriately titrated to the patient's needs and have boluses been given for pain escalation?	Consider adding adjuvant analgesic drugs Discuss the situation with the acute pain service or anaesthetist
Multiple *bad tries* with PCA	Does the child understand how to use the PCA optimally?	Re-educate if necessary
	Is the bolus dose adequate?	Consider addition of a background infusion or increase in bolus size
	Is the lockout time appropriate?	Consider addition of other analgesic drugs
	Is a background infusion required?	Address and manage non-pain issues
	Is the analgesia adequate for the pain severity?	
	Consider other causes: anxiety, confusion, inappropriate use	

Source: Ragg and McKenzie (1997); Ellis et al. (1999); Macintyre (2001)

7.8.1　Transition to oral analgesics after specialist analgesia techniques

The transition from specialist analgesia techniques can be problematic if not planned carefully (Brislin and Rose 2005). As the child's pain decreases and medical condition improves oral medications are generally tolerated, which allows the specialist analgesia techniques to be weaned or ceased. If the child needs to remain fasting for extended period of time some step 1 and step 2 analgesic drugs (e.g. paracetamol, tramadol) can be given via the intravenous route, enabling cessation of step 3 analgesics.

It is important not to remove step 3 analgesic drugs too soon as this will slow recovery if the child becomes reluctant to mobilise or cough due to pain. It is far more helpful to encourage active mobilisation while keeping specialist analgesia techniques for an additional day, than ceasing because it is the *expected day* the technique should finish. Ensuring a *safety net* of rescue doses of step 3 analgesic drugs is available also allays child and parental anxiety.

Most children self-wean from PCA, using it less as the pain improves, thus making a natural progression to simple analgesics. If the child is reluctant to cease using the PCA it may be helpful to negotiate an extended period of demand-only use on the PCA (Brislin and Rose 2005). This is particularly useful for children after major thoracic or orthopaedic surgery (e.g. chest wall reconstruction or scoliosis surgery) that have required large doses of intravenous analgesia as it allows the healthcare professional to leave the PCA for additional analgesia *rescues* while deciding if the prescribed oral analgesia is adequate. This population of children will commonly need to stay on oral step 3 analgesics for an extended period (see Table 7.3) following discharge from hospital.

Once the child is ready for discharge from hospital it is essential that parents are given clear instructions about pain management and medications, the expected time analgesia is required and what to do if the pain is not well controlled (Brislin and Rose 2005). Figure 7.4 outlines an analgesia decision algorithm for weaning analgesia and Figure 7.5 outlines an easy approach to managing acute pain in children.

Analgesia decision algorithm

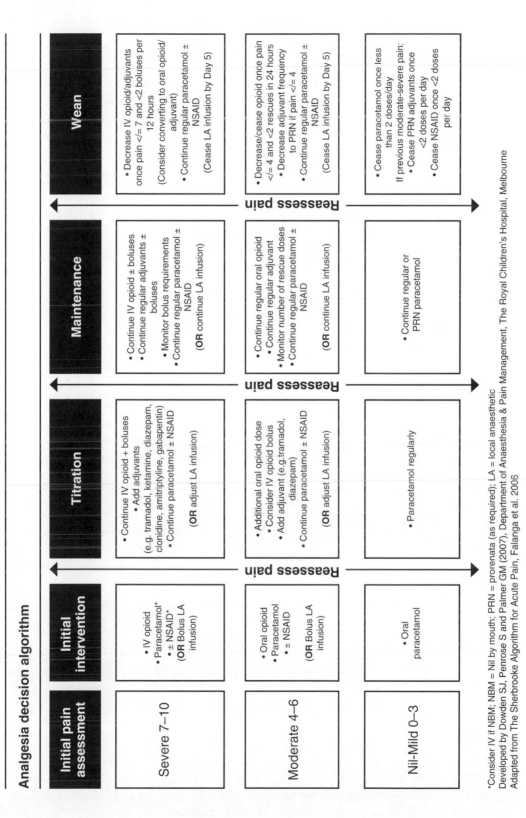

Initial pain assessment	Initial intervention	Titration	Maintenance	Wean
Severe 7–10	• IV opioid • Paracetamol* ± NSAID* (**OR** Bolus LA infusion)	• Continue IV opioid + boluses • Add adjuvants (e.g. tramadol, ketamine, diazepam, clonidine, amitriptyline, gabapentin) • Continue paracetamol ± NSAID (**OR** adjust LA infusion)	• Continue IV opioid ± boluses • Continue regular adjuvants ± boluses • Monitor bolus requirements • Continue regular paracetamol ± NSAID (**OR** continue LA infusion)	• Decrease IV opioid/adjuvants once pain <= 7 and <2 boluses per 12 hours (Consider converting to oral opioid/adjuvant) • Continue regular paracetamol ± NSAID (Cease LA infusion by Day 5)
Moderate 4–6	• Oral opioid • Paracetamol ± NSAID (**OR** Bolus LA infusion)	• Additional oral opioid dose • Consider IV opioid bolus • Add adjuvant (e.g.tramadol, diazepam) • Continue paracetamol ± NSAID (**OR** adjust LA infusion)	• Continue regular oral opioid • Continue regular adjuvant • Monitor number of rescue doses • Continue regular paracetamol ± NSAID (**OR** continue LA infusion)	• Decrease/cease opioid once pain <= 4 and <2 rescues in 24 hours • Decrease adjuvant frequency to PRN if pain <= 4 • Continue regular paracetamol ± NSAID (Cease LA infusion by Day 5)
Nil-Mild 0–3	• Oral paracetamol	• Paracetamol regularly	• Continue regular or PRN paracetamol	• Cease paracetamol once less than 2 doses/day If previous moderate-severe pain: • Cease PRN adjuvants once <2 doses per day • Cease NSAID once <2 doses per day

Reassess pain (between Initial intervention and Titration)
Reassess pain (between Titration and Maintenance)
Reassess pain (between Maintenance and Wean)

*Consider IV if NBM; NBM = Nil by mouth; PRN = prorenata (as required); LA = local anaesthetic
Developed by Dowden SJ, Penrose S and Palmer GM (2007), Department of Anaesthesia & Pain Management, The Royal Children's Hospital, Melbourne
Adapted from The Sherbrooke Algorithm for Acute Pain, Falanga et al. 2006

Figure 7.4   Analgesia decision algorithm.

Five-point plan for pain management:

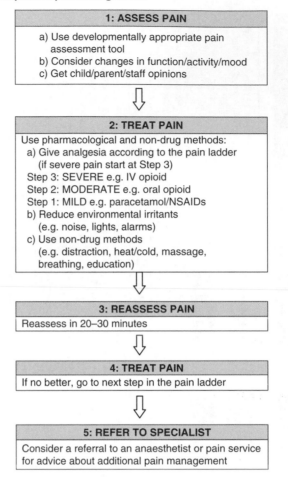

Figure 7.5 Five-point plan for pain management.
Source: Department of Anaesthesia and Pain Management, RCH, Melbourne (used with permission).

Summary

- Acute pain is a common childhood experience. It is generally of short duration and resolves completely.
- There are multiple causes of acute pain ranging from childhood illnesses to trauma, surgery or exacerbation of pre-existing medical conditions.
- Children with developmental disabilities experience significant pain in their daily life from a variety of causes.
- Opioids are the mainstay for the management of severe acute pain, but should be given with simple analgesics as these have an opioid-sparing effect.
- Multimodal analgesia allows for optimal pain management, while minimising adverse effects by utilising combinations of analgesics at lower doses.
- Epidurals offer superior pain relief to most other analgesic techniques, however they are not without risk.
- Close monitoring is key to prevention of serious adverse effects related to opioid and epidural administration.

- Using lateral thinking and problem-solving can assist nurses to improve the pain management of their patients.
- Any pain disproportional to the surgery or medical condition should always be investigated as it may indicate serious medical or surgical complications.
- Transition to oral analgesia following specialist analgesia techniques requires planning to ensure optimal pain management.
- Parents should be given clear instructions about managing pain at home following their child's discharge from hospital.

Useful web resources

Department of Anaesthesia and Pain Management, Royal Children's Hospital, Melbourne Pain Clinical Practice Guidelines: www.rch.org.au/anaes/pain

Great Ormond Street Hospital for Children, NHS Trust, Clinical Practice Guideline, Epidural Analgesia: http://www.ich.ucl.ac.uk/clinical_information/clinical_guidelines/cpg_guideline_00079

References

American Society for Pain Management Nursing (ASPMN) (2006) Authorized and Unauthorized ('PCA by Proxy') Dosing of Analgesic Infusion Pumps, Position Statement, American Society for Pain Management Nursing, www.aspmn.org (accessed 26/12/2007).

Anderson, B.J. and Palmer, G.M. (2006) Recent developments in the pharmacological management of pain in children, *Current Opinion in Anaesthesiology*, 19: 285–292.

Ansermino, M., Basu, R., Vandebeek, C. and Montgomery, C. (2003) Non-opioid additives to local anaesthetics for caudal blockade in children: a systematic review, *Paediatric Anaesthesia*, 13(7): 561–573.

Australian and New Zealand College of Anaesthetists and Faculty of Pain Medicine [ANZCA] (2005) *Acute Pain Management: Scientific Evidence*, 2nd edition, Australian and New Zealand College of Anaesthetists, Melbourne.

Aydin, O.N., Ugur, B., Ozgun, S., Eyigor, H. and Copcu, O. (2007) Pain prevention with intraoperative ketamine in outpatient children undergoing tonsillectomy or tonsillectomy and adenotomy, *Journal of Clinical Anesthesia*, 19: 115–119.

Bertin, L., Pons, G., d'Athis, P., Duhamel, J.F., Mandelonde, C., Lasfargues, G., Guillot, M., Marsac, A., Debregeas, B. and Olive, G. (1996) A randomized double blind multicentre controlled trial of ibuprofen versus acetaminophen and placebo for symptoms of acute otitis media in children, *Fundamentals in Clinical Pharmacology*, 10: 387–392.

Borland, M.L., Jacobs, I. and Geelhoed, G. (2002) Intranasal fentanyl reduces acute pain in children in the emergency department: a safety and efficacy study, *Emergency Medicine Australasia*, 14(3): 275–280.

Borland, M.L., Jacobs, I., King, B. and O'Brien, D. (2007) A randomized controlled trial comparing intranasal fentanyl to intravenous morphine for managing acute pain in children in the emergency department, *Annals of Emergency Medicine*, 49(3): 335–40.

Bouwmeester, N.J., van den Anker, J.N., Hop, W.C.J., Anand, K.J.S. and Tibboel, D. (2003) Age- and therapy-related effects on morphine requirements and plasma concentrations of morphine and its metabolites in postoperative infants, *British Journal of Anaesthesia*, 90(5): 642–652.

Bozkurt, P. (2005) Use of tramadol in children, *Pediatric Anesthesia*, 15: 1041–1047.

Brady-Fryer, B., Wiebe, N. and Lander, J.A. (2004) Pain relief for neonatal circumcision, *Cochrane Database Systematic Review*, Oct 18(4): CD004217.

Brislin, R.P. and Rose, J.B. (2005) Pediatric Acute Pain Management, *Anesthesiology Clinics of North America*, 23: 789–814.

Cunliffe, M. and Roberts, S.A. (2004) Pain Management in Children, *Current Anaesthesia & Critical Care*, 15: 272–283.

Dal, D., Celebi, N., Elvan, E.G., Celiker, V. and Aypar, U. (2007) The efficacy of intravenous or peritonsillar infiltration of ketamine for postoperative pain relief in children following adenotonsillectomy, *Pediatric Anesthesia*, 17: 263–269.

Davies, S.C. and Oni, L. (1997) Management of patients with sickle cell disease, *British Medical Journal*, 315: 656–660.

De Negri, P., Ivani, G., Visconti C. and De Vivo, P. (2001) How to prolong postoperative analgesia after caudal anaesthesia with ropivacaine in children: S-ketamine versus clonidine, *Paediatric Anaesthesia*, 11: 679–683.

Duedal, T.H. and Hansen, E.H. (2007) A qualitative systematic review of morphine treatment in children with postoperative pain, *Pediatric Anesthesia*, 17: 756–774.

Ellis, J.A., Blouin, R. and Lockett, J. (1999) Patient-controlled analgesia: optimising the experience, *Clinical Nursing Research*, 8(3): 283–294.

Engelhardt, T., Steel, E. Johnston, G. (2002) Tramadol for pain relief in children undergoing tonsillectomy: a comparison with morphine, *Paediatric Anaesthesia*, 13: 249–252.

Falanga, I.J., Lafrenaye, S., Mayer, S.K and Tetrault, J-P. (2006) Management of acute pain in children: safety and efficacy of a nurse-controlled algorithm for pain relief, *Acute Pain*, 8(2): 45–54.

Gan, T.J. and Meyer, T. (2006a) Revised consensus guidelines: management of postoperative vomiting in pediatric patients, [abstract no. A-971], *Anesthesiology*, 105: A971.

Gan, T.J., Meyer, T. and Apfel C.C. (2006) Revised consensus guidelines: pediatric POV [poster], *American Society of Anesthesiologists*, 14–18 October 2006, Chicago, IL.

Gatti, J.M., Perez-Brayfield, M., Kirsch, A.J., Smith, E.A., Scherz, H.C. Massad, C.A. and Broecker, B.H. (2001) Acute urinary retention in children, *Journal of Urology*, 165: 918–921.

Gazal, G. and Mackie, I.C. (2007) A comparison of paracetamol, ibuprofen or their combination for pain relief following extractions in children under general anaesthesia: a randomized controlled trial, *International Journal of Paediatric Dentistry*, 7(3): 169–177.

Gold, J.I., Townsend, J., Jury, D.L., Kant, A.J., Gallardo, C.C. and Joseph, M.H. (2006) Current trends in pediatric pain management: from preoperative to the postoperative bedside and beyond, *Seminars in Anesthesia, Perioperative Medicine and Pain*, 25(3): 159–171.

Goldman, R.D. (2006) Intranasal drug delivery for children with acute illness, *Current Drug Therapy*, 1(1): 127–130.

Greco, C. and Berde, C. (2005) Pain management for the hospitalised pediatric patient, *Pediatric Clinics of North America*, 52: 995–1027.

Harrop, J.E. (2007) Management of pain in children, *Archives of Disease in Childhood, Education and Practice Edition*, 92: ep101-ep108.

Hiller, A., Meretoja, O.A., Korpela, R., Piiparinen, S. and Taivainen, T. (2006) The analgesic efficacy of acetaminophen, ketoprofen, or their combination for pediatric surgical patients having soft tissue or orthopedic procedures, *Anesthesia and Analgesia*, 102(5): 1365–1371.

Hoberman, A., Paradise, J.L., Reynolds, E.A. and Urkin, J. (1997) Efficacy of Auralgan for treating ear pain in children with acute otitis media, *Archives of Pediatric and Adolescent Medicine*, 151: 675–678.

Johnston, C.C., Gagnon, A.J., Pepler, C.J. and Bourgault, P. (2005) Pain in the emergency department with one-week follow-up of pain resolution, *Pain Research and Management*, 10(2): 67–70.

Kendall, J.M., Reeves, B.C. and Latter, V.S. (2001) Multicentre randomised controlled trial of nasal diamorphine for analgesia in children and teenagers with clinical fractures, *British Medical Journal*, 322: 261–265.

Kokinsky, E. and Thornberg, E. (2003) Postoperative pain control in children: a guide to drug choice, *Pediatric Drugs*, 5(11): 751–762.

Kokki, H., Rasnanen, I., Lasalmi, M., Lehtola, S., Ranta, V.P., Vanamo, K. and Ojanpera, I. (2006) Comparison of oxycodone pharmacokinetics after buccal and sublingual administration in children, *Clinical Pharmacokinetics*, 45(7): 745–754.

Kovac, A.L. (2007) Management of postoperative nausea and vomiting in children, *Pediatric Drugs*, 9(1): 47–69.

Lehmann, K.A. (2005) Recent developments in patient-controlled analgesia, *Journal of Pain and Symptom Management*, 29(5): S72-S89.

Lin, C. and Durieux, M.E. (2005) Ketamine and kids: an update, *Paediatric Anaesthesia*, 15: 91–97.

Llewellyn, N. and Moriarty, A. (2007) The national pediatric epidural audit, *Pediatric Anesthesia*, 17: 520–533.

Locatelli, B., Ingelmo, P., Sonzogni, V., Zanella, A., Gatti, V., Spotti, A., Di Marco, S. and Fumagalli, R. (2005) Randomized, double-blind, phase III, controlled trial comparing levobupivacaine 0.25%, ropivacaine 0.25% and bupivacaine 0.25% by the caudal route in children. *British Journal of Anaesthesia*, 94(3): 366–371.

Lönnqvist, P.-A. and Morton, N.S. (2005) Postoperative analgesia in infants and children, *British Journal of Anaesthesia*, 95(1): 59–68.

Lönnqvist, P.-A., Ivani, G. and Moriarty, T. (2002) Use of caudal-epidural opioids in children: still state of the art or the beginning of the end? *Paediatric Anaesthesia*, 12: 747–749.

Macintyre, P.E. (2001) Safety and efficacy of patient-controlled analgesia, *British Journal of Anaesthesia*, 87(1): 36–46.

Malviya, S., Voepel-Lewis, T., Tait, A.R., Merkel, S., Tremper, K. and Naughton, N. (2002) Depth of sedation in children undergoing computed tomography: validity and reliability of the University of Michigan Sedation Scale (UMSS), *British Journal of Anaesthesia*, 88(2): 241–245.

McClain, B.C. (2006) Pediatric hospital-based pain care. In Finley, G.A., McGrath, P.J. and Chambers, C.T (eds.) *Bringing Pain Relief to Children: Treatment Approaches*, Humana Press, Totowa, pp 1–30.

McDonald, A.J. and Cooper, M.G. (2001) Patient-controlled analgesia: an appropriate method of pain control in children, *Paediatric Drugs*, 3(4): 273–284.

Morton, N.S. (2007) Management of postoperative pain in children, *Archives of Disease in Childhood Education and Practice Ed*, 92: ep14-ep19.

Morton, N.S. and O'Brien, K. (1999) Analgesic efficacy of paracetamol and diclofenac in children receiving PCA morphine, *British Journal of Anaesthesia*, 82: 715–717.

Murat, I., Gall, O. and Tourniaire, B. (2003) Procedural pain in children, evidence-based best practice and guidelines, *Regional Anesthesia and Pain Medicine*, 28: 561–572.

Naja, M.Z., El-Rajab, M., Kabalan, W., Ziade, M.F., and Al-Tannir, M.A. (2005) Pre-incisional infiltration for pediatric tonsillectomy: a randomized double-blind clinical trial, *International Journal of Pediatric Otorhinolaryngology*, 69(10): 1333–1341.

Oberlander, T.F. and Symons, F.L. (2006) *Pain in Children and Adults with Developmental Disabilities*, Paul Brookes Publishing Co., Baltimore, Maryland.

Oztekin, S., Hepağuşlar, H., Kar, A.A., Ozzeybek, D., Artikaslan, O., and Elar, Z. (2002) Preemptive diclofenac reduces morphine use after remifentanil-based anaesthesia for tonsillectomy, *Paediatric Anaesthesia*, 12(8): 694–699.

Pasero, C. and McCaffery, M. (2002) Monitoring sedation, *American Journal of Nursing*, 102(2): 67–69.

Pasero, C., Portenoy, R. and McCaffery, M. (1999) Opioid analgesics. In McCaffery, M. and Pasero, C. (1999) *Pain: Clinical Manual*, 2nd edition, Mosby, St Louis, pp. 161–299.

Pendeville, P.E., Von Montigny, S., Dort, J.P. and Veyckemans, F. (2000) Double-blind randomised study of tramadol vs. paracetamol in analgesia after day-case tonsillectomy in children, *European Journal of Anaesthesiology*, 17: 576–582.

Pickering, A.E., Bridge, H.S., Nolan, J. and Stoddart, P.A. (2002) Double-blind placebo-controlled analgesic study of ibuprofen or rofecoxib in combination with paracetamol for tonsillectomy in children, *British Journal of Anaesthesia*, 88(1): 72–77.

Polkki, T., Pietila, A-M. and Vehvilamen-Julkunen, K. (2003) Hospitalized children's descriptions of their experiences with postsurgical pain-relieving methods, *International Journal of Nursing Studies*, 40: 33–44.

Purday, J.P., Reichert, C.C. and Merrick, P.M. (1996) Comparative effects of three doses of intravenous ketorolac or morphine on emesis and analgesia for restorative dental surgery in children, *Canadian Journal of Anaesthesia*, 43(3): 221–225.

Pyati, S. and Gan, T.J. (2007) Perioperative pain management, *CNS Drugs*, 21(3): 185–211.

Ragg, P. (1997a) Epidural analgesia in children. In McKenzie, I.M., Gaukroger, P.B., Ragg, P.G. and Brown, T.C.K. (eds.) *Manual of Acute Pain Management in Children*, Churchill Livingstone, New York, pp. 47–61.

Ragg, P. (1997b) Safety and monitoring of analgesic techniques. In McKenzie, I.M., Gaukroger, P.B., Ragg, P.G. and Brown, T.C.K. (eds.) *Manual of Acute Pain Management in Children*, Churchill Livingstone, New York, pp. 91–96.

Ragg, P. and McKenzie, I.M. (1997) Management of common problems. In McKenzie, I.M., Gaukroger, P.B., Ragg, P.G. and Brown, T.C.K. (eds.) *Manual of Acute Pain Management in Children*, Churchill Livingstone, New York, pp. 109–114.

Ready, L.B. and Edwards, W.T. (eds.) (1992) *Management of Acute Pain: A Practical Guide*, Task Force on Acute Pain, International Association for the Study of Pain, IASP Publications, Seattle.

Rose, M. (2007) Systemic analgesics for children, *Anaesthesia and Intensive Care Medicine*, 8(5): 184–188.

Royal Children's Hospital, Melbourne. (2007) Acute Pain Management Clinical Practice Guidelines 2007, http://ww.rch.org.au/anaes/pain/index.cfm?doc_id=2384 (accessed 2 November /2007).

Rusy, L.M. and Weisman, S.J. (2002) Acute postoperative pediatric pain management: pearls from a busy children's hospital, *Techniques in Regional Anesthesia and Pain Management*, 6(2): 66–69.

Schechter, N.L. (2006) Treatment of acute and chronic pain in the outpatient setting. In Finley, G.A., McGrath, P.J. and Chambers, C.T (eds.) *Bringing Pain Relief to Children: Treatment Approaches*, Humana Press, Totowa, pp. 31–58.

Telfer, P., Coen, P., Chakravorty, S., Wilkey, O., Evans, J., Newell, H., Smalling, B., Amos, R., Stephens, A., Rogers, D. and Kirkham, F. (2007) Clinical outcomes in children with sickle cell disease living in England: a neonatal cohort in East London, *Haematology*, 92: 905–912.

Thomas, J. (2008) Opioid-induced bowel dysfunction, *Journal of Pain and Symptom Management*, 35(1): 103–113.

Vessey, J.A. and Carlson, K.L. (1996) Nonpharmacological interventions to use with children in pain, *Issues in Comprehensive Pediatric Nursing*, 19:169–182.

Viitanen, H., Tuominen, N., Vaaraniemi, H., Nikanne, E. and Annila, P. (2003) Analgesic efficacy of rectal acetaminophen and ibuprofen alone or in combination for paediatric day-case adenoidectomy, *British Journal of Anaesthesia*, 91: 363–367.

Vincent, C.V.H. and Denyes, M.J. (2004) Relieving children's pain: nurses' abilities and analgesic administration practices, *Journal of Pediatric Nursing*, 19(1): 40–50.

Wennström, B. and Reinsfelt, B. (2002) Rectally administered diclofenac (voltaren) reduces vomiting compared with opioid (morphine) after strabismus surgery in children, *Acta Anaesthesiologica Scandanavica*, 46(4): 430–434.

Williams, D.G. and Howard, R.F. (2003) Epidural analgesia in children: a survey of current opinions and practices amongst UK paediatric anaesthetists, *Paediatric Anaesthesia*, 13: 769–776.

World Health Organization (1996) *Cancer Pain Relief*, 2 nd edition, World Health Organization, Geneva.

World Health Organization (1998) *Cancer Pain Relief and Palliative Care in Children*, World Health Organization, Geneva.

Wrede-Seaman, L. (2005) *Pediatric pain and symptom management algorithms for palliative care*, Intellicard Inc, Yakima, Washington.

CHAPTER 8

Chronic Pain in Children

Jennifer Stinson and Elizabeth Bruce

Introduction

This chapter provides an overview of chronic pain in children. It defines and describes the main types of chronic pain experienced by children and adolescents and discusses the impact of this on the child and family. Key factors that have been found to influence the development and maintenance of chronic pain are outlined. The principles of treatment are discussed and the role of the multidisciplinary team in the management of children's chronic pain is described.

8.1 What is Chronic Pain?

Chronic pain is a term used to describe persistent or recurrent pain. Chronic pain in children and adolescents is commonly defined as any prolonged pain that lasts a minimum of three months, or any recurrent pain that occurs at least three times throughout a minimum period of three months (Van Den Kerkhof and Van Dijk 2006). No definition of chronic pain exists for infants (Stevens and Pillia Riddell 2006).

BOX 8.1

APS Position Statement on chronic pain in children

'Chronic pain in children is the result of a dynamic integration of biological processes, psychological factors, and socio-cultural context, considered within a developmental trajectory. This category of pain includes persistent (ongoing) and recurrent (episodic) pain with possible fluctuations in severity, quality, regularity, and predictability. Chronic pain can occur in single or multiple body regions and can involve single or multiple organ systems.'

Source: Bursch et al. 2006a, p.1

The Pediatric Chronic Pain Task Force, which is part of the American Pain Society (APS), has provided a description of chronic pain in children (Box 8.1).

Chronic pain in children is a serious health problem due to its complex nature and can result in significant disability (Roth-Isigkeit et al. 2005; Gauntlett-Gilbert and Eccleston 2007; Martin et al. 2007). Table 8.1 outlines the main differences between acute and chronic pain. Unlike acute pain which usually has an identifiable cause, most chronic pain conditions in children are idiopathic in nature or unexplained. This often results in patients and families continuing their search for an underlying cause for the pain, which leads to

Table 8.1   Differences between acute and chronic pain

Characteristic	Acute pain	Chronic pain
Cause	Usually single obvious cause (e.g. tissue damage due to surgery)	Usually multiple causative or triggering factors Neuronal or CNS abnormality (plasticity, sensitisation)
Type	Nociceptive and or neuropathic	Nociceptive, neuropathic or mixed; psychosocial factors
Purpose	Protective; activation of sympathetic nervous system	No protective function; rarely accompanied by signs of activation of sympathetic nervous system
Duration	Short-lived (days to weeks)	Long lasting (> 3 months) or recurring beyond time of normal healing, may be associated with chronic disease
Pain intensity	Usually proportionate to severity of injury	Often out of proportion to objective physical findings
Treatment	Usually easy to treat with single modalities (pharmacological or physical)	More difficult to treat, requiring multidisciplinary, multimodal treatment approach
Outcome	Expected to resolve with healing	Pain persists in significant proportion (30–62%) (Hunfield et al. 2002; Perquin et al. 2003; El-Metwally et al. 2005; Martin et al. 2007); with smaller proportion developing pain-associated disability syndrome (Bursch et al. 1998)

Source: Adapted from Goldman (2002)

multiple medical investigations in a vicious cycle of doctor shopping to find a diagnosis and cure. During this process the child often receives little, if any, appropriate pain management. This cycle elevates the child's fear and the parent's stress and anxiety, which may further contribute to pain symptoms and disability (Eccleston and Malleson 2003).

Practice point

Acute and chronic pain may occur concurrently. Acute pain that is not properly treated may become chronic.

Children with chronic pain respond differently to those with acute pain and may not seem to be in pain. They may appear withdrawn and unresponsive, or have a seemingly exaggerated response to a usually non-painful stimulus such as light touch.

Source: Eccleston et al. (2006)

8.2 How Common is Chronic Pain in Children?

Little is known about the epidemiology of chronic pain in children (McGrath, 1999; Van Den Kerkhof and van Dijk 2006). Table 8.2 provides information regarding the nature and prevalence of chronic pain in children from 16 studies carried out between 1999–2004 (Van Den Kerkhof and Van Dijk 2006). Prevalence estimates range from 3.7% for back pain (Groholt et al. 2003) to 97% for non-migraine headaches (Bandell-Hoekstra et al. 2001). These findings indicate that chronic pain is common in children and adolescents. The most common chronic pain conditions are headaches, abdominal pain and musculoskeletal pain. A subgroup of children with recurrent and persistent pain

Table 8.2 Prevalence of chronic pain in children

Pain sites	Prevalence (range)
Abdominal pain	Female = 11–53% Male = 6.1–35% All = 8.3–43%
Back pain	Female = 5.6–43% Male = 3.7–38% All = 4.7–40%
Headache (non-migraine)	Female = 12–95% Male = 7.9–92% All = 9.8–97%
Headache (migraine)	Female = 11–53% Male = 6.1–35% All = 8.3–43%
Limb	Female = 29% Male = 32% All = 22–30%
Neck and shoulder	Female = 23–24% Male = 12% All = 17%
Overall or general pain	Female = 24–36% Male = 23–30% All = 24–80%

Source: Van Den Kerkhof and Van Dijk (2006)

(30–40%) will develop significant pain-related disability that increases with age (Perquin et al. 2000; Roth-Isigkeit et al. 2005; Martin et al. 2007). Chronic pain has been reported in children as young as three years, but is most prevalent in early teens and is more commonly reported by girls (Wilder et al. 1992; Perquin et al. 2000; Lynch et al. 2007).

Practice point

Despite the relatively high prevalence of chronic pain in children and its significant physical, psychological, social and economic impact on children and their families, it is often under-recognised and undertreated by clinicians.

The lack of objective signs (no sympathetic nervous system arousal, no overt distress) often leads the inexperienced clinician to diagnose the pain as functional or psychosomatic.

Viewing pain as organic or non-organic is harmful because it leads to over-medicalisation (inappropriate investigations, procedures, and interventions) or insufficient acknowledgement of the child's multidimensional experience and underlying neurophysiology.

Source: Bursch et al. (2006a)

8.3 Aetiology or Causes of Chronic Pain

Chronic pain may be part of a chronic medical condition, develop following surgery, illness or injury, or have no obvious cause (Table 8.3).

• Chronic pain conditions can be nociceptive, neuropathic, or mixed (combination of nociceptive and neuropathic) in nature and/or associated with psychological factors. (For definitions of nociceptive and neuropathic pain see Chapter 2.)

- Idiopathic musculoskeletal (bone, joint and muscle) pain is common (experienced by 10–35% of children) and is often associated with rheumatological conditions such as juvenile idiopathic arthritis and systemic lupus erythmatosus (El-Metwally et al. 2004). One in four children referred to paediatric rheumatology clinics present with idiopathic musculoskeletal pain (McGhee et al. 2002).
- Children with cancer can experience multiple sources of pain including: distension or infiltration of tissue by bone and tumour; inflammation (mucositis), infection and necrosis; and neuropathic pain (tumour infiltration, side effects of chemotherapy and radiation) (Hooke et al. 2002). Wolfe et al. (2000) found that in children at the palliative stage of illness, 82% of parents believed that their children suffered greatly from persistent pain.
- Children with cognitive, motor and communication impairments are at particular risk of experiencing chronic pain. For example, children with cerebral palsy commonly have musculoskeletal and abdominal pain (Castle et al. 2007).
- Pain is common in children with somatoform disorders. Mullick (2002) found that in 112 patients who met the criteria for somatoform disorder; pain was the most common symptom. Children had significantly higher rates of abdominal complaints, whereas adolescents had higher rates of headaches.

Pain disorders associated with psychological factors were previously referred to as psychogenic pain (that is, real pain caused by psychological problems). They are now referred to as *somatoform disorders* (American Psychiatric Association 2000).

> **Somatisation** is the communication of emotional distress, troubled relationships and personal predicaments through bodily symptoms in the absence of clear physical pathology (Taylor and Garralda 2003).

Table 8.3   Types of chronic pain in children

Category/Aetiology	Examples
Disease-related pain	Sickle cell disease Haemophilia Epidermolysis bullosa Osteogenesis imperfecta Rheumatological conditions Post-viral (e.g. herpes) Cancer and treatment-related pain (e.g. chemotherapy, radiotherapy)
Injury-related pain	Burns Sprains, fractures Post-surgery (e.g. phantom limb pain, scar tissue, nerve damage) Complex regional pain syndrome (e.g. post-fracture or sprain)
Non-specific (unexplained/chronic benign pain)	Headache Recurrent abdominal pain Complex regional pain syndrome Low back pain Widespread chronic pain Chronic fatigue syndrome
Somatoform disorders	Pain disorder Conversion disorder

Psychological factors are judged to have a major role in the onset, severity, exacerbation or maintenance of certain somatoform disorders. Pain that is solely psychological in nature is rare (<2%) (Taylor and Garralda 2003). The explanation of pain as psychogenic is often considered unhelpful, partly due to the misconceptions attached to such a diagnosis and because all pain has psychological, social and biological components (McGrath et al. 2003).

8.3.1 Common chronic pain conditions in children and adolescents

Headache

> Headaches are distinguished and defined largely on the basis of their clinical features.
>
> Headaches have been classified by the International Headache Society (see http://216.25.100.131/ihscommon/guidelines/pdfs/ihc_II_main_no_print.pdf).
>
> The most common types in children are migraine with and without aura (Table 8.4) and tension-type headaches. Migraine headaches may transform into tension-type headaches and vice versa; and these two types may co-exist in the early phases (Grazzi 2004).
>
> Chronic daily headache is a relatively new diagnostic category to categorise those individuals who do not meet the criteria for episodic tension or migraine headaches. It is defined as an almost continual headache (>15 days per month) in the absence of a serious underlying medical condition (McGrath 2006a).

Headaches are the most commonly reported chronic pain in children. For the most common types of headaches in children, the actual causes are not known. Other causes of headaches include:

- epilepsy;
- migraine;

Table 8.4   Types of paediatric migraines

Paediatric migraine without aura	Paediatric migraine with aura
At least 5 distinct attacks	Fulfils criteria for migraine without aura
Headache attack lasting 1–48 h	At least 3 of the following:
	• One or more fully reversible aura symptoms indicating focal cortical and or brainstem dysfunction • At least one aura developing gradually over more than 4 min or two or more symptoms occurring in succession • No aura lasting more than 60 minutes • Headache follows in less than 60 minutes
Headache has at least 2 of the following: • Bilateral location (frontal/temporal) or unilateral location • Pulsating quality • Moderate to severe intensity • Aggravated by routine physical activity During headache, at least one of the following: • Nausea and/or vomiting • Photophobia and/or phonophobia (heightened sensitivity to sound)	
Source: Van Den Kerkhof and Van Dijk (2006)	

- ophthalmologic and dental causes;
- psychological factors;
- post-traumatic syndrome (e.g. post-traumatic headache);
- sinusitis;
- trauma;
- tumours and raised intracranial pressure;
- systemic diseases (e.g. arteriovenous malformation);
- drugs (e.g. chronic opioid use);
- sleep apnoea.

(Hämäläinen and Masek 2003)

Practice point

It is imperative to rule out serious neurological or neurosurgical causes for the headaches (e.g. cerebral haemorrhage, shunt malfunction) before implementing chronic pain management strategies.

Chronic abdominal pain

Chronic abdominal pain is defined as three or more bouts of abdominal pain and associated gastrointestinal symptoms over a period of at least three months that are severe enough to interfere with normal activities. Chronic abdominal pain is common (10–15%) in childhood, usually affecting children between 5 and 15 years of age. Females appear to be affected slightly more than males. The majority of children with chronic abdominal pain have no obvious underlying cause for their pain and therefore are classified as having functional abdominal pain (Jones and Walker 2006).

Functional abdominal pain (FAP) is defined as abdominal pain without obvious pathology and includes functional dyspepsia (indigestion), irritable bowel syndrome, abdominal migraine and functional abdominal pain syndrome (Subcommittee on Chronic Abdominal Pain 2005). Table 8.5 outlines diagnosis criteria and estimated incidence within the four subgroups of FAP. Until recently the term recurrent abdominal pain (RAP) was used to describe this condition, but is now considered outdated. It is estimated that nearly one-third of children with FAP will continue to experience symptoms and disability into adulthood (Jones and Walker 2006).

The lack of an obvious cause for abdominal pain can result in considerable distress for the child and family and it is essential that children are not subjected to unnecessary tests. The signs and symptoms that may indicate underlying pathology and thus the need for further investigation include:

- weight loss;
- pain that wakes the child at night;
- abdominal pain that is not near the umbilicus;
- fever;
- dysuria;
- abnormal stools;
- abnormal blood test results.

(Scharff et al. 2003)

Musculoskeletal pain

Common chronic musculoskeletal pain conditions include complex regional pain syndrome (described under neuropathic pain), juvenile primary fibromyalgia, idiopathic chronic limp (growing pains) and back pain syndromes (El-Metwally et al. 2005; Connelly and Schanberg 2006).

Juvenile primary fibromyalgia syndrome (JPFS) is characterised by diffuse chronic musculoskeletal pain with numerous tender points on palpation in the absence of an underlying condition. Etiology is unknown and it is more common in females during adolescence. Other common symptoms include sleep disturbances, chronic anxiety and/or tension, fatigue and abdominal pain (Anthony and Schanberg 2001).

Idiopathic chronic limb pain in children is often referred to as *growing pains*. Growing pains typically present as recurrent bilateral non-articular pain in the lower extremities that occur late in the day or at night. In severe cases, pain can occur daily and have a significant impact on the child and family (Connelly and Schanberg 2006).

Chronic low back pain in children was thought to be relatively uncommon. However, recent epidemiological evidence suggests that it has a marked impact on daily activities and is an increasing problem in school-age children and adolescents (Watson et al. 2002; Bejia et al. 2005). Psychosocial factors (Kopek and Sayre 2005; Diepenmaat et al. 2006),

Table 8.5   Types of functional abdominal pain

Diagnosis	Criteria
Irritable bowel syndrome (44.9%)	1 Abdominal discomfort or pain with 2 of 3 features: • Relieved with defecation • Onset associated with change in stool frequency • Onset associated with change in stool form/appearance 2 No structural or metabolic abnormalities to explain symptoms
Functional dyspepsia (15.9%)	1 Persistent or recurrent pain or discomfort centred in the upper abdomen 2 No evidence that organic disease is likely to explain symptoms 3 No evidence that dyspepsia is relieved by defecation or associated with change in stool frequency/form 4 May be characterised by abdominal fullness, bloating, nausea, early satiety
Functional abdominal pain syndrome (7.5%)	1 Continuous or nearly continuous abdominal pain in school-age children or adolescent 2 No or only occasional relation of pain to physiological events (e.g. eating) 3 Some loss of daily functioning 4 The pain is not malingering or feigned 5 Insufficient criteria for other functional GI disorders that would explain pain 6 No structural, inflammatory or metabolic abnormalities to explain symptoms
Abdominal migraine (4.7%)	1 Three or more episodes, in preceding 12 months, of midline abdominal pain lasting several hours to days, paroxysmal in nature 2 No evidence of metabolic, structural or CNS disease 3 Two of the following features: • headaches during episodes • photophobia during episodes • family history of migraines • headache confined to one side of head • sensory, visual or motor aura preceding episodes

Source: Jones and Walker (2006)

as well as physical activity and body positioning during repeated activities have been shown to increase the risk of low back pain (Bejia et al. 2005; Kopek and Sayre 2005; Diepenmaat et al. 2006).

Neuropathic pain

What is neuropathic pain?

Neuropathic pain is often described as burning, stabbing or shooting and may be spontaneous or *evoked* (that is, having a trigger factor such as touch or change in temperature).

Neuropathic pain conditions may also be characterised by sensory disturbances such as *allodynia, dysaesthesia, hyperalgesia, hyperpathia and paraesthesia* (Box 8.2).

There may also be motor abnormalities such as tremor, spasms, atrophy, dystonia and weakness and autonomic disturbances such as cyanosis, erythema, mottling, increased sweating, swelling and poor capillary refill (Berde et al. 2003; Johnson 2004).

BOX 8.2

Terms associated with neuropathic pain

Allodynia: Severe pain triggered by innocuous (non-harmful) stimuli such as stroking, the touch of clothing on the affected area, or changes in temperature.

Dysaesthesia: An unpleasant abnormal sensation, which may be spontaneous or evoked (e.g. shooting, tingling sensations).

Hyperalgesia: A reduced threshold to pain.

Hyperpathia: Increased pain from stimuli which are normally painful (e.g. increased sharpness from a pin prick).

Paraesthesia: An abnormal sensation, which may be spontaneous or evoked (e.g. pins and needles).

Further information about the anatomy and physiology of neuropathic pain can be found in Chapter 2.

Examples of neuropathic pain in children include complex regional pain syndrome (CRPS) and phantom limb pain, which is pain that is felt in the area of a limb that has been amputated. Children with cancer also experience neuropathic pain, which may either be due to the cancer treatment (e.g. chemotherapy or radiotherapy) or the underlying cancer itself (e.g. due to the tumour impinging on a spinal nerve root).

8.3.2　Common types of neuropathic pain conditions

Complex regional pain syndrome

What is complex regional pain syndrome?

Complex regional pain syndrome (CRPS) is a syndrome of chronic neuropathic pain associated with dysfunction of the autonomic nervous system.

CRPS is further classified into two types: type 1 manifests following injury without a definable nerve lesion and type 2 occurs following damage to an identifiable nerve.

The pathophyisology of CRPS is not well understood; however, it is believed to be a systemic disease involving both the central and peripheral nervous systems (Jäing and Baron 2004).

Both types of CRPS are also known by other names: CRPS I is referred to as reflex sympathetic dystrophy (RSD), while CRPS II is referred to as causalgia.

The incidence of CRPS in children is not well defined, but it is more common in females in later childhood and adolescence. CRPS in children is seen more commonly in the lower limbs and often follows a minor injury or traumatic event (Wilder et al. 1992; Dangel 1998; Low et al. 2007). The pain is persistent and is disproportionate to the initiating injury (Connelly and Schanberg 2006).

A clinical diagnosis of CRPS requires:

- the report of at least two symptoms of persistent neuropathic pain, for example: burning, dysaesthesia, paraesthesia, mechanical allodynia, hyperalgesia to cold; and
- at least two physical signs of autonomic nervous system dysfunction, for example: cyanosis, mottling, oedema, cooling of the affected area, hyperhydrosis (excessive sweating) (Low et al. 2007).

Children with CRPS have a better prognosis than adults (Berde et al. 2003). Most children will have complete resolution of symptoms with non-invasive treatment; however a small proportion will continue to have pain or relapse (20%) (Low et al. 2007). Early recognition and treatment are associated with the best chance of good outcomes.

Phantom limb pain

Congenital or traumatic (accidental or surgical) loss of a limb can result in sensations in the missing limb; some that are painful (*phantom limb pain;* described as burning, cramping, shooting) and some that are not (*phantom limb sensation;* described as tingling or itchy). In addition, there can be pain in the stump (*stump pain*). These sensations tend to begin within days of amputation and they usually decrease in frequency and duration over time (Wilkins et al. 1998). Wilkins et al. (1998) in a retrospective survey of children (*n* = 66) with congenital or traumatic amputation found that less than half the sample experienced phantom sensations or pain; however, those with traumatic amputation were more likely to experience these sensations.

8.3.3 Factors triggering and maintaining chronic pain

As outlined in Chapter 3 there are many factors that influence a child's perception of pain and ways they behave when in pain. Many studies have provided evidence (primarily using cross-sectional studies) that a few isolated biological, physical, psychological, family and social factors play an important role in chronic pain in children (Figure 8.1). However, little is known about which factors or combination of factors predispose children to chronic pain and disability:

- Certain situational factors can intensify pain and distress, while others can eventually trigger pain episodes and prolong pain-related disability or maintain the cycle of repeated pain episodes in recurrent pain syndromes (McGrath 2006b).
- Miró et al. (2007) conducted a Delphi poll to establish consensus on the factors that predict chronic pain in children. Excessive use of healthcare services, a tendency to somatise, and children's catastrophising had the greatest influence on pain.
- Age, sex and psychosocial factors are now recognised as important factors in the development of persistent pain and pain-related disability (McGrath 2006b).
- In a recent population-based Canadian study, being female and having high levels of depressive and anxiety symptoms at age 10 years were highly predictive of the likelihood to develop and maintain pain across adolescence (Stanford et al. 2008).
- There is evidence that chronic pain in childhood persists throughout adolescence and into adulthood (Perquin et al. 2003; Martin et al. 2007).
- Early identification of risk factors for development of chronic pain may influence outcome (Miró et al. 2007).

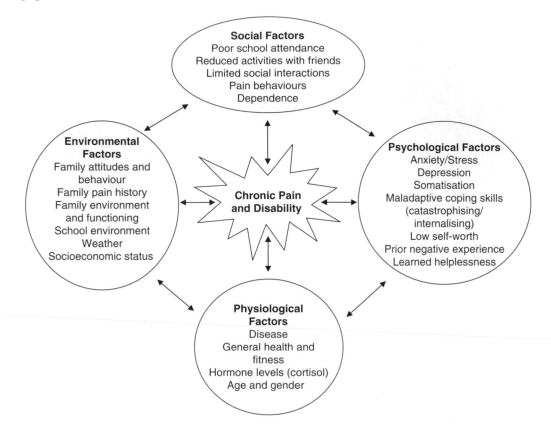

Figure 8.1   Factors associated with children's chronic pain.

Coping styles of the child, parents and family as a whole have a huge influence on chronic pain:

- Maladaptive or ineffective coping styles have been linked to anxiety, depression and functional disability in children with chronic pain (Kashikar-Zuck et al. 2001, 2002; Eccleston et al. 2004).
- Pain catastrophising, or describe pain as awful, horrible and unbearable, is recognised as an important factor in chronic pain in children and adults (Sullivan and Adams 2006).
- Pain catastrophising is a multidimensional construct that includes: rumination (excessive focus on pain sensations), magnification (exaggerating the threat value of pain sensations) and helplessness (perceiving oneself as unable to cope with pain symptoms) (Sullivan and Adams 2006).
- Studies have found associations between catastrophising and increased pain, disability, depression and emotional distress in children and adolescents with chronic pain (Kashikar-Zuck 2001; Crombez et al. 2003; Merlijn et al. 2006; Vervoort et al. 2006; Lynch et al. 2007).

Practice point

Education of both the child *and* family is essential to reduce fear and misconceptions related to chronic pain and to teach appropriate coping strategies (relaxation and cognitive restructuring).

As outlined in Chapter 3, *gender differences* are apparent in relation to chronic pain in older school-age children and adolescents. Chronic pain is more common in girls, who also report more intense, more frequent and more prolonged pain than boys (Perquin et al. 2000; Hunfield et al. 2001; Martin et al. 2007). Differences in coping styles also exist, with girls using more emotional coping styles such as catastrophising (Keogh and Eccleston 2006; Lynch et al. 2007). Differences in self-reported trigger factors are also present between boys and girls (Roth-Isigkeit et al. 2005).

> Due to lack of knowledge of the psychosocial aspects and complexity of chronic pain, children with unexplained or persistent chronic pain are sometimes viewed as malingerers or attention seekers, or made to feel that the problem is *all in their head*.
>
> This can further exacerbate the pain and increases the family's distrust of health professionals and leads them to doubt healthcare professionals' ability to diagnose and treat the pain.

Practice point

Once serious or treatable physical causes are ruled out, most children and parents need and are willing to accept an explanation based on both physical (sensitisation of pain receptors) and psychological (stress or worry) factors. This helps prevent or reduce the continued search for the cause of the pain (von Baeyer 2006).

8.4 Pain-Related Disability

Many children and adolescents experience persistent or recurrent pain; however only a small proportion become disabled by it (Gauntlett-Gilbert and Eccleston 2007):

- Chronic pain may include varying degrees of disability, from none to severe, and may be independent of the amount of tissue damage and perceived severity (Melzack and Wall 1965).
- Scharff et al. (2005) used a statistical technique to identify three levels of disability in children and adolescents ($n = 117$) with chronic pain. Of the sample 30% were classified as highly distressed (high anxiety, depression and escape/avoidance) and disabled, 18% were in the moderately distressed/disabled group, and 52% were comparatively well functioning and not distressed.
- Biological, psychological, social, cultural and developmental factors can impact pain-related functioning (Bursch et al. 2006b).
- In the Delphi poll mentioned earlier in this chapter, Miró et al. (2007) explored the factors that predict pain-related disability in children. They found that the factors that had the greatest influence on long-term disability were children's self-concept as being disabled, a hesitance to perform exercise because of fear of potential injury, and children's catastrophising.
- A recent study suggests that higher levels of functional disability are associated with greater pain intensity and depression (Gauntlett-Gibert and Eccleston 2007).
- Perceptions of self-worth seem to be important in reducing the relationship between pain and functional disability in children with chronic pain (Guite et al. 2007).

> The term **pain-associated disability syndrome** (PADS) is used to describe chronic pain in patients who, regardless of the location or cause of their pain, are unable to function effectively.
>
> This model of disability is particularly useful for children with unexplained pain, as it enables the clinician to focus attention away from the pain and its possible causes to concentrate on the factors that maintain it (Bursch et al. 1998; Hyman et al. 2002).

8.5 The Impact of Chronic Pain

Chronic pain negatively impacts all aspects of the child's life (Hunfield et al. 2001; Merlijn et al. 2006) and results in frequent use of healthcare services (Perquin et al. 2001; Sleed et al. 2005). It is associated with significant levels of functional impairment in areas such as academic performance and school attendance, emotional functioning, sleep disturbance, peer and social functioning, and parental burden (parenting stress and dysfunctional family roles).

Recent studies demonstrate that chronic pain can severely affect the lives of children and their families:

- Children describe living with chronic pain as a constant challenge that takes over all aspects of their lives (Carter et al. 2002; Castle et al. 2007).
- Roth-Isigkeit et al. (2005) explored the impact of pain on the daily lives and activities of children and adolescents ($n = 749$) with chronic pain. More than two-thirds of the sample reported restrictions in activities of daily living due to pain and 30–40% reported moderate effects of their pain on school attendance, participation in hobbies, maintenance of social contacts, appetite and sleep, and increased use of healthcare services due to pain.
- Konijnenberg et al. (2005) studied the impact of chronic pain in children ($n = 149$) with chronic pain of unknown origin. They found that 72% suffered impairment in sport activities, 51% had school absenteeism, 40% experienced restrictions in social functioning, and 34% had problems with sleep.
- Hunfield et al. (2002) studied the impact of physically unexplained chronic pain on children and their families ($n = 77$ child-parent dyads). Overall, they found that the pain had a mild impact on children and their families. However, pain showed a negative impact on family life in terms of restrictions in social activities and personal strain.
- Hunfield et al. (2001) studied the impact of chronic pain on quality of life in adolescents ($n = 128$) and their families. They found that pain had a negative impact on quality of life (physical and psychological functioning) and negatively impacted family life (restrictions in mother's social life).
- Depression, emotional distress and anxiety are common in children with chronic pain (Kashikar-Zuck et al. 2001; Merlijn et al. 2003; Konijnenberg et al. 2006).
- Family functioning can be affected and parents report a life dominated by uncertainty, fear, distress and loss (Eccelston 2005; Jordan et al. 2007).
- Parents report marital and financial problems and experience feelings of helplessness, despair and depression (Hunfield et al. 2001; Eccleston et al. 2004).

The parent–child relationship has a huge influence on the child's response to pain. Chronic pain often occurs in early teens, a stressful period for any parent–child relationship, and parents of children with chronic pain report high levels of parenting stress (Eccleston et al. 2004). Research has shown that the parent–child relationship affects the child's perception of and ability to cope with pain (Reid et al. 2005; Logan et al. 2006). Chronic pain is also more common in children who have a parent with a chronic condition (Evans et al. 2006; Evans and Keenan 2007; Saunders et al. 2007). Furthermore, children of mothers with chronic pain have been found to have more physical and psychological problems compared to having a father with chronic pain or parents without chronic pain (Evans and Keenan 2007).

8.6 The Cost of Chronic Pain

Chronic pain in adults has been shown to be extremely costly to society in terms of both treatment and lost working days. There has, however, been little research in this area in regard to children. Parents of children with chronic pain often have to take time off work to care for their child, which also has an effect on the workforce and the economy.

- Perquin et al. (2000) conducted a large (n = 6636) population-based cross-sectional survey to determine physician consultation and medication use in children with chronic pain. A total of 57% had consulted a physician and 39% had used medications for the pain.
- Perquin et al. (2001) examined the utilisation of healthcare resources for children and adolescents with benign chronic pain (n = 254). Over a three-month period, 53.4% used medication for pain, and general practitioners (31.1%) and specialists (13.9%) were consulted for pain. Physiotherapists (11.5%), psychologists (2.8%) and alternative health practitioners (4.0%) were also consulted. During the previous year, 6.4% had been hospitalised due to the pain. The most important factors linked to healthcare utilisation were gender, various pain characteristics, school absenteeism and disability.
- The cost of adolescent chronic pain in the UK has been estimated to be £3,840 million per year or £8,000 per adolescent per year, including direct and indirect costs (Sleed et al. 2005).
- Children with chronic pain often have long periods of absence from school and their social and emotional functioning is affected. This can impact their long-term development and future role within society (Eccleston 2005).

8.7 Management of Chronic Pain

The management of chronic pain involves the use of a range of psychological, physical and pharmacological interventions (Table 8.6):

- The main goal of treatment is to return the child to a functional state that will enable them to participate in daily activities and return to school, rather than focusing solely on reducing or controlling the pain.
- As has been discussed earlier in this chapter and in Chapter 3, pain is a bio-psycho-social phenomenon and hence a multidisciplinary, multimodal approach that incorporates the three Ps (physical, psychological and pharmacological interventions) is likely to be most effective.
- Decisions regarding the most appropriate treatments should be individualised and based on the assessment of the child.
- Interventions should be aimed at treating any trigger factors, as well as the underlying cause(s) of the pain wherever possible.
- Many children and adolescents with chronic pain can be managed effectively by their family doctor.
- Referral to a multidisciplinary paediatric pain programme should be considered for children with complex or ongoing chronic pain.
- There is a lack of studies involving children for many areas of treatment. In children, physical and psychological interventions are the mainstay of treatment for many types of chronic pain; with drug treatments being used only when physical and psychological interventions are insufficient.

- Treatment should also address pain-related disability with the goal of maximising functioning and improving quality of life. This approach includes specific treatment targeting possible underlying pain mechanisms, as well as symptom-focused management addressing pain, sleep disturbance, anxiety, or depressive feelings.

The general goals of treatment are outlined in Box 8.3.

BOX 8.3

General treatment goals

1 Increasing independent function in terms of activities of daily living, school, social and physical activities.
2 Facilitating adaptive problem-solving, communication and coping skills.
3 Reducing specific symptoms, deficits, or problems revealed in a comprehensive bio-psycho-social assessment (e.g. anxiety, depression, poor sleep).
4 Helping children and their families to understand the nature of pain, the pain condition and its treatment from a holistic perspective.

Source: Stinson (2006)

Practice point

'Controlling pain is not merely *drug versus non-drug therapy* but rather an integrated approach' of pharmacological, physical and psychological therapies to reduce or block ascending and/or descending pain pathways as well as modifying situational factors that exacerbate pain.

Source: M'Grath (2006b, p. 1668)

Non-drug methods of pain relief

Pharmacological strategies are often insufficient in alleviating pain and increasing functioning. Non-drug methods of pain relief are discussed in Chapter 5. The methods that have been shown to be most effective in the management of chronic pain are outlined in Figure 8.2.

Physical therapies

Chronic pain often leads children to avoid physical activities due to fear of re-injury or because it exacerbates the pain. Lack of muscle use leads to loss of muscle strength, flexibility, endurance and overall de-conditioning. Therefore, physiotherapy (physical therapy) is an integral component (Table 8.6), and in certain instances, (e.g. with CRPS) it is the cornerstone of treatment for children with chronic pain (Engel and O'Rourke 2006). Physiotherapy is usually administered on an outpatient basis with the ultimate goal of teaching the child to continue the programme at home. Regular exercise (e.g. 20 minutes three times per week) can also help improve sleep, mood, self-esteem and energy levels (McCarthy et al. 2003; Engel and O'Rourke 2006; Stinson 2006).

Physiotherapists and occupational therapists are primarily, although not exclusively, involved in rehabilitation programmes for children with chronic musculoskeletal pain.

Physiotherapists apply a wide range of physical and behavioural interventions to reduce pain, prevent impairment and disability as well as to promote function.

Occupational therapists are primarily concerned with the psychosocial and environmental factors that contribute to pain and have an impact on the individual's daily activities and participation (Engel and O'Rouke 2006).

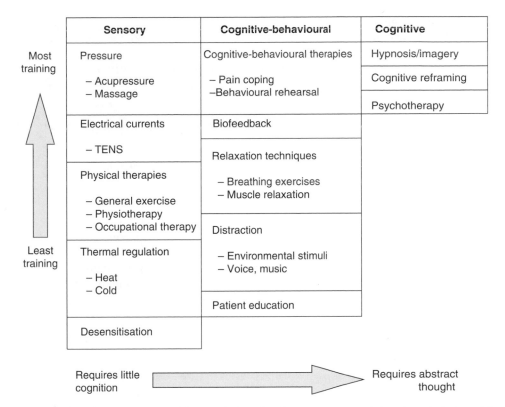

	Sensory	Cognitive-behavioural	Cognitive
Most training	Pressure – Acupressure – Massage	Cognitive-behavioural therapies – Pain coping –Behavioural rehearsal	Hypnosis/imagery
			Cognitive reframing
			Psychotherapy
	Electrical currents – TENS	Biofeedback	
		Relaxation techniques – Breathing exercises – Muscle relaxation	
	Physical therapies – General exercise – Physiotherapy – Occupational therapy		
		Distraction – Environmental stimuli – Voice, music	
Least training	Thermal regulation – Heat – Cold		
		Patient education	
	Desensitisation		

Requires little cognition → Requires abstract thought

Figure 8.2 Non-drug interventions of pain relief used in the management of chronic pain (adapted from Vessey and Carlson 1996).

Table 8.6 An overview of interventions for chronic pain management in children

Pharmacological interventions	Physical interventions	Psychological interventions
Simple analgesic drugs	Exercise	Education (about pain experience and pain problem)
Opioid analgesic drugs	Thermal stimulation (heat, cold, desensitisation)	Sleep hygiene
Anticonvulsants	Physiotherapy	Relaxation
Antidepressants	Occupational therapy	Biofeedback
Antiarrhythmics (alpha-adrenergic blockers)	Massage	Behavioural therapies
Anxiolytics	TENS	Cognitive therapies
Hypnotics	Acupuncture	Cognitive behavioural therapy (CBT)
Anaesthetic agents	Nerve blocks	Acceptance and commitment therapy (ACT)
Cannabinoids		Family therapies
		Psychotherapy

Psychological therapies

There are many psychological therapies available to treat chronic pain in children (Table 8.6). Often these therapies are integrated into a comprehensive cognitive behavioural therapy (CBT) programme that is directed at identifying and ameliorating trigger factors that affect the child's pain and disability. Such programs usually include:

- education about the pain;
- learning cognitive behavioural pain-coping skills (e.g. imagery, distraction and relaxation);
- stress management (e.g. identifying and coping with stressful situations, using thought stopping, cognitive restructuring, assertiveness and problem solving);
- relapse prevention.

(Hermann 2006)

A systematic review documented the efficacy of CBT for chronic headache and abdominal pain in children (Eccleston et al. 2003b). There is strong evidence that these psychological therapies can be administered without a therapist being physically present (Elgar and McGrath 2003), using alternative models of service delivery such as the internet (Stinson 2008) or on computer disks (CD-ROMs) (Connelly et al. 2006). Biofeedback has also been found to be effective for the treatment of headaches in children (Hermann and Blanchard 2002). (CBT and biofeedback are discussed in more detail in Chapter 5.)

More recently, acceptance and commitment therapy (ACT) is being adopted as a treatment approach in chronic pain programmes (Wicksell 2007). This approach emphasises the acceptance of or willingness to experience pain and other interfering experiences (fear of pain with activities) rather than trying to control or reduce symptoms. The goal is to achieve functionality even in the presence of interfering pain and distress. There is early evidence of the effectiveness of this approach in children with chronic pain (Wicksell et al. 2005, 2007).

Sleep hygiene

Sleep disturbances are common in children with chronic pain (Lewin and Dahl 1999; Palermo and Kiska 2005). Pain can interfere with the quality and quantity of sleep and insufficient sleep can cause daytime sequelae (behavioural and emotional changes) that undermine the coping skills necessary for effective pain management. Therefore, efforts should be directed towards improving the sleep hygiene (good sleep habits) of children with chronic pain.

For specific strategies to improve sleep hygiene see the National Sleep Foundation at http://www.sleepfoundation.org.

Pharmacological interventions

Pharmacological interventions are of benefit for certain types of chronic pain, although research involving children is extremely limited. Few medications are specifically created or licensed for use in children, especially for the treatment of chronic pain (Grégoire and Finley 2007). The clinical use of these medications in children is extrapolated from the research evidence in adults with chronic pain. The evidence currently available is summarised in Box 8.4. See Chapter 4 for additional information.

Invasive therapies

Non-invasive therapies are the mainstay of treatment of paediatric chronic pain conditions. However, intravenous regional analgesia (single regional anaesthesia blocks or continuous lumbar sympathetic blocks) can be a useful adjunct in children with CRPS who do not respond to treatment with non-invasive therapies (Dangel 1998). More recently, spinal cord stimulation has been reported to be effective in a case series of seven female adolescents with severe, incapacitating and therapy-resistant CRPS type I (Olsson et al. 2008).

BOX 8.4
Evidence for pharmacological interventions

Anticonvulsants

Gabapentin, pregabalin, carbamazepine, phenytoin are effective for the management of adult neuropathic pain (Wiffen et al. 2000; Mellegers et al. 2001; Moulin et al. 2007).

Gabapentin has been reported to be effective in single case studies of children with complex regional pain syndrome (Tong and Nelson 2000; Wheeler et al. 2000) and in a study of seven children with phantom limb pain (Rusy et al. 2001).

Gabapentin and pregabalin are licensed for use in adult neuropathic pain and although not licensed, both are used for the management of chronic pain in children.

Oxycarbazepine was reported to be effective in a singe case study of an adolescent with therapy-resistant CRPS (Lalwani et al. 2005).

Despite the frequent use of anticonvulsants (especially gabapentin) for the treatment of migraines and neuropathic pain in children, there is insufficient data regarding their efficacy in children and adolescents (Golden et al. 2006).

Antispasmodic drugs or muscle relaxants

For disease-related chronic pain, treatment of the underlying cause or condition (e.g. muscle relaxants for spasms) is effective.

Bisphosphonates

Bisphosphonates have been used to improve low bone density associated with bone pain in conditions such as osteogenesis imperfecta (Glorieux 2000; Vyskocil et al. 2005).

Cannabinoids

Cannabinoids have been found to be effective in treatment of neuropathic pain related to multiple sclerosis in adults (Burns and Ineck 2006; Iskedjian et al. 2007). There is no research on their use in children with chronic pain.

Rudich et al. (2003) report on the use of dronabinol in two adolescents with intractable neuropathic pain.

Opioids

Opioids have been shown to have some efficacy for the management of adult neuropathic pain (Moulin et al. 2007).

There is relatively little clinical or laboratory data on the use of opioids in the management of chronic pain in children (Anderson and Palmer 2006).

Tramadol has been used successfully to treat persistent pain related to Ehlers-Danlos syndrome (hypermobility type) in two siblings (Brown and Stinson 2004).

Transdermal fentanyl was found to be a safe and well-tolerated alternative to oral opioid treatment for children ($n = 199$) with malignant and non-malignant chronic pain (Finkel et al. 2005). In a recent systematic review, transdermal fentanyl was found to be a promising option for chronic pain control in children due to lower incidence of side effects (especially constipation) (Zernikow et al. 2007).

There remains a reluctance to use strong opioids in the treatment of chronic pain in children. Kimura et al. (2006) surveyed paediatric rheumatologists and found that despite the fact that children with rheumatic conditions can have persistent pain, even with treatment; two-thirds disagreed with using opioids for those patients.

BOX 8.4 Continued

Simple analgesics

Paracetamol (acetaminophen) and ibuprofen have been shown to be effective in the management of paediatric migraine (Damen et al. 2005).

Non-steroidal anti-inflammatory drugs (NSAIDs) are the first choice for the treatment of pain associated with juvenile idiopathic arthritis (Maunuksela and Olkkola 2003).

Topical NSAIDs have been shown to be effective for adult rheumatological pain (Moore et al. 1998).

Serotonin selective reuptake inhibitors (SSRIs)

Selective serotonin reuptake inhibitors (SSRIs) are less effective in adult neuropathic pain and their use in children is not recommended (Mehta 2007; Moulin et al. 2007).

Duloxetine has been used with good effect in two children with severe depression associated with chronic pain (Meighen 2007).

Lignocaine (lidocaine)

In the form of a patch or gel lignocaine has been shown to be effective in a number of adult studies of localised neuropathic pain and *antiarrhythmics* such as intravenous lignocaine and oral mexiletine have also been used, although there is less evidence of their effectiveness (Moulin et al. 2007).

Intravenous lignocaine and oral mexiletine have been reported to be effective in a case study involving an 11-year-old boy with erythromelalgia, a rare condition characterised by redness, warmth and severe burning pain of the hands and feet (Nathan et al. 2005).

Tricyclic antidepressants (TCAs)

Amitriptyline, imipramine, desipramine and nortriptyline have been shown to be effective for the management of adult neuropathic pain (McQuay et al. 1996).

TCAs not only have analgesic properties, but are useful for the management of associated symptoms such as mild depression and disturbed sleep (Chambliss et al. 2002).

Multidisciplinary approach

The key to the success of chronic pain management in children is adopting a multidisciplinary, multimodal rehabilitation approach (Kashikar-Zuck 2006). Because of the complexity of chronic pain, no single discipline has the expertise to assess and manage it independently. While not all children require a multidisciplinary approach, the services provided by multidisciplinary pain treatment programmes (chronic pain clinics) are considered the optimal therapeutic model for the management of chronic pain in children (Peng et al. 2007).

Chronic pain clinics

Specialised interdisciplinary chronic pain teams are now the standard of care for children with complex chronic pain conditions (Stinson 2006). These generally include specialist physicians (e.g. anaesthetists, neurologists and psychiatrists), nurses and allied health professionals (e.g. psychologists, occupational therapists and physiotherapists) (Peng et al. 2007). More recently, teams may also include complementary and alternative therapists (e.g. acupuncturists and/or massage therapists). The specific team members involved in any one case depend on the individual needs of the child and family (Stinson 2006).

A child's initial consultation includes either a joint interview and physical examination or separate interviews with each healthcare professional. Comprehensive physical and psychosocial assessments may typically last a few hours to a full day, depending on the child's previous diagnostic tests and the team's set of core assessment measures (e.g. standardised sensory testing, questionnaires). The team then meets to formulate the child's diagnosis and treatment plan (Figure 8.3).

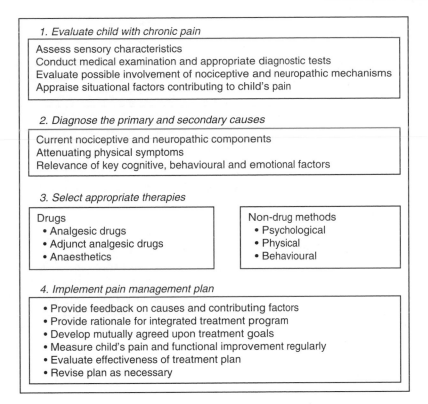

1. *Evaluate child with chronic pain*

Assess sensory characteristics
Conduct medical examination and appropriate diagnostic tests
Evaluate possible involvement of nociceptive and neuropathic mechanisms
Appraise situational factors contributing to child's pain

2. *Diagnose the primary and secondary causes*

Current nociceptive and neuropathic components
Attenuating physical symptoms
Relevance of key cognitive, behavioural and emotional factors

3. *Select appropriate therapies*

Drugs
• Analgesic drugs
• Adjunct analgesic drugs
• Anaesthetics

Non-drug methods
• Psychological
• Physical
• Behavioural

4. *Implement pain management plan*

• Provide feedback on causes and contributing factors
• Provide rationale for integrated treatment program
• Develop mutually agreed upon treatment goals
• Measure child's pain and functional improvement regularly
• Evaluate effectiveness of treatment plan
• Revise plan as necessary

Figure 8.3 Treatment algorithm for children with chronic pain.
Source: Adapted from Brown (2006).

The treatment plan should include:

• diagnosis (underlying causes and contributing factors);
• rationale for rehabilitation approach with a clear description of the specific treatment options;
• opportunity for the family to help fine-tune the plan.

(Stinson 2006)

There are a limited number of chronic pain services for children internationally (Peng et al. 2007). For example, a recent survey found only five multidisciplinary chronic pain programmes in Canada and all were located in large urban centres (Peng et al. 2007). Children's chronic pain services typically offer outpatient programmes, however some centres offer inpatient, day or residential treatment programmes (Berde and Solodiuk 2003). The Bath Pain Management Unit in the UK (www.bath.ac.uk/pain-management/) provides a residential programme of pain management based on the principles of cognitive behavioural therapy. Three months after attending the programme, adolescents report reduced anxiety, pain and depression, many had returned to normal activities and had improved school attendance (Eccleston et al. 2003a, 2006).

Ongoing assessment and re-evaluation of the treatment plan is essential. One way to monitor children with chronic pain is through the use of electronic pain diaries. Diaries can be used to obtain a better understanding of the impact of pain on children's daily lives and activities as well as the pain intensity (Stinson et al. 2007). Diaries can also be a useful way to help children and adolescents keep track of improvements in their physical, social and psychological functioning. (Pain assessment is discussed in detail in Chapter 6).

> **Practice point**
>
> Nurses play a key role in educating children and their families about the nature of chronic pain and the factors that intensify it, as well as pharmacological and non-drug strategies used to control the pain.

Long-term outcomes

Little research has been conducted on long-term outcomes of children treated for chronic pain conditions. While clinic waiting lists for children are shorter than for adults with chronic pain, some children may wait up to nine months to be seen in a multidisciplinary clinic (Peng et al. 2007). Chalkiadis (2001) reported on the outcomes of children (n = 207) who were treated at a multidisciplinary chronic pain clinic (outpatient and inpatient programmes) over a two-year period. The outcome was considered good for 65% of patients, with significant improvement reported in school attendance, sleep and participation in sports. Conversely, Martin et al. (2007) interviewed children (n = 143) with chronic pain three years following their last visit at a large metropolitan multidisciplinary paediatric pain clinic. A total of 62% were found to still have pain and the frequency of pain episodes increased with age. Females were found to be at higher risk for continuing pain and reported greater use of healthcare, medication and non-drug methods of pain control.

Summary

- Chronic pain in children is the result of a dynamic integration of biological processes, psychological factors, and socio-cultural context, considered within a developmental trajectory.
- Chronic pain can occur as a result of a chronic medical condition, develop following surgery, illness or injury, or have no obvious cause.
- Persistent and recurrent pains in children are common.
- Chronic pain can negatively impact all aspects of life and lead to pain-related disability.
- Children's chronic pain can impact family functioning and result in significant economic costs.
- Management of chronic pain in children is best achieved using a multidisciplinary, multimodal rehabilitative approach.
- Most chronic pain conditions can be treated using a combination of pharmacological, physical and psychological therapies.

> **Useful web resources**
>
> Great Ormond Street Hospital. Helping children with musculoskeletal chronic pain conditions. http://www.ich.ucl.ac.uk/factsheets/families/F050225/index.html
> National Children's Pain Centre: http://www.pediatricpain.org/home.php
> National Sleep Foundation: http://www.sleepfoundation.org
> Pediatric Chronic Pain: A Position Statement from the American Pain Society: http://www.ampainsoc.org/advocacy/pediatric.htm

References

American Psychiatric Association (2000) *Diagnostic and Statistical Manual of Mental Disorders, Fourth Edition, Text Revision.* http://www.behavenet.com/capsules/disorders/dsm4tr.htm (accessed 6 January 2008).

Anderson, B.J. and Palmer, G.M. (2006) Recent developments in the pharmacological management of pain in children, *Current Opinion in Anaesthesiology*, 19: 285–292.

Anthony, K.K, and Schanberg, L.E. (2001) Juvenile primary fibromyalgia syndrome, *Current Rheumatology Reports*, 3: 165–171.

Bandell-Hoekstra, I.E., Abu-Saad, H.H., Passchier, J., Frederiks, C.M., Feron, F.J. and Knipschild, P. (2001) Prevalence and characteristics of headache in Dutch schoolchildren, *European Journal of Pain*, 5: 145–153.

Bejia, I., Abid, N., Ben Salem, K., Letaief, M., Younes, M., Touzi, M. and Bergaoui, N. (2005) Low back pain in a cohort of 622 Tunisian school children and adolescents: an epidemiological study, European Spine Journal, 14: 331–336.

Berde, C.B., and Solodiuk, J. (2003) Multidisciplinary programs for management of acute and chronic pain in children. In Schechter, N.L., Berde, C.B., Yaster, M. (eds) *Pain in Infants, Children and Adolescents.* Lippincott Williams & Wilkins. Baltimore, pp. 471–486.

Berde, C.B., Lebel, A.A. and Olsson, G. (2003) Neuropathic pain in children. In Schechter, N.L., Berde, C.B. and Yaster, M. (eds.) *Pain in Infants, Children and Adolescents*, 2nd edition, Lippincott, Williams & Wilkins, Baltimore, pp. 620–641.

Brown, S.C. (2006) Cancer pain: palliative care in children. In Schmidt, R.F. and Willis, W.D. (eds.) *Encyclopaedia Reference of Pain*, Springer-Verlag, Heidelberg, pp. 220–224.

Brown, S.C. and Stinson, J. (2004) Treatment of pediatric chronic pain with tramadol hydrochloride: siblings with Ehlers-Danlos syndrome – hypermobility type, *Pain Research & Management*, 9: 209–211.

Burns, T.L. and Ineck, J.R. (2006) Cannabinoid analgesia as a potential new therapeutic option in the treatment of chronic pain, *Annals of Pharmacotherapy*, 40: 251–260.

Bursch, B., Walco, G.A. and Zeltzer, L. (1998) Clinical assessment and management of chronic pain and pain-associated disability syndrome, *Journal of Developmental & Behavioral Pediatrics*, 19: 45–53.

Bursch, B., Collier, J., Joseph, M., Kuttner, L., McGrath, P., Sethna, N., Walco, G. and Zeltzer, L. (Pediatric Chronic Pain Task Force) (2006a) *Pediatric Chronic Pain – A Position Statement from the American Pain Society.* Available from: http://www.ampainsoc.org/advocacy/pediatric.htm (accessed 11 December 2007).

Bursch, B., Tsao, J.C., Meldrum, M. and Zeltzer, L.K. (2006b) Preliminary validation of a self-efficacy scale for child functioning despite chronic pain (child and parent versions), *Pain*, 125(1–2): 35–42.

Carter, B., Lambrenos, K. and Thursfield, J. (2002) A pain workshop: an approach to eliciting the views of young people with chronic pain, *Journal of Clinical Nursing*, 11(6): 753–762.

Castle, K., Imms, C. and Howie, L. (2007) Being in pain: a phenomenological study of young people with cerebral palsy, *Developmental Medicine and Child Neurology*, 49(6): 445–449.

Chalkiadis, G.A. (2001) Management of chronic pain in children, *Medical Journal of Australia*, 175: 476–479.

Chambliss, C.R., Heggen, J., Copelan, D.N., and Pettignano, R. (2002) The assessment and management of chronic pain in children, *Paediatric Drugs*, 4: 737–746.

Connelly, M. and Schanberg, L. (2006) Latest developments in the assessment and management of chronic musculoskeletal pain syndromes in children, *Current Opinion in Rheumatology*, 18(5): 496–502.

Connelly, M., Rapoff, M.A., Thompson, N. and Connelly, W. (2006) Headstrong: a pilot study of a CD-ROM intervention for recurrent pediatric headache, *Journal of Pediatric Psychology*, 31: 737–747.

Crombez, G., Bijttebier, P., Eccleston, C., Mascagni, T., Mertens, G., Goubert, L. and Verstraeten, K. (2003) The child version of the pain catastrophizing scale (PCS-C): a preliminary validation, *Pain*, 104(3): 639–446.

Damen, L., Bruijn, J.K.J., Verhagen, A.P., Berger, M.Y., Passchier, J. and Koes, B.W. (2005) Symptomatic treatment of migraine in children: a systematic review of medication trials, *Pediatrics*, 116: 295–302.

Dangel, T. (1998) Chronic pain management in children. Part II: Reflex sympathetic dystrophy, *Paediatric Anaesthesia*, 8: 105–112.

Diepenmaat, A.C.M., Van der Wal, M.F., de Vet, H.C.W. and Hirasing, R.A. (2006) Neck/shoulder, low back, and arm pain in relation to computer use, physical activity, stress, and depression among Dutch adolescents, *Pediatrics*, 117: 412–416.

Eccleston, C. (2005) Managing chronic pain in children: the challenge of delivering chronic care in a 'modernising' health care system, *Archives of Disease in Childhood*, 90: 332–333.

Eccleston, C. and Malleson, P. (2003) Managing chronic pain in children and adolescents, *British Medical Journal*, 326: 1408–1409.

Eccleston, C., Malleson, P.N., Clinch, J., Connell, H. and Sourbut, C. (2003a) Chronic pain in adolescents: evaluation of a programme of interdisciplinary cognitive behaviour therapy, *Archives of Disease in Childhood*, 88: 881–885.

Eccleston, C., Yorke, L., Morley, S., Williams, A.C. and Mastroyannopoulou, K. (2003b) Psychological therapies for the management of chronic and recurrent pain in children and adolescents, *Cochrane Database Systematic Reviews*, CD003968.

Eccleston, C., Crombez, G., Scotford, A., Clinch, J and Connell, H. (2004) Adolescent chronic pain: patterns and predictors of emotional distress in adolescents with chronic pain and their parents, *Pain*, 108(3): 207–208.

Eccleston, C., Jordan, A.L., and Crombez, G. (2006) The impact of chronic pain on adolescents: a review of previously used measures, *Journal of Pediatric Psychology*, 31(7): 684–697.

Elgar, F.J. and McGrath, P.J. (2003) Self-administered psychosocial treatments for children and families, *Journal of Clinical Psychology*, 59:321–339.

El-Metwally, A., Salminen, J.J., Auvinen, A., Kautiainen, H. and Mikkelsson, M. (2004) Prognosis of non-specific musculoskeletal pain in preadolescents: a prospective 4-year follow-up study til adolescence, *Pain*, 110: 550–559.

El-Metwally, A., Salminen, J.J., Auvinen, A., Kautiainen, H. and Mikkelsson, M. (2005) Lower limb pain in a preadolescent population: prognosis and risk factors for chronicity – a prospective 1- and 4-year follow-up study, *Pediatrics*, 116: 673–681.

Engel, J.M. and O'Rouke, D.A. (2006) Chronic pain in children, physical medicine and rehabilitation. In Schmidt, R.F., Willis, W.D. (eds.) *Encyclopaedia Reference of Pain*, Springer-Verlag, Heidelberg, pp. 368–371.

Evans, S. and Keenan, T.R. (2007) Parents with chronic pain: Are children equally affected by fathers as mothers in pain? A pilot study, *Journal of Child Health*, 11; 143–157.

Evans, S., Shipton, E.A. and Keenan, T. (2006) The relationship between maternal chronic pain and child adjustment: the role of parenting as a mediator, *Journal of Pain*, 7: 236–243.

Finkel, J.C., Finley, A., Greco, C., Weisman, S.J. and Zeltzer, L. (2005) Transdermal fentanyl in the management of children with chronic severe pain: results from an international study, *Cancer*, 104: 2847–2857.

Gauntlett-Gilbert, J. and Eccleston, C. (2007) Disability in adolescents with chronic pain: patterns and predictors across different domains of functioning, *Pain*, 131: 132–141.

Glorieux, F.H. (2000) Bisphosphonate therapy for severe osteogenesis imperfecta, *Journal of Pediatric Endocrinology*, 13 Suppl 2: 989–992.

Golden, A.S., Haut, S.R. and Moshé, S.L. (2006) Nonepileptic use of antiepileptic drugs in children and adolescents, *Pediatric Neurology*, 34: 421–432.

Goldman, B. (2002) Acute pain. In Jovey, R.D. (ed.) *Managing Pain: The Canadian Healthcare Professional's Reference*, Healthcare and Financial Publishing, Toronto, pp. 87–102.

Grazzi, L. (2004) Headache in children and adolescents: conventional and unconventional approaches to treatment, *Neurological Science*, 25: S223–S225.

Grégoire, M.C. and Finley, G.A. (2007) Why were we abandoned? Orphan drugs in pediatric pain, *Paediatrics and Child Health*, 12: 95–96.

Groholt, E.K., Stigum, H., Nordhagen, R. and Kohler, L. (2003) Recurrent pain in children, socio-economic factors and accumulation in families, *European Journal of Epidemiology*, 18: 965–975.

Guite, J.W., Logan, D.E., Sherry, D.D. and Rose, J.B. (2007) Adolescent self-perception: associations with chronic musculoskeletal pain and functional disability, *Journal of Pain*, 8(5): 379–386.

Hämäläinen, M. and Masek, B.J. (2003) Diagnosis, classification and medical management of headache in children and adolescents. In Schechter, N.L., Berde, C.B. and Yaster, M. (eds.) *Pain in Infants, Children and Adolescents*, 2nd edition, Lippincott, Williams & Wilkins, Baltimore, pp. 707–718.

Hermann, C. (2006) Psychological treatment of pain in children. In: Schmidt R.F. and Willis, W.D. (eds.) *Encyclopaedia Reference of Pain*, Springer-Verlag, Heidelberg, pp. 2037–2039.

Hermann, C. and Blanchard, E.B. (2002) Biofeedback in the treatment of headache and other childhood pain, *Applied Psychophysiology Biofeedback*, 27: 143–162.

Hooke, C., Hellsten, M.B., Stutzer, C., Forte, K. (2002) Pain management for the child with cancer in end-of-life care: APON position paper, *Journal of Pediatric Oncology Nursing*, 19: 43–47.

Hunfield, J.A.M., Perquin, C.W., Duivenvoorden, H.J., Hazebroek-Kampschreur, A.A.J.M., Passchier, J., van Suijlekom-Smit, L.W.A. and van der Wouden, J.C. (2001) Chronic pain and its impact on quality of life in adolescents and their families, *Journal of Pediatric Psychology*, 26:145–153.

Hunfield, J.A.M., Perquin, C.W, Bertina, W., Hazebroek-Kampschreur, A.A.J.M, van Suijlekom-Smit, L.W.A., Koes, B.W., van de Wouden, J.C. and Passchier, J. (2002) Stability of pain parameters and pain-related quality of life in adolescents with persistent pain: a three year follow-up, *Clinical Journal of Pain*, 18: 99–106.

Hyman, P.E., Bursch, B., Sood, M., Schwankovsky, L., Cocjin, J. and Zeltzer, L.K. (2002) Visceral pain-associated disability syndrome: a descriptive analysis, *Journal of Pediatric Gastroenterology and Nutrition*, 35: 663–668.

Iskedjian, M., Bereza, B., Gordon, A., Piwko, C. and Einarson, T.R. (2007) Meta-analysis of canna-bis-based treatments for neuropathic and multiple sclerosis-related pain, *Current Medical Research & Opinion*, 23:17–24.

Jäing, W. and Baron, R. (2004) Experimental approach to CRPS, *Pain*, 108: 3–7.

Johnson, L. (2004) The nursing role in recognizing and assessing neuropathic pain, *British Journal of Nursing*, 13(18): 1092–1097.

Jones, D.S. and Walker, L.S. (2006) Recurrent abdominal pain in children. In Schmidt, R.F., Willis, W.D. (eds.) *Encyclopaedia Reference of Pain*, Springer-Verlag, Heidelberg, pp. 359–363.

Jordan, A.L., Eccleston, C. and Osborn, M. (2007) Being a parent of the adolescent with complex chronic pain: an interpretative phenomenological analysis, *European Journal of Pain*, 11(1): 49–56.

Kashikar-Zuck, S. (2006) Treatment of children with unexplained chronic pain. *Lancet*, 367: 380–382.

Kashikar-Zuck, S., Goldschneider, K.R., Powers, S.W., Vaught, M.H. and Hershey, A.D. (2001) Depression and functional disability in chronic pediatric pain, *Clinical Journal of Pain*, 17: 341–349.

Kashikar-Zuck, S., Vaught, M.H., Goldschneider, K.R., Graham, T.B. and Miller, J.C. (2002) Depression, coping, and functional disability in juvenile primary fibromyalgia syndrome, *Journal of Pain*, 3(5): 412–419.

Keogh, E. and Eccleston, C. (2006) Sex differences in adolescent chronic pain and pain-related coping, *Pain*, 123(3): 275–284.

Kimura, Y., Walco, G.A. Sugarman, E., Conte, P.M. and Schanberg L.E. (2006) Treatment of pain in juvenile idiopathic arthritis: a survey of pediatric rheumatologists. *Arthritis & Rheumatism*. 55: 81–85.

Konijnenberg, A.Y., de Graeff-Meeder, E.R., van der Hoeven, J., Kimpen, J.L., Buitelaar, J.K. and Uiterwaal, C.S. (2006) Pain of Unknown Origin in Children Study Group. Psychiatric morbidity in chil-dren with medically unexplained chronic pain: diagnosis from the pediatrician's perspective, *Pediatrics*, 177(3): 889–897.

Konijnenberg, A.Y., Uiterwaal, C.S., Kimpen, J.L., van der Hoeven. J., Buitelaar, J.K. and de Graeff-Meeder, E.R. (2005) Children with unexplained chronic pain: substantial impairment in everyday life, *Archives of Disease in Childhood* 90(7): 680–686.

Kopek, J.A. and Sayre, E.C. (2005) Stressful experiences in childhood and chronic back pain in the gen-eral population, *Clinical Journal of Pain*, 21: 478–483.

Lalwani, K., Shoham, A., Koh, J.L. and McGraw, T. (2005) Use of oxcarbazepine to treat a pediatric patient with resistant CRPS. *Journal of Pain*, 6: 704–706.

Lewin, D.S. and Dahl, R.E. (1999) Importance of sleep in the management of pediatric pain, *Journal of Developmental and Behavioural Pediatrics*, 20: 244–252.

Logan, D.E., Guite, J.W., Sherry, D.D. and Rose, J.B. (2006) Adolescent-parent relationships in the con-text of adolescent chronic pain conditions, *Clinical Journal of Pain* 22(6): 576–583.

Low, A.K., Ward, K. and Wines, A.P. (2007) Pediatric complex regional pain syndrome. *Journal of Pediatric Orthopedics*, 27: 567–572.

Lynch, A.M., Kashikar-Zuck, S., Goldschneider, K.R. and Jones, B.A. (2007) Sex and age differences in coping styles among children with chronic pain, *Journal of Pain and Symptom Management*, 33(2): 208–216.

Martin, A.L., McGrath, P.A., Brown, S.C. and Katz, J. (2007) Children with chronic pain: impact of sex and age on long-term outcomes, *Pain*, 128: 13–19.

Maunuksela, E. and Olkkola, K.T. (2003) Nonsteroidal anti-inflammatory drugs in pediatric pain man-agement. In Schechter, N.L., Berde, C.B. and Yaster, M. (eds.) *Pain in Infants, Children and Adolescents*, 2nd edition, Lippincott, Williams & Wilkins, Baltimore, pp. 171–180.

McCarthy, C.F., Shea, A.M. and Sullivan, P. (2003) Physical therapy management of pain in chil-dren. In Schechter, N.L., Berde, C.B. and Yaster, M. (eds.) *Pain in Infants, Children and Adolescents*, 2nd edition, Lippincott, Williams & Wilkins, Baltimore, pp. 434–448.

McGhee, J.L., Burks, F.N. and Sheckles, J.L. (2002) Identifying children with chronic arthritis based on chief complaints: absence of predictive value for musculoskeletal pain as an indicator of rheumatic disease in children, *Pediatrics*, 110: 354–359.

McGrath, P.A. (1999) Chronic pain in children. In Crombie, I.K. (ed.) *Epidemiology of Pain*, IASP Press, Seattle, pp. 81–101.

McGrath, P.A. (2006a) Chronic daily headache in children. In Schmidt. R.F. and Willis, W.D. (eds.) *Encyclopaedia Reference of Pain*, Springer-Verlag, Heidelberg, pp. 359–363.

McGrath, P.A. (2006b) Pain in children. In Schmidt. R.F. and Willis, W.D. (eds.) *Encyclopaedia Reference of Pain*, Springer-Verlag, Heidelberg, pp. 1665–1669.

McGrath, P.J., Hetherington, R. and Finley, G.A. (2003) Chronic pain in children. In Jensen, T.S., Wilson, P.R. and Rice, A.S.C. (eds.) *Clinical Pain Management: Chronic Pain/Practical Applications & Procedures,* Arnold Publishing: London, pp. 637–646.

McQuay, H.J., Tramèr, M., Nye, B.A., Carroll, D., Wiffen, P.J. and Moore, R.A. (1996) A systematic review of antidepressants in neuropathic pain, *Pain*, 68(2–3): 217–227.

Mehta, D.K. (ed.) (2007) *British National Formulary for Children*, BMJ Publishing, London.

Meighen, K.G. (2007) Duloxetine treatment of pediatric chronic pain and co-morbid major depressive disorder, *Journal of Child and Adolescent Psychopharmacology*, 17(1): 121–127.

Mellegers, M.A., Furlan, A.D. and Mailis, A. (2001) Gabapentin for neuropathic pain: systematic review of controlled and uncontrolled literature, *Clinical Journal of Pain*, 17(4): 284–295.

Melzack, R. and Wall, P.D. (1965) Pain mechanisms: a new theory, *Science*, 50: 971–979.

Merlijn, V.P.B.M., Hunfield, J.A.M., van der Wouden, J.C., Hazebroek-Kamschreur, A.A.J.M., Passchier, J. and Koes, B.W. (2006) Factors related to quality of life in adolescents with chronic pain, *Clinical Journal of Pain*, 22: 306–315.

Merlijn, V.P., Hunfield, J.A., van der Wouden, J.C., Hazebroek-Kampschreur, A.A., Koes, B.W. and Passchier, J. (2003) Psychosocial factors associated with chronic pain in adolescents, *Pain*, 101(1–2): 33–43.

Miró, J., Huguet, A. and Nieto, R. (2007) Predictive factors of chronic pediatric pain and disability, *Journal of Pain*, 8: 774–792.

Moore, R.A., Tramèr, M.R., Carroll, D., Wiffen, P.J. and McQuay, H.J. (1998) Quantitative systematic review of topically applied non-steroidal anti-inflammatory drugs, *British Medical Journal*, 316(7128): 333–338.

Moulin, D.E., Clark, A.J., Gilron, I., Ware, M.A., Watson, C.P., Sessle, B.J., Coderre, T., Morley-Forster, P.K., Stinson, J., Boulanger, A., Peng, P., Finley, G.A., Taenzer, P., Squire, .P, Dion, D., Cholkan, A., Gilani, A., Gordon, A., Henry, J., Jovey, R., Lynch, M., Mailis-Gagnon, A., Panju, A., Rollman, G.B. and Velly, A. (2007) Pharmacological management of chronic neuropathic pain – consensus statement and guidelines from the Canadian Pain Society, *Pain Research Management*, 12(1): 13–21.

Mullick, M.S.I. (2002) Somatoform disorders in children and adolescents, *Bangladesh Medical Research Council Bulletin*, 28: 112–122.

Nathan, A., Rose, J.B., Guite, J.W., Hehir, D. and Milovcich, K. (2005) Primary erythromelalgia in a child responding to intravenous lidocaine and oral mexiletine treatment, *Pediatrics*, 115(4): 504–507.

Olsson, G.L., Meyerson, B.A. and Linderoth, B. (2008) Spinal cord stimulation in adolescents with complex regional pain syndrome type 1 (CRPS-I), *European Journal of Pain*, 12: 53–59.

Palermo, T.M. and Kiska, R. (2005) Subjective sleep disturbances in adolescents with chronic pain: relationship to daily functioning and quality of life, *Journal of Pain*, 6: 201–207.

Pearlman, E.M. (2006) Migraine, childhood syndromes. In Schmidt, R.F., Willis, W.D. (eds) *Encyclopaedia Reference of Pain*, Springer-Verlag, Heidelberg, pp. 1136–1138.

Peng, P., Stinson, J., Choiniere, M., Dion, D., Intrater, H., Lefort, L.M., Ong, M., Rshig, S., Tkachuk, G., Veilltette, Y. and STOP PAIN Investigator Group. (2007) Dedicated multidisciplinary pain management centres for children in Canada: the current status, *Canadian Journal of Anesthesia*, 54: 963–968.

Perquin, C.W., Hazebroek-Kampschreur, A.A.J.M., Hunfield, J.A.M., Bohen, A.M., van Suijlekom-Smit, L.W.A., Passchier, J. and van der Wouden, J.C. (2000) Pain in children and adolescents: a common experience, *Pain*, 87: 51–58.

Perquin, C.W., Hazebroek-Kampscheur, A.A.J.M., Hunfield, J.A.M., van Suijlekom-Smit, L.W.A., Passchier, J. and van der Wouden, J.C. (2001) Chronic pain among children and adolescents: physician consultation and medication use, *Clinical Journal of Pain*, 16: 229–235.

Perquin, C.W., Hunfled,, J.A.M., Hazebroek-Kampschreur, A.A.J.M, van Suijlekom-Smit, L.W.A., Passchier, J., Koes, B.W. and van der Wouden, J.C. (2003) The natural course of chronic benign pain in childhood and adolescence: a two-year population-based follow-up study, *European Journal of Pain*, 7(6): 551–559.

Reid, G.J., McGrath, P.J. and Lang, B.A. (2005) Parent–child interactions among children with juvenile fibromyalgia, arthritis, and healthy controls, *Pain*, 113(1): 201–210.

Roth-Isigkeit, A., Thyen, U., Stoven, H., Schwarzenberger, J. and Schumaker, P. (2005) Pain among children and adolescents: restrictions in daily living and triggering factors, *Pediatrics*, 115(2): 152–162.

Rudich, Z., Stinson, J., Jeavons, M. and Brown, S.C. (2003) Treatment of chronic intractable neuropathic pain with dronabinol: case report of two adolescents, *Pain Research & Management*, 8: 221–224.

Rusy, L.M., Troshynski, T.J. and Weisman, S.J. (2001) Gabapentin in phantom limb pain management in children and young adults: report of seven cases, *Journal of Pain and Symptom Management* 21(1): 78–82.

Saunders, K., Korff, M.V., LeResche, L. and Mancl, L. (2007) Relationship of common pain conditions in mothers and children, *Clinical Journal of Pain*, 23(3): 204–213.

Scharff, L., Leichtner, A.M. and Rappaport, L.A. (2003) Recurrent abdominal pain. In Schechter, N.L., Berde, C.B. and Yaster, M. (eds.) *Pain in Infants, Children and Adolescents,* 2nd edition, Lippincott, Williams & Wilkins, Baltimore, pp. 719–731.

Scharff, L., Langan, N., Rotter, N., Scott-Sutherland. J., Schenck, C., Tayor, N., McDonald-Nolan, L. and Masek, B. (2005) Psychological, behavioural and family characteristics of pediatric patients with chronic pain: a 1-year retrospective study and cluster analysis, *Clinical Journal of Pain*, 21: 432–438.

Sleed, M., Eccleston, C., Beecham, J., Knapp, M. and Jordan, A. (2005) The economic impact of chronic pain in adolescence: methodological considerations and a preliminary costs-of-illness study, *Pain*, 119(1–3): 183–190.

Stanford, E.A., Chambers, C.T., Biesanz, J.C. and Chen, E. (2008) The frequency, trajectories and predictors of adolescent recurrent pain: a population-based approach, *Pain* (in press).

Stevens, B.J. and Pillia Riddell, R. (2006) Looking beyond acute pain in infancy, *Pain*, 124: 11–12.

Stinson, J.N. (2006) Complex chronic pain in children, interdisciplinary treatment. In Schmidt, R.F. and Willis, W.D. (eds.) *Encyclopaedia Reference of Pain*. Springer-Verlag, Heidelberg, pp. 431–434.

Stinson, J. (2008) Self-management interventions on the internet: can they have an impact on JIA? *Arthritis Practitioner*, 4(1). Available at http://www.arthritispractitioner.com/article/8271

Stinson, J.N., Stevens, B.J., Feldman, B.M., Streiner, D., McGrath, P.J., Dupuis, A., Gill, N. and Petroz, G.C. (2007) Construct validity of a multidimensional electronic pain diary for adolescents with arthritis, *Pain*, 136(3): 281–292.

Subcommittee on Chronic Abdominal Pain (2005) Chronic abdominal pain in children, *Pediatrics*, 115(3): 812–815.

Sullivan, M.J.L. and Adams, H. (2006) Castrophizing. In Schmidt, R.F and Willis, W.D. (eds.) *Encyclopaedia Reference of Pain*, Springer-Verlag, Heidelberg, pp. 297–298.

Taylor, S. and Garralda, E. (2003) The management of somatoform disorder in childhood, *Current Opinion in Psychiatry*, 16: 2227–2231.

Tong, H.C. and Nelson, V.S. (2000) Recurrent and migratory reflex sympathetic dystrophy in children, *Pediatric Rehabilitation*, 4(2): 87–89.

Van Den Kerkhof, E. and van Dijk, A. (2006) Prevalence of chronic pain disorders in children. In Schmidt, R.F. and Willis W.D. (eds.) *Encyclopaedia Reference of Pain*, Springer-Verlag, Heidelberg, pp. 1972–1974.

Vervoort, T., Goubet, L., Eccleston, C., Bijttebier, P. and Crombez, G. (2006) Catastrophic thinking about pain is independently associated with pain severity, disability and somatic complaints in school children and children with chronic pain, *Journal of Pediatric Psychology*, 31: 674–683.

Vessey, J.A. and Carlson, K.L. (1996) Nonpharmacological interventions to use with children in pain, *Issues in Comprehensive Pediatric Nursing*, 19: 169–182.

Von Baeyer, C. (2006) Understanding and managing children's recurrent pain in primary care: a biopsychosocial perspective, *Paediatrics and Child Health*, 12: 121–125.

Vyskocil, V., Pikner, R. and Kutilek, S. (2005) Effect of alendronate therapy in children with osteogenesis imperfecta, *Joint, Bone, Spine: Revue du Rhumatisme*, 72(5): 416–423.

Watson, K.D., Papageorgiou, A.C., Jones, G.T., Taylor, S., Symmons, D.P.M., Silman, A.J. and Macfarlane, G.J. (2002) Low back pain in schoolchildren: occurrence and characteristics, *Pain*, 97: 87–92.

Wheeler, D.S., Vaux, K.K. and Tam, D.A. (2000) Use of gabapentin in the treatment of childhood reflex sympathetic dystrophy, *Pediatric Neurology*, 22: 220–221.

Wicksell, R. (2007) Values-based exposure and acceptance in the treatment of pediatric chronic pain: from symptom reduction to valued living, *Pediatric Pain Letter*, 9: 13–20.

Wicksell, R., Dahl, J., Magnusson, B. and Olsson, G. (2005) Using acceptance and commitment therapy in the rehabilitation of an adolescent female with chronic pain: a case example, *Cognitive Behavioural Practitioner*, 12: 415–423.

Wicksell, R., Melin, L. and Olsson, G. (2007) Exposure and acceptance in the rehabilitation of adolescents with idiopathic chronic pain – a pilot study, *European Journal of Pain*, 11: 267–274.

Wiffen, P., Collins, S., McQuay, H., Carroll, D., Jadad, A. and Moore, A. (2000) Anticonvulsant drugs for acute and chronic pain, *Cochrane Database of Systematic Reviews*, (3): CD001133.

Wilder, R.T., Berde, C.B., Wolohan, M., Vieyra, M.A., Masek, B..J. and Micheli, L.J. (1992) Reflex sympathetic dystrophy in children: clinical characteristics and follow-up of seventy patients, *Journal of Bone Joint Surgery of America*, 74: 910–919.

Wilkins, K.L., McGrath, P.J., Finley, G.A. and Katz, J. (1998) Phantom limb sensations and phantom limb pain in child and adolescent amputees, *Pain*, 78: 7–12.

Wolfe, J., Grier, H., Klar, N., Levin, S.B., Ellenbogen, J.M., Salem-Schatx, S., Emanuel, E.J. and Weeks, J.C. (2000) Symptoms at end of life in children with cancer, *New England Journal of Medicine*, 342: 326–333.

Zernikow, B., Michel, E. and Anderson, B. (2007) Transdermal fentanyl in childhood and adolescence: a comprehensive literature review, *Journal of Pain*, 8: 187–207.

CHAPTER 9

Palliative Care in Children

Stephanie J. Dowden

Introduction

This chapter will provide an overview of palliative care for children, with a particular focus on control of pain and other symptoms. After defining paediatric palliative care there will be a review of the history of palliative care with discussion of how paediatric services evolved from adult models. Causes of death in childhood will be examined with the current status of family preference versus reality of location of death. The current evidence base for best practice in palliative care will be reviewed together with the key aims for quality outcomes. Different models of paediatric palliative care provision will be considered. Finally, there will be detailed discussion about pain and symptom management during the palliative phase and at end of life. Both pharmacological and non-drug methods of symptom management will be discussed.

9.1 What is Palliative Care?

The World Health Organization (WHO 2006) defines palliative care as encompassing the following beliefs. Palliative care:

- provides relief of pain and other distressing symptoms;
- affirms life and regards dying as a normal process;
- intends to neither hasten nor postpone death;
- integrates psychological and spiritual aspects of care;
- supports people to live fully before they die;
- uses a team approach to address the needs of patients and their families;
- supports the family to cope during the illness and after the death.

Paediatric palliative care is a separate but closely related entity to adult palliative care, combining the key palliative care beliefs with a paediatric focus. The emergence of interest in paediatric palliative care gained impetus following the publication of the WHO booklet *Cancer Pain Relief and Palliative Care in Children* (WHO 1998). This booklet presented the expectation that all children worldwide should have access to a minimum standard of pain relief and palliative care (Collins and Frager 2006). Two definitions of paediatric palliative care can be seen in Box 9.1.

BOX 9.1

Definitions of paediatric palliative care

WHO (1998) definition

- Palliative care is the active total care of the child's body, mind and spirit, and also involves giving support to the family
- It begins when illness is diagnosed and continues *regardless* of whether or not a child receives treatment directed at the disease
- Healthcare providers must evaluate and alleviate a child's physical, psychological and social distress
- Effective palliative care requires a broad multidisciplinary approach that includes the family and makes use of available community resources
- It can be provided in tertiary care facilities, in community health centres and in children's homes
- The goal of palliative care is the achievement of the best quality of life for patients and their families

American Academy of Pediatrics (2000) definition

Palliative care seeks to enhance the quality of life in the face of an ultimately terminal condition. Palliative treatments focus on the relief of symptoms (e.g. pain, dyspnoea) and conditions (e.g. loneliness) that cause distress and detract from the child's enjoyment of life. It also seeks to ensure that bereaved families remain functional and intact.

9.2 History and Evolution of Paediatric Palliative Care

The modern *hospice* movement began in the United Kingdom in the late 1960s when Cicely Saunders, aiming to give people an alternative to dying in hospital, established St Christopher's Hospice. Saunders' focus on the patient and family unit, interdisciplinary care and connection of home and community established the foundations of palliative care as we know it today. Growing interest in the previously taboo subject of death and dying followed with Elisabeth Kubler-Ross publishing the first of many texts on the subject in 1969 (Abu-Saad and Courtens 2003).

The term *palliative care* was coined in 1975 to further differentiate what care was given. Over time the terms hospice and palliative care have merged in meaning and are now used interchangeably as their aims have combined. Hospice care tends to be more focused on end of life care, while palliative care encompasses the broader range of care. Palliative care models currently exist on every continent; however, many countries still only have models at early development stage or absent, particularly in the most resource-poor countries. The establishment of palliative care services in some countries has been driven by the HIV/AIDS pandemic, with some of these models now extending care to other diagnoses (Harding 2006).

Palliative care for children grew out of the adult hospice and palliative care movement and was established in the USA and UK during the late 1970s and early 1980s (Goldman et al. 2006a). Paediatric palliative care follows the ideals of adult palliative care while acknowledging paediatric-specific considerations (Canadian Hospice Palliative Care Association [CHPCA] 2006):

- developmental concerns (e.g. the breadth of ages and stages of children);
- child-specific issues (e.g. pharmacokinetics, drugs not licensed for children);
- ethical and legal differences (e.g. legal minors, parental decision-making);
- children have rare conditions and diseases not seen in adult populations;

- parental involvement and the family unit;
- parental and sibling consequences of the death of a child.

In the past 5–10 years paediatric palliative care has evolved further with the recognition of two key issues, that:

- most families prefer their children to receive end of life care at home rather than in a hospital or hospice;
- the population of children that have palliative care needs is quite different to the adult population, with only about one-third having cancer-related diseases.

> The majority of children with palliative care needs have congenital and progressive, degenerative conditions with an uncertain time course, leading to a multiplicity of issues and a *great diversity in the process of dying* (Bartell and Kissane 2005).

9.3 Death in Childhood

9.3.1 Causes of death in childhood

Accidents are the primary cause of death (30–43%) for *all* children, aged 0–19 years, with the majority of remaining deaths caused by congenital anomalies, deformities, nervous system disorders and cancers (Bartell and Kissane 2005; Himelstein 2005; Department of Health (DH) 2007a). The causes of death for children with *life-limiting illnesses* (LLI) aged 0–19 years (Association for Children with Life-Threatening or Terminal Conditions and their Families [ACT] 2003a) are:

- 40% cancer;
- 20% cardiac;
- 40% other life-limiting illnesses.

Palliative care terminology is defined in Table 9.1.

9.3.2 Where do children die?

Despite the growing evidence that families would prefer their children to die at home (Collins et al. 1998; Vickers 2000; ACT 2003a; Himelstein 2006), most children die in hospital.

- Bartell and Kissane (2005) found 72% of children died in hospital, 11% at home and 17% in other areas (including emergency departments).
- There is an increased likelihood for infants under one year to die in hospital (up to 75%) and for those children over one year to die at home (Himelstein 2005).
- Almost all (98%) neonatal deaths occur in hospital (DH 2007b).
- Of the in-hospital deaths fewer than 15% of children die in ward areas, with 80–90% dying in critical care areas (e.g. in paediatric or neonatal intensive care units [ICUs]), commonly receiving high levels of invasive interventions (McCallum et al. 2000; Carter et al. 2004; Himelstein 2005; Ramnarayan et al. 2007).

Children who die in ICUs receive large numbers of interventions even when they have life-limiting illnesses:

- In a study reviewing pain and symptom management in children ($n = 108$) at end of life by Carter et al. (2004), up to 90% of patients received pain medication, 55% received additional comfort measures, 98% were mechanically ventilated and 45% received CPR in the last 72 hours before death.
- Of the deaths in paediatric ICUs, 60–70% occurred following withdrawal of life-sustaining treatment (Garros et al. 2003; Carter et al. 2004).

Table 9.1   Terminology in paediatric palliative care

Life-limiting illness (LLI) *or life-limiting condition (LLC)*	An illness or condition where premature death is inevitable
Life-sustaining treatment (LST)	Medical treatment directed at sustaining life (e.g. mechanical ventilation, cardiopulmonary resuscitation [CPR])
Life-threatening illness (LTI) or *life-threatening condition (LTC)*	An illness or condition that the child may survive, but that is life threatening for varying lengths of time or has the potential to cause death
Premature death	Where the child is expected to die before their parents (e.g. in childhood or early adulthood)
Technology-dependent children	Children who are dependent on technology for survival and to prevent a premature death (most of these children have LTI, but do not necessarily need palliative care)

Source: Field and Behrman (2003); Goldman et al. (2006a)

- A 10-year study by Ramnarayan et al. (2007) of in-hospital deaths of children with life-limiting illness ($n = 1127$) at a tertiary paediatric hospital in the UK found that ICU was the most common place of death (87%). LLI diagnosis at death included congenital malformations (22%), perinatal disease (18%), cardiovascular anomalies (15%) and cancers (12%).
- Feudtner et al. (2002) reviewed three cohorts of deaths in US children's hospitals in 1991, 1994 and 1997 ($n = 13761$). Of these children, 60% had LLI diagnoses: they were also more likely to have been mechanically ventilated prior to death and ventilated for longer periods than the non-LLI group.
- Despite the high rate of accidental death in childhood, the majority of paediatric ICU deaths occur in children with chronic conditions including LLI, suggesting that earlier referral to palliative and supportive care services might allow some of these children a more peaceful death (Feudtner et al. 2002; Carter et al. 2004).

> There is growing awareness that a palliative care approach should be encouraged within paediatric ICU and neonatal ICU settings, ensuring the focus is on the best interests of the child at the end of life.

9.3.3 How many children need palliative care?

The commonly quoted figure of the number of children per year with palliative care needs (in developed countries) is 10 per 10,000 children aged 0–19 years (ACT 2003a). So, for example, in a population of 250,000 (with a child population of ~50,000) there would be 5 deaths per year, 50 children with life-limiting conditions and 25 children actively needing palliative care. The figures are difficult to accurately calculate but an English Department of Health paper released in May 2007 suggests the actual figure might be significantly higher, with as many as 16 per 10,000 children aged 0–19 years requiring palliative care each year (DH 2007b).

9.3.4 Conditions requiring paediatric palliative care

A joint working party of ACT and the Royal College of Paediatrics and Child Health (RCPCH) identified four groups of conditions (Table 9.2) for which children and young people will require palliative care (ACT 2003a).

Table 9.2   Conditions requiring paediatric palliative care

Group 1	Life-threatening conditions for which curative treatment may be feasible, but can fail (e.g. cancer, organ failure of heart, liver or kidney, infections)
Group 2	Conditions requiring long periods of intensive treatment aimed at prolonging life, but where premature death is still possible (e.g. cystic fibrosis, HIV/AIDS, cardiovascular anomalies, extreme prematurity)
Group 3	Progressive conditions without curative options, where treatment is palliative after diagnosis (e.g. neuromuscular or neurodegenerative disorders, progressive metabolic disorders, chromosomal abnormalities, advanced metastatic cancer on first presentation)
Group 4	Irreversible, non-progressive conditions with severe disability causing extreme vulnerability to health complications (e.g. severe cerebral palsy, genetic disorders, congenital malformations, prematurity, brain or spinal cord injury)

Source: ACT and RCPCH (2003a)

BOX 9.2

Challenges to carrying out research in palliative care

- Ethics of doing research with dying people
- Societal attitudes to death
- Fear of intruding in a person's last weeks or days
- Burden of research participation by researchers and participants
- Attrition rates due to early death
- Definition of end of life/palliative phase
- Recruitment issues due to overprotective clinicians, families and ethics committees
- Low questionnaire compliance
- Heterogeneity of many clinical groups (adult and children)
- Small patient numbers
- Difficulty defining outcome measures or research end points
- Randomisation issues and lack of ability to have a control group

Source: Abu-Saad (2000); Collins and Frager (2006); Kendall et al. (2007)

9.3.5 Evidence base for palliative care

Currently there are no *gold standard* measures to evaluate adult or paediatric palliative care (Abu-Saad 2000; Goldman et al. 2006a). However, to prove their effectiveness and maintain funding and support it is vital that *all* palliative care programmes show good evidence of their achievements and outcomes. Obtaining evidence about care at the end of life raises many dilemmas for researchers and clinicians alike (Box 9.2), which makes this a difficult area to research both methodologically and ethically (Abu-Saad 2000; Kendall et al. 2007; Mongeau and Liben 2007). Randomised controlled trials (RCTs) are both impractical and possibly unethical; instead research designs using non-RCTs with matched controls are more common. Standard research methodologies can be effective and may be enhanced by using a range of innovative methods (Abu-Saad 2000; Kendall et al. 2007), such as:

- combining qualitative and quantitative approaches;
- chart audits;
- population-based studies;

- surveys of users, families and carers;
- comparing different types of palliative care service delivery.

> The key to effectiveness in palliative care is family and patient satisfaction with quality of care, quality of life and symptom management (Abu-Saad 2000). Evidence based palliative care will only become a reality once these issues are addressed.

9.4 Quality in Palliative Care

Measuring quality in paediatric palliative care is also difficult as there are limited tools to assess best practice (Abu-Saad and Courtens 2003; Goldman et al. 2006a). Widger and Wilkins (2004) undertook a literature review to develop a questionnaire to measure the quality of paediatric end of life care. They found no reliable or validated survey tools, although some were at development stage. The challenges in researching end of life care (mentioned in the previous section) are part of the reason for this, combined with paediatric palliative care being a relatively new field of clinical specialty and the added challenge of research with children. (See Chapter 11 for more information about undertaking research with children.)

To date insufficient attention has been paid to these issues by government and non-government funding bodies. However, given the imperative for adult palliative care providers to prove their worth to maintain funding and clinical accreditation (Goldman et al. 2006a), it is reasonable to assume the same will happen soon in paediatric palliative care. Rather than viewing this as a burden, Goldman et al. (2006a) suggests that paediatric palliative care programmes should see this as an opportunity to deliver best practice and then to share their knowledge with the wider paediatric palliative care community. A growing number of paediatric palliative care standards and guidelines have been published that have a strong basis in quality assurance and quality improvement processes, which could be used to ensure minimum standards or to promote best practice guidelines (Table 9.3).

9.5 Principles of Paediatric Palliative Care

The principles and aims of paediatric palliative care can be seen in Box 9.3.

BOX 9.3

Principles of paediatric palliative care

- Child and family-centred care addressing and meeting their actual needs
- Child participation in decisions whenever possible
- Provision of symptom management that addresses the relief of suffering in all its forms
- Emotional, physical, psychological and spiritual support for the child and whole family
- Knowledge-based, reflective and evidence-based care
- Open and honest communication
- Accessible, coordinated and equitable care
- Continuity of care across all settings

Source: ACT (2003a); CHPCA (2006); Goldman et al. (2006a)

Table 9.3 Paediatric palliative and hospice care standards, policies and guidelines

Organisation	Document type
AAP 2000 *(USA)* *Palliative Care for Children*www.aap.org	Policy statement, standards and recommendations for care
ACT 2003a *(UK)* ACT/RCPCH: *A Guide to the Development of Children's Palliative Care Services* www.act.org.uk	Palliative care definitions, service plan recommendations, family needs and standards of care
ACT 2003c *(UK)* *Assessment of children with life-limiting conditions and their families: A guide to effective care planning.* Available from: www.act.org.uk	Framework for assessment and care coordination for children with LLI
ACT 2004a *(UK)* *A framework for the development of integrated multi-agency care pathways for children with life-threatening and life-limiting conditions.* Available from: www.act.org.uk	Care pathways to integrate multi-agency care for children with LLI and LTI
ACT 2007a *(UK)* *ACT Integrated Palliative Care Pathway Standards: Service self assessment tool* Available from: www.act.org.uk	Tool to identify best practice in palliative care within a local area
ACT 2007b *(UK)* *ACT Transition Care Pathway Standards: Service self assessment tool* Available from: www.act.org.uk	Tool to identify best practice in transition to adult care within a local area
ACT 2004b *(UK)* *The ACT Charter.* Available from: www.act.org.uk	14 point charter setting out standards of paediatric palliative care support
ACH 2004a *(UK)* *Guidelines for Best Practice in a Children's Hospice Service.* Available from: www.childhospice.org.uk	Guidelines for paediatric hospice care
ACH 2004b *(UK)* *Are we getting it right? A tool to measure the quality of children's hospice services.* Available from: www.childhospice.org.uk	QA tools to measure paediatric hospice care
NCP 2004 *(USA)* *Clinical practice guidelines for quality palliative care.* Available from: www.nationalconsensusproject.org	Clinical Practice Guidelines for palliative care across the life span
CHPCA 2006 *(Canada)* *Pediatric Hospice Palliative Care: Guiding principles and norms of practice.* Available from: www.chpca.net/	Standards of practice and principles to guide paediatric hospice and palliative care
IMPaCCT 2007 *(Europe)* International Meeting for Palliative Care in Children, Trento (IMPaCCT): *Standards for paediatric palliative care in Europe* (Craig et al. 2007)	Core standards for paediatric palliative care
DH 2007a *(England)* *Palliative Care Services for children and young people in England.* Available from: www.dh.gov.uk/publications	Recommendations for best practice in paediatric palliative care

Association for Children with Life-threatening or Terminal Conditions and their Families (ACT) is now known as the Association for Children's Palliative Care (ACT).

9.5.1 Where is palliative care for children delivered?

Palliative care for children has a combined hospital, hospice and community focus for care delivery (Table 9.4). Active home-based palliative care originated from oncology outreach nursing models of care (Goldman et al. 2006a) and this model is increasingly being embraced by paediatric palliative care providers. Although in the UK the trend is for increasing numbers of children to die at home, this is not yet the case elsewhere in the world. In the UK deaths occurring at home in children with LLI range from 15–77%, in Poland 23%, in the USA 20%, in Germany 40% and in Italy 5% (Dangel 2002; Friedrichsdorf et al. 2005). At-home death is strongly influenced by diagnosis and the availability of comprehensive paediatric community-based services:

- Friedrichsdorf et al. (2005) surveyed 71 (of 73) German paediatric oncology departments. Of 488 deaths, 60% of children died in hospital and 40% at home. Community palliative care services were limited with the likelihood of children dying at home being dependent on the oncology department's ability to offer outreach and home-based support.
- Vickers et al. (2007) studied place of death for a group of children (n = 164) with cancer in the UK. The preferred place of death was home in 68–80% of families, with 80% of deaths occurring at their preferred place.
- Widger et al. (2007) surveyed all eight paediatric palliative care programmes in Canada. In 2002 the programmes cared for 317 children. During that year 123 children died: 44% died at home, 40% died in hospital, 8% died in a hospice. At-home deaths varied between 18% and 86% per programme, depending on the extent of home care services available.
- In England during 2002–2005 the number of paediatric deaths that occurred at home from all causes requiring palliative care ranged from 14.5% to 25% of deaths in children (DH 2007b).

Table 9.4   Types of palliative care for children

Place of care	Services offered
Hospital care	in-patient acute care, respite, or dedicated hospice beds availability of full range of hospital services specialist palliative medicine/symptom control teams paediatric hospital, community hospital, general hospital
Home care	domiciliary services (cleaning, shopping, washing, child-minding) respite care, home care teams, liaison nurses, community nurses volunteer sitters or lay carers, family support outreach specialist teams, crisis intervention teams, hospice teams, district nurses, Diana community teams (nurse-led home-based care)
Consultative care	hospital-based outreach specialist teams tele-video and tele-audio conference link-ups advice-based services
Hospice care	hospice at home or residential hospice respite care, emergency care, end of life care sibling/family support bereavement care staff, family and community education and training
Community care	school, child care, play groups at-home respite, residential respite

Source: Abu Saad (2000); Goldman et al. (2006a)

- The number of at-home deaths for patients of a London paediatric tertiary hospital increased from 22% to 77% once a symptom care team was established (Friedrichsdorf et al. 2005)
- Only about 20% of children using hospice services will die there, instead dying at home or in hospital (Goldman et al. 2006b).
- If cure-based treatment is ceased it is more likely that the child will die at home or hospice; if cure-based treatment continues it is more likely the child will die in hospital (receiving intensive care) (Goldman et al. 1990; Abu-Saad 2000).

For home-based care to be successful it must be desired by the child and parents and be supported by their healthcare team. Ideally families should be offered home, hospice or hospital care and be able to change from one to another as needed (Liben and Goldman 1998).

If the family opts for home-based palliative care several factors need considering:

- Is 24-hour expertise in paediatric/family care available?
- Is there 24-hour access to paediatric palliative care experts?
- Is there a key worker to coordinate care?
- Are respite facilities available? (home and residential)
- Is immediate access to hospital available (if required)?

Source: Goldman 1996; Liben and Goldman 1998; Abu-Saad and Courtens 2003; ACT 2003a

---

There are many hidden costs and challenges of providing *at-home palliative care* including:

- emotional and psychological cost to family and carers (e.g. sleep disruption/deprivation, fatigue, anxiety, grief and stress);
- balancing need for assistance with loss of privacy (e.g. impact of carers, health professionals and domiciliary staff coming into the home);
- financial costs (e.g. loss of family wages, cost of consumables and hiring equipment, child care);
- skills and knowledge required and the burden of these (e.g. learning *nursing tasks*, managing medications, managing technology, dual role of being a nurse and a parent).
  (Abu-Saad and Courtens 2003; Hynson et al. 2003; Goldman et al. 2006a)

9.5.2 When should palliative care be implemented?

When considering whether a palliative care referral should be made there are a number of factors that need to be considered. These are outlined in Table 9.5.

9.5.3 What are the child's and their family's needs?

Different family members have different palliative care needs that are not related solely to end of life issues. These needs depend on the child's diagnosis, symptoms, disability, quality of life and the degree of disruption to family life (Table 9.6).

9.5.4 Symptoms and their prevalence in children with palliative care needs at the end of life

Children with palliative care needs experience a number of symptoms, outlined in Table 9.7. From the studies presented the most common symptoms irrespective of diagnosis are *fatigue* and *pain*. The management of pain and non-pain symptoms will be discussed in turn.

Table 9.5 Factors to consider before making a palliative care referral

Factor	Points to consider
Timeliness	Recognising opportunities to discuss referral to palliative care Making referral at most useful and helpful time for the child and family – not too soon or too late Early referral leads to improved symptom control and reduction in invasive clinical interventions
Illness trajectory	Is a slow or rapid decline expected? Change in course of illness Increasing episodes of serious illness
Goals of care	Acknowledging cure is unlikely Discussion about prognosis Balancing cure-based care versus comfort care with symptom management focus Quantity versus quality of life Allowing open discussions about risks versus benefits of treatment Exploring the possible outcomes with or without interventions Discussion about end of life preferences
Maintaining hope	Hoping for the best while preparing for the worst Encouraging families to view palliative care not as giving up but as offering different hopes Allowing reality to be accepted and new openness between child, family and healthcare professionals

Source: Hutton et al. (2006); Mack and Wolfe (2006)

Table 9.6 Family needs

Parent's needs	Child's needs	Sibling's needs
Honest and complete information	Socialising (school/friends/play)	Emotional support
24-hour access to paediatric staff	Symptom management	Respite from the situation
Community based services	Supported parents	School support and regular communication with the school
Communication and care coordination	Aids for activities of daily living (ADL) and medical supplies	Information about what is happening
Respite facilities/services	Emotional support	Bereavement support
Emotional expression and support by staff	Support in the community	Parental presence
Preservation of the integrity of the parent-child relationship	Integration at school and in community	
Faith	Pets, toys and special items	
Financial support	To feel safe and cared for	
Privacy	To not feel abandoned	
Choice and control	Parental presence	
Practical support: transport, household tasks, household adaptations, child care, ADL supplies and medical equipment	Respite	
Bereavement support for self and other children		

Source: Liben and Goldman (1998); Vickers and Carlisle (2000); ACT (2003b, 2004b); CHCPA (2006); DH (2007a)

Table 9.7   Most prevalent symptoms in children receiving palliative and/or end of life care

Symptom	Study								
	Hunt (1990) All diagnoses (n = 30)	Robinson et al. (1997) Cystic fibrosis (n = 44)	Collins et al. (2000) Cancer (n = 160)	Wolfe et al. (2000) Cancer (n = 130)	Goldman (2000) Cancer (n = 152)	Collins et al. (2002) Cancer (n = 149)	Drake et al. (2003) All diagnoses (n = 30)	Goldman et al. (2006b) Cancer (n = 185)	Jalmsell et al. (2006) Cancer (n = 449)
Pain	83%	86%	49%	76%	92%	32%	53%	71%	73%
Fatigue and/or drowsiness			48%	96%	52%	36%	70%	29%	86%
Dyspnoea and/or cough	40%	Dyspnoea*	16%/41%	65%	41%		47%	~15%	38%
Anorexia and/or weight loss			40%/27%		72%	22%		48%	71%
Sadness, depression or psychological distress	30%		36%			10%		41%	48%
Nausea and/or vomiting			45%/28%		57%	13%		37%	63%/49%
Constipation and/or diarrhoea			13%/20%		58%			38%	39%
Secretions and/or swallowing difficulty	25%		13%					17%	47%
Sweating and/or skin changes			20%			Itch 25%	57%		46%
Seizures	30%		37%				53%	14%	
Agitation and/or irritability			35%						
Fear and/or anxiety			35%			20%		40%	36%
Other		Headache*	Itch 33%		Weakness 91%	Sleep problems 31%	Swelling of arms/legs 50%	Weakness 66%	Reduced mobility 76%

* % not stated

9.6 Pain and Symptom Management

Symptom management is a fundamental component of palliative care (Poltorak and Benore 2006). In palliative care, more than most other areas of pain management, there is a strong interconnection between physical and psychological symptoms with one having considerable effect on the other. Thus it is vital to combine both non-drug and pharmacological approaches. The core principles of symptom management are outlined in Box 9.4.

BOX 9.4

Core principles of symptom management

- Treat the underlying cause of a symptom and/or provide symptom control
- Non-drug therapies should be combined with pharmacological therapies
- Persistent symptoms should be treated around the clock
- Severe/uncontrolled symptoms are a medical emergency
- Invasive or painful routes of drug administration should be avoided if possible
- Adverse effects of medications should be anticipated and promptly treated

Source: Craig et al. (2007)

9.6.1 Pain

> There are many different reasons for children to experience pain at end of life.
>
> Further information about pain at end of life can be found in McCulloch and Collins (2006) and Freidrichsdorf and Kang (2007).

Pain assessment

The assessment of pain is discussed in Chapter 6. Children's self-report about their pain is considered the gold standard. Many of the pain history questions identified in Table 6.1 for children with chronic pain will also be appropriate for children with palliative care needs. For some children the additional use of multidimensional pain tools (Table 6.3 and Figure 6.6) or pain diaries may be helpful. However, for many children requiring palliative care, self-report is not possible. For these non-verbal and/or cognitively impaired children the Non-Communicating Children's Pain Checklist – Revised (Figure 6.9) provides a useful way of evaluating pain.

To ensure that a global pain assessment is completed, a number of parameters need to be considered, encompassing direct and indirect causes of pain (Wrede-Seaman 2005; Collins and Frager 2006), including:

- child report (where possible);
- carer and/or clinician report;
- behavioural components (e.g. impact on activities of daily life (ADL) and self care, sleep and activity, energy levels);
- physiological components (e.g. liver and renal function, physical consequences of illness or treatment);
- affective components (e.g. emotions, self-image, relationships);
- cognitive components (e.g. understanding of current situation, past experience, developmental stage, beliefs and coping abilities, sense of control, meaning of pain);
- sensory components (e.g. pain aetiology, location, quality, relieving and aggravating factors, duration, frequency);

- previous and current pain management (e.g. experience, efficacy, acceptability, preferences);
- use of non-drug methods of pain relief;
- social factors (e.g. family structure, family and friends support systems and functioning, community support and resources available).

Practice point

Emotions such as anxiety, depression, helplessness, hopelessness, sadness and anger can have a considerable effect on pain.

Choosing pain-relieving interventions

The pain-relieving interventions chosen will depend on:

- findings from the global assessment;
- the cause of the pain;
- pain type and severity;
- stage of disease or condition;
- other medications the child is receiving;
- possibility of drug interactions;
- past successful and less successful pain management;
- nearness to death.

The core principles and aims of pain management in paediatric palliative care are outlined in Boxes 9.5 and 9.6.

BOX 9.5

Core principles of pain management

- Unnecessary painful procedures should be avoided; procedural pain should be anticipated and prevented (see Chapter 10)
- The WHO analgesic ladder should be used, starting at step 3 if required (see Chapter 4)
- Analgesia should be administered around the clock with provision for breakthrough dosing as needed (see Chapter 4)
- Appropriate dosing and formulations should be utilised to allow the child and family restful, pain-free sleep
- The appropriate opioid dose is the one that is effective to relieve pain
- Opioid analgesia will not lead to addiction but opioid tolerance should be anticipated (see Chapter 4)
- Non-drug therapies are an integral part of pain management (see Chapter 5)

Source: Craig et al. (2007)

BOX 9.6

Aims of pain management

The aims of pain management are:

- to provide optimal analgesia
- to allow and/or maintain daily life activities
- to minimise side effects
- to have early detection, prevention and treatment of adverse effects of medications
- to have safe delivery of analgesic drugs
- to educate the child and/or family to identify and manage pain exacerbations

These aims outlined in Box 9.6 can be achieved by:

- working together with child and family;
- explaining pain assessment findings and options;
- addressing sensory issues first, prior to addressing other issues;
- developing a plan based on *all* the information gathered.

(Wrede-Seaman 2005)

The different analgesic and adjuvant drugs available are discussed in Chapters 4 and 7. Once a decision has been made about which analgesic drugs should be given, the routes of delivery need considering. The following principles should be adopted.
Use:

- the simplest route;
- the route preferred by child or family;
- the route that will have the least impact on life.

Practice point

If the pain or medical condition changes the route of administration may need to be changed.

9.6.2 Management of persistent pain

For persistent pain with or without periods of exacerbation, it is imperative to have:
- around-the-clock dosing of analgesia to keep pain away, preferably using long-acting medications to minimise the frequency of dosing;
- additional doses of analgesia (rescue doses) for breakthrough pain, usually one-sixth of the daily dose;
- regular pain assessment.

Explaining palliative care analgesia terminology

- **Breakthrough pain** is episodic pain that 'breaks through' the regular analgesia.
- **A rescue dose** of analgesia is given to enable rapid control of breakthrough pain, instead of having to wait for the next dose of regular analgesia.
- **Opioid switching** or **opioid rotation** is when a patient is changed from one opioid to another to improve analgesia effects or reduce adverse effects.

Paediatric palliative care analgesia regimes commonly consist of combining a *long-acting opioid* administered two times per day (e.g. slow release morphine) with a *short-acting* version of the same opioid (e.g. normal-release morphine tablets or morphine mixture) used as a rescue dose, administered as needed 1–4 hourly. Depending on the type of pain, other analgesics (e.g. paracetamol or adjuvant analgesic drugs) may be administered as well.

For children on *around-the-clock* analgesia, regular assessment needs to be made to determine when more analgesia is required. The child and/or family should be asked:

- Is the current analgesia sufficient for normal function?
- Does the child wake overnight or limit activities due to pain?
- Does the long-acting dose wear off before the next dose is due?
- Does the child need rescue doses?
- Is the rescue dose sufficient?
- How many rescue doses are needed in 24 hours?

Before any changes are made to the analgesia regime, check:

- Is the child taking all their doses?
- Is the analgesia regime easy to understand and follow?
- Has the pain changed?
- Is there a need for different medications?
- Is there a need for adjuvant analgesia?

Source: Wrede-Seaman, 2005

Adjusting analgesia regimes

If the analgesia regime is insufficient to ensure good relief of pain and the child is requiring more than one or two doses per day of rescue analgesia for breakthrough pain, the following changes should be made (Frager 1997; Drake et al. 2004):

- If using four rescue doses/day the total daily dose of long-acting opioid should be increased by 30–50%.
- The rescue dose should be increased also, keeping it one-sixth of the new total daily dose.
- Consider changing to another opioid if dose escalation is frequent.
- Consider the addition of adjuvant analgesics, such as ketamine or clonidine.

When caring for a child receiving palliative care occasionally a **pain crisis** will occur. McCulloch and Collins (2006) suggest that, when this happens, the following steps are taken:
- Treat the crisis as an emergency.
- Diagnose the primary cause of pain if possible.
- Titrate IV bolus doses of opioid at 10–15 minute intervals until relief of pain is achieved.
- Increase the bolus dose by 50 to 100% if no response.
- Adjust analgesia regime to meet the new needs, including addition of adjuvant analgesics.
- Consider invasive approaches to treat the pain if the above steps are insufficient (e.g. neuraxial [intrathecal, epidural] or neurosurgical techniques).

Intractable pain

Pain that is resistant to standard analgesia regimes is referred to as intractable pain (McCulloch and Collins 2006). The incidence of intractable pain in children at the end of life is low, most commonly occurring in children with cancer. As paediatric pain management has become more sophisticated the need to resort to techniques such as palliative sedation has diminished, although this is still required in rare situations (McCulloch and Collins 2006).

Misconceptions about using opioids in palliative care

There are several common misconceptions relating to the use of opioids in palliative care. These are discussed later in this chapter in addition to other misconceptions that affect care for children at the end of life.

9.6.3 Other pain-relieving interventions

Radiotherapy

- Used to palliate pain, bleeding and obstruction or compression caused by cancers (Zaki 2005).
- Commonly used for pain caused by bony metastases, spinal cord compression, solid tumours, brain metastases and headache from brain tumours.

- Opioid doses may need to be considerably reduced following radiotherapy, as significant pain relief is usually achieved (Goldman et al. 2006a).

Palliative chemotherapy

- Used to reduce pain by reduction of tumour size or to slow the rate of medullary distension in long bones caused by proliferation of immature cancer cells in the bone marrow (Goldman et al. 2006a).
- The desired outcome needs to be balanced against the adverse effects, which may entail further medical interventions and hospitalisation.

Regional anaesthesia

- Regional anaesthesia techniques such as epidural, intrathecal or regional nerve blocks can be used to target pain in specific areas of the body. These may be administered as short-term infusions or implantable delivery devices can be used for long-term management (Collins and Frager 2006).
- While these techniques often provide significant improvement in analgesia, their benefits need to be weighed against the requirement for invasive procedures, additional monitoring and supervision, and reduction in mobility.

9.6.4 Management of non-pain symptoms

The varied causes of non-pain symptoms commonly seen in paediatric palliative care and both pharmacological and non-drug strategies for their management are reviewed in Table 9.8.

Assessing non-pain symptoms

There are limited instruments for assessing and measuring symptoms other than pain in children. Simple strategies, such as using a 5-point Likert rating scale (a Likert scale rates from complete agreement to complete disagreement, with a neutral middle point) to rate severity and frequency of the symptoms can be useful (Goldman et al. 2006a). There are only a very small number of formal paediatric tools, such as the Memorial Symptom Assessment Scale: a 30-point patient-rated scale to rate the severity, prevalence and impact of cancer-related symptoms (Collins et al. 2000) and the Children's Fatigue Scale: a patient-rated scale to measure the severity and impact of fatigue on life activities (Goldman et al. 2006a). Utilising the strategies discussed earlier in this chapter to enable global assessment of pain may assist in the assessment of non-pain symptoms also.

When to treat non-pain symptoms

When considering which symptoms need treating the following points should be considered:

- impact of the symptoms (e.g. physical and emotional impact);
- interference with life (e.g. with activities of daily life, sleep and quality of life);
- degree of disruption or distress the symptoms cause to the child, parent or family;
- the impact of the child's symptoms on parental mood and coping.

9.6.5 Non-drug methods of symptom management

Detailed discussions about non-drug methods of pain relief can be found in Chapter 5. Many of these strategies are useful for non-pain symptoms as well, although research

Table 9.8 Management of non-pain symptoms

Symptom	Possible causes	Considerations	Pharmacological	Non-drug
Fatigue and/or drowsiness	Disease process Raised intracranial pressure (ICP) Anaemia Hypoxia Medication Mood related Inactivity Deconditioning Renal/hepatic failure	Review activity and sleep regime	Adjust medications Add non-opioids Consider morning psychostimulants Consider medication to restore sleep cycle Trial of melatonin	Educate that opioid tolerance improves in time Schedule am activities & pm naps Keep active/mild exercise & avoid inactivity Review mood Consider trial of caffeinated beverages
Dyspnoea and/or cough	Disease process Anxiety Anaemia Secretions Medication Pulmonary oedema Hypoxia Infection Ascites Pain Organ failure	Reduce anxiety	Trial low dose opioid (25% analgesic dose) Topical local anaesthetic Benzodiazepines Trial drying agents, e.g. glycopyrrolate Consider antibiotics Treat anaemia	Educate and reassure Try fan, breeze Trial waiting/blow-by oxygen Relaxation, music Sip iced water Breathing exercises Position upright Humidification
Anorexia and/or weight loss (cachexia)	Disease process Medication Bowels/nausea related Ileus/Obstruction Pain Mucositis Inactivity Depressed mood Metabolic	This may be a normal part of disease process Review current food intake Review mood	Consider appetite stimulants or steroids Consider food supplements or hydration depending on goals of care	Educate Calm and reassure Small, frequent, high caloric meals as desired Mouth care Relaxation, hypnosis Emotional support

Table 9.8   Continued

Symptom	Possible causes	Considerations	Pharmacological	Non-drug
Seizures	Disease process Metabolic Raised ICP Infection Tumour growth Hypoglycaemia Missed medications Acute drug withdrawal	Ensure seizure management plan Ensure safe environment	Adjust/review anticonvulsant doses Benzodiazepines for prolonged seizures, e.g. rectal diazepam, buccal midazolam or clonazepam	Educate about seizures and safety Consider use of helmet Calm and reassure
Restlessness Agitation Confusion	Medications Disease process Pain Raised ICP Infection Metabolic Hypoxia Renal/hepatic failure Fear/anxiety Urinary retention Acute drug withdrawal	Assess family mood Review environment stimulus Review medications	Rotate opioids Consider: Benzodiazepines, e.g. lorazepam, diazepam Neuroleptics, e.g. haloperidol Antipsychotics, e.g. respiridone, chlorpromazine Other medications: clonidine, chloral hydrate	Educate and reassure Decrease environmental stimulation Regular orientation Relaxation, massage Calm and safe environment Music Aromatherapy
Anxiety Distress Sadness and/or Depression	Pain Hypoxia Sleep Mood Secrecy Poor communication Loss of hope Collusion Spiritual distress	Assess family mood Assess child's and family knowledge of the situation	Consider mood elevating drugs Consider benzodiazepines for anxiety, e.g. lorazepam, diazepam	Educate and reassure Calm and safe environment Open communication Emotional support Relaxation, hypnosis Massage Music, aromatherapy Psychological support Prayer

Symptom	Causes	Assessment/Prevention	Pharmacological	Non-pharmacological
Nausea and/or Vomiting	Medications Constipation Reduced motility Tumour growth Disease process Neurological Raised ICP Metabolic Renal/hepatic failure Pain Anxiety Secretions Ileus/obstruction	Review environmental stimulus Assess hydration status	Antiemetics, e.g. metoclopramide, ondansetron, dexamethasone, promethazine Anticholinergics, e.g. scopolamine Sedation e.g. benzodiazepines, haloperidol, clonidine Opioid rotation Surgical review	Peppermint Ginger Ginger ale Acupressure bands Iced drinks Acupuncture Relaxation Distraction Hypnosis Small, bland meals Minimise environmental smells Mouth care
Constipation	Medication Inactivity Muscle weakness Neurological Tumour growth Reduced intake Metabolic Ileus/obstruction	Prevention is the best treatment Begin anti-constipation regime as soon as opioids are started Monitor frequency of bowel actions	Stool softeners, e.g. docusate Bowel stimulants, e.g. senna or bisacodyl Osmotic agents, e.g. lactulose Bulking agents Enema	Increase fluid and diet intake High fibre Activity Abdominal massage Heat packs
Secretions and/or swallowing difficulty	Disease process Medication Cough Intake Bulbar palsy Neurological Infection	Assess if safe to have oral intake	Trial drying agents if secretion-related Saline nebs Artificial saliva Sedation if distressed	Suctioning Mouth care Ice chips Diet as desired Citrus sweets Position upright or on side

Source: Frager (1997); Sourkes et al. (2005); Wrede-Seaman (2005); Poltorak and Benore (2006); Santucci and Mack (2007); Wusthoff et al. (2007); Kersun and Shemesh (2007)

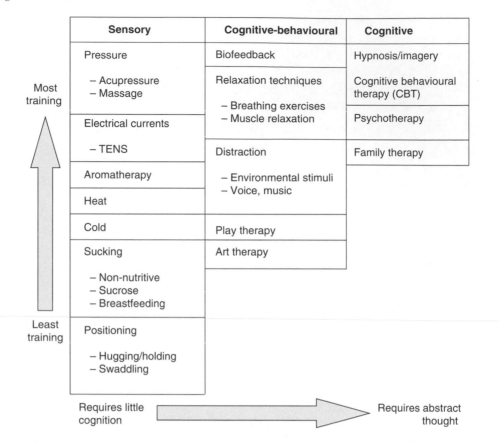

Figure 9.1 Non-drug interventions of pain relief in paediatric palliative care (adapted from Vessey and Carlson 1996).

into safety and efficacy for paediatric palliative care is limited (Kelly 2007). Specific non-drug methods for managing different paediatric palliative care symptoms are outlined in Figure 9.1.

Although the research is sparse there are several authors with extensive experience in paediatric palliative care who recommend various non-drug methods for this population, such as cognitive-behavioural approaches and sensory therapies:

- Vickers et al. (2007) reviewed palliative care provision for children with cancer (*n* = 160) including symptom management and treatment. Of the children at end of life 66% used non-drug methods of pain relief: relaxation 30%, massage 43%, physiotherapy 30%, hypnosis 2.5%. And 54% of children used more than one method at time of death with 32% using more than two. Only 34% used *no* non-drug methods during palliative care.
- Kelly (2007) noted prevalence rates of non-drug methods of pain relief in the past decade had increased from the previous two decades and now ranged from 24% to 90% in children with cancer. Non-drug methods were primarily used for symptom management.
- CHPCA (2006) recommend the following non-drug methods of pain relief to be useful in palliative care: music, art, books, journaling, guided imagery, clowns, play and hypnosis.
- Cognitive behavioural therapies (CBT) are well researched in chronic illness, with less research in palliative care populations (Poltorak and Benore 2006). Effective therapies

are: controlled breathing, progressive muscle relaxation, yoga, acupuncture and biofeedback.

- Russell and Smart (2007) in a small case series (*n* = 4) found hypnosis and guided imagery a useful tool in paediatric hospice to augment other analgesic strategies.
- Brown and Sourkes (2006) considered that the child receiving palliative care (and any siblings) should have psychological evaluation (± parents) to enable optimal care to be planned.
- Brown and Sourkes (2006) nominated relaxation, guided imagery and hypnosis (e.g. the 'pain switch') as useful strategies to give the child a sense of control over anxiety, nausea and pain, to decrease emotional and physical distress and increase their sense of well-being.

> Sourkes et al. (2005) and Wrede-Seaman (2005) provide an overview of different non-drug methods and their application to treating different end of life symptoms.

9.6.6 Misconceptions relating to paediatric palliative care

Several misconceptions exist in relation to paediatric palliative care. These are discussed in Table 9.9. To overcome these misconceptions and enable delivery of optimal palliative care, these issues must be dealt with openly, involving the child, family and healthcare professionals, by:

- addressing the fears;
- clarifying the misconceptions;
- explaining the current knowledge and understanding about opioids;
- having proformas or templates to enable rapid titration of medication to manage symptoms;
- the use of policies and guidelines to direct practice.

Practice point

Reassure parents:
- Saving opioids until pain is worse is unnecessary.
- The child is **not** a drug addict.
- There is **no need** for the child to suffer severe and prolonged pain.
- Strong opioids are best for severe pain.
- The correct dose is the one that relieves the pain.
- Inadequate doses of analgesia will make the child suffer, request more drugs and watch the clock.

9.7 Managing the End of Life Phase

Aims at the end of life are to:

- put the child's needs first and foremost;
- have respect for the family's wishes;
- meet the family's needs;
- ensure healthcare professionals needs are secondary to the child's needs.

Table 9.9   Misconceptions affecting care at end of life

Issue	Reason	Consequence	Reality
Pain is often under treated at end of life (EOL) due to misconceptions about the use of opioids	Healthcare professionals': fear of giving too much analgesia; fear of hastening death with opioids; uncertainty about correct dosing for analgesia and sedation at EOL; Healthcare professionals and family fear of opioid addiction or tolerance	Pain is poorly treated Underuse of opioids High levels of family anxiety The child suffers unnecessarily Increased likelihood of family suffering after the death	There is no upper dose limit for opioids – titration to effect is the aim The disease process is the cause of the child's death, not the medication The risk of addiction is extremely low (Chapter 4) Exaggerated fears of adverse effects minimise opioid use Utilising pain management and palliative care experts enables best outcomes at EOL
Philosophical or religious reasons (of healthcare professionals or family)	Fear of giving up too soon	Refusal to consider palliative care services	Giving up on curative therapy does not imply failure
	Belief that opioids should be reserved until all curative treatments have failed	Avoidance of opioids The child suffers unnecessarily	Relief of pain and suffering does not need to mean the treatment team has given up
	Causing drug-induced respiratory depression is the same as euthanasia	The intent of analgesia is to reduce pain and suffering, not cause death	Respiratory depression is rare in opioid tolerant patients
	Suffering brings you closer to God	The child suffers unnecessarily	Parents' beliefs should not be used to allow suffering Involving religious advisors is vital to resolve the impasse
Clinician 'expertise' issues	'I am the expert and don't need to refer to palliative or pain management services'	Impedes clinicians from seeking advice Parents assume all is being done or nothing more can be done	Evidence does not support this claim – pain and other symptoms are often undertreated by primary clinicians Parents should be encouraged to *always* ask for pain relief *if they consider it is needed*
	Refusal to acknowledge or accept the child's impending death	No open discussions held with family No referral to palliative care	Clinical burden of failure Acknowledging that a cure is not likely frees the family to consider other choices
	Futile treatment at all cost	Focus on goal of cure Inability to accept reality	Curative goals should never override the child's best interest

Source: McGrath and Finley (1996); Galloway and Yaster (2000); Houlahan et al. (2006); Hutton et al. (2006)

9.7.1 Talking with children about death

Children's knowledge of their impending death is often far more advanced than adults around them appreciate. However, children realise that this knowledge is a taboo subject, particularly to their parents. Many children, therefore, collude with their parents to maintain the secrecy or *mutual pretence* but may select other individuals to talk about it (Bluebond-Langner 1978; Liben and Goldman 1998). In a study of parents (*n* = 429) of children who died of cancer almost half the parents (47%) sensed their child knew of their impending death. Thirty-four percent of the parents talked with their children about their impending death and *none* regretted doing this. Of the 258 parents (66%) who did *not* talk with their children 69 (27%) regretted not having done so (Kreicbergs et al. 2004).

9.7.2 Ethical and legal issues in paediatric palliative care

Clinical management of children with life-limiting illness presents a number of ethical issues to healthcare professionals in caring for children at end of life. Different views about value of life, quality of life and beliefs and moral standards can lead to conflict between individual healthcare professionals and between healthcare professionals and families (Goldman et al. 2006a).

> The *Oxford Textbook of Palliative Care for Children* provides an excellent overview and discussion about ethical issues in paediatric palliative care (Goldman et al. 2006a).

Futility in medical management

- The difficulty that some healthcare professionals and families have in accepting the untimely death of a child can lead to futile medical treatments being continued, sometimes until the moment of death.
- Uncertainty about illness trajectory, the outcome of interventions, the child's prognosis, legal implications, defining the terminal phase, illnesses with mixed phases (e.g. cystic fibrosis) can play a key role also (Levetown 1996).
- The consequence of continuing futile treatments can lead to the child's best interests being overlooked and the parents' requests being overridden, which can be compounded by healthcare professionals with poor skills in decision-making and the ability to be objective (Liben and Goldman 1998).

Euthanasia versus double effect

It is important that healthcare professionals clearly understand the differences between *euthanasia* and *treatment to relieve pain and suffering* and *the principle of double effect.*

- Assisted suicide or euthanasia is an intentional or deliberate act with the *primary intent* being to cause death and the *secondary effect* being pain relief or end to suffering. In many countries of the world euthanasia is regarded as a criminal act.
- Palliative care practice does *not* include euthanasia, even if requested by the patient or family.
- In palliative care the *primary intent* is to give pain relief and comfort and the *secondary effect* of this may be risk of respiratory depression or apnoea or early death. Analgesia given in this situation is thus considered a morally good and legally justified act.
- There is a philosophical and legal difference between the intended and unintended outcomes of these actions, known as the *principle of double effect.*

- The principle of double effect is defined as: *the actions resulting in unfavourable results are forgiven if the consequences are foreseen but unintended* (Harrington Jacobs 2005).
- A final ethical and moral difficulty facing healthcare professionals is the withholding or withdrawing of medical treatment, which may be considered by some to be *passive* euthanasia. The debate over this will no doubt continue for a considerable time (Goldman et al. 2006a).

Further information and detailed discussion about decisions to withhold or withdraw medical treatment can be found in the RCPCH (2004) document: *Withholding or Withdrawing Life Sustaining Treatment in Children: A framework in practice.*
A useful education module about decision-making in paediatric palliative care by McConnell and Frager (2004) can be found at: http://www.cme.utoronto.ca/endoflife/default.html.

9.7.3 End of life care

Diagnosis of dying

The diagnosis and physical process of dying causes enormous distress to many healthcare professionals, who in their attempts to make things better for families or reduce their own anxiety, can unwittingly make the situation worse (Ellershaw and Ward 2003). The family is often unaware that death is imminent due to confusing and conflicting information and poor communication by healthcare professionals (Ellershaw and Ward 2003). This leads to:

- false hopes;
- decreased trust of healthcare professionals;
- concerns about withholding or withdrawing treatment;
- uncontrolled symptoms;
- inappropriate decisions for unrealistic and futile interventions;
- inappropriate CPR;
- the patient's and family's needs not being met;
- family regrets after the death.

All these factors place families at increased risk of complex bereavement (Ellershaw and Ward 2003).

Ellershaw and Ward (2003) recommend overcoming these issues by healthcare professionals:

- identifying and regularly reporting signs of dying to the family;
- communicating clearly and unambiguously;
- planning care based on the clinical findings.

Kuttner (2007) provides an excellent overview about talking to families of dying children.

Management of the final stages

During the final stages the following steps should be taken:

- Regular assessment of symptoms.
- Regular identification of the patient's and family's needs and desires.
- Regular discussion and update about the clinical condition with the family.

- Have clear rescue plans for symptom control (adequate for severe escalation) for: pain and sedation (e.g. for dyspnoea/agitation/uncontrolled bleeding).
- Have a key contact person for 24-hour support (regardless of the location of death).
- Convert analgesics to the most simple *and* effective route: nasogastric or PEG (only if gut is functioning); subcutaneous; intravenous.
- Discontinue less-necessary medications, e.g. simple analgesics, laxatives, antibiotics, steroids and cardiac drugs.
- Stop or minimise tests, observations, interventions, monitoring, turning regimes.
- Continue comfort care: mouth care, repositioning.
- Consider 'do not resuscitate' (DNR) or 'allow natural death' (AND) orders, if necessary.
- Offer discussions about autopsy, organ or tissue donation, dying phase and funerals.

'Rule of 3' for monitoring deterioration

- Hour by hour deterioration: review in 3 hours.
- Day by day deterioration: review in 3 days.
- If further deterioration has occurred, treat for comfort.
- If no further deterioration, consider treating or set another review time or date.

Source: Dean et al. 2006

Family bereavement care

The death of a child or sibling causes profound grief and distress for the whole family. Parental grief may be more severe, profound and longer lasting than other types of grief. This makes the psychosocial care of families during the palliative phase of a child's illness particularly important. It has recently become apparent that it is the time *leading up to* the child's death, rather than the time following the death when support may be crucial (Bartell and Kissane 2005).

No consensus has been reached about the best way to manage bereavement, but factors that promote recovery (Bartell and Kissane 2005; Kreicbergs et al. 2007) are:

- family-focused psychological support prior to the death;
- providing information about normal grief and what to expect;
- encouraging strong social support systems;
- offering additional support for those with very high levels of distress and at risk for complicated grief (Box 9.7).

BOX 9.7

Risk factors for complicated grief

- Death of a child
- Long illness prior to the death
- Sudden, unexpected death
- Difficult or traumatic death
- Feelings of regret related to the death
- Lack of social support
- History of previous losses
- Multiple stressors in life
- Physical or mental illness
- Very high distress after the death
- Isolated, alienated individuals
- Being a parent of a child that dies
- Lack of sense of control over life

Source: Aranda and Milne (2000)

Staff support

Healthcare professionals involved in paediatric palliative care experience trauma responses, particularly secondary traumatic stress (Rourke 2007). A major occupational hazard of working in this field is *compassion fatigue*. This encompasses three key areas: psychological, interpersonal and cognitive (Rourke 2007):

- Psychological effects (e.g. strong emotions, intrusive thoughts, numbness, somatic complaints, isolation).
- Interpersonal effects (e.g. withdrawal from colleagues, withdrawal from relationships, skewed boundaries, emotional detachment, being easily irritated).
- Cognitive effects (e.g. mistrust, grandiose ideas, cynicism, increased sense of responsibility or blame, feeling that no one understands).

To continue working in such a high stress area, paediatric palliative care staff need to look after themselves in a systematic way (Table 9.10) for self-preservation, satisfaction and most importantly to ensure their patients and families are being cared for in the best possible way.

Summary

- Palliative care encompasses relief of pain and other symptoms by providing total care of the child and the family while aiming to achieve the best possible quality of life.
- 60% of children die from life-limiting conditions such as cancers, congenital abnormalities and nervous system disorders.
- Despite the evidence that most families would prefer their children to die at home, most die in hospital, receiving high levels of invasive medical care.
- The most common symptoms at end of life are fatigue and pain, regardless of diagnosis.
- Providing holistic family-centred care involving comprehensive pharmacological and non-drug techniques are the most useful ways to manage symptom control.
- Severe pain should be treated as an emergency and dealt with rapidly.

Table 9.10　Prevention of compassion fatigue for staff involved in paediatric palliative care

Personal	Professional	Organisational
Appropriate sleep, nutrition and exercise	Peer support networks	Acknowledge compassion fatigue
Add relaxation into day via tools such as meditation or massage	Maintain clear boundaries	Ensure the physical environment is conducive to decrease stress
Do non-work activities to restore, refocus and revitalise	Balanced workload and adequate time not on-call	Ensure adequate resources for the team to function
Keep a good work-life balance	Staff support: debriefing, clinical supervision	Respect for the work of the team and the importance of their work
Acknowledge losses and responses to these	Education and information sharing	Develop a connected, supportive team unit
Develop healthy coping skills Attend to own spiritual needs		

Source: Rourke (2007)

- The appropriate dose of an opioid is the one that is effective to relieve pain.
- Misconceptions about pain control and end of life care should be dealt with openly and promptly to avoid these impacting negatively on the child's terminal phase.
- Open, honest discussions about death and dying reduce inappropriate medical decisions, relieve family distress and decrease the risk of complex bereavement.
- Family bereavement issues should be addressed both before and after the death of a child.
- Healthcare professionals involved in paediatric palliative care risk burnout unless preventive interventions are implemented at personal, professional and institutional levels.

Useful web resources

The Association of Children's Hospices (ACH): www.childhospice.org.uk
The Association for Children's Palliative Care (ACT): http://www.act.org.uk
The Canadian Network for Palliative Care for Children: www.cnpcc.ca
Center for Palliative Studies, San Diego Hospice: www.cpsonline.info/
Children's International Project on Palliative/Hospice Services (ChIPPS): www.nhpco.org
Initiative for Pediatric Palliative care: http://www.ippcweb.org/
The Royal Children's Hospital, Melbourne, Paediatric Palliative Care program: http://www.rch.org.au/rch_palliative/index.cfm?doc_id=1650
World Health Organization Cancer Programme: www.who.int/cancer/en/

Other useful resources

Carter, B.S. and Levetown, M. (eds.) (2004) *Palliative Care for Infants, Children and Adolescents*, The Johns Hopkins University Press, Baltimore, Maryland.
Hilden, J., Tobin, D.R. and Lindsey, K. (2003) *Shelter from the Storm: Caring for the Child with a Life-threatening Condition*, Perseus Books Group, Cambridge, Massachusetts.
Jassal, S.S. (ed) (2008) *Basic symptom control in paediatric palliative care: The Rainbow Children's Hospice Guidelines*, 7th edition: www.library.nhs.uk/childhealth/ViewResource.aspx?resID=276035
Noyce, M. and Irving, H. (2002) *Palliative Care for Children with Cancer – A Guide for Parents*, Royal Children's Hospital, Brisbane, Queensland Health, Australia.
Sourkes, B. (1995) *Armfuls of time: The Psychological Experience of the Child with a Life-threatening Illness*, University of Pittsburgh Press, Pittsburgh.
Turner, M. (2006) Talking with children and young people about death and dying, Jessica Kingsley Publishers, London, UK.

References

Abu-Saad, H.H. (2000) Palliative care: an international view, *Patient Education and Counseling*, 41: 15–22.
Abu-Saad, H.H. and Courtens, A. (2003) *Evidence-based palliative care – across the life span*, Blackwell Science Ltd, Oxford, UK.
American Academy of Pediatrics (AAP) Committee on Bioethics and Committee on Hospital Care (2000) Palliative Care for Children, *Pediatrics*, 106(2) 351–357.
Aranda, S. and Milne, D. (2000) *Guidelines for the assessment of bereavement risk in family members of people receiving palliative care*, Centre for Palliative Care, Melbourne.
Association of Children's Hospices (ACH) (2004a) *Guidelines for Best Practice in a Children's Hospice Service*, ACT, Bristol.
Association of Children's Hospices (ACH) Hurd, E. (2004b) *Are we getting it right? A tool to measure the quality of children's hospice services*, ACT, Bristol.
Association for Children with Life-threatening or Terminal Conditions and their Families (ACT) and the Royal College of Paediatrics and Child Health (RCPCH) (2003a) *A Guide to the Development of*

Children's Palliative Care Services, (2nd edition), Report of a Joint Working party of ACT and RCPCH, ACT, Bristol.

Association for Children with Life-threatening or Terminal Conditions and their Families (ACT) Hunt, A., Elston, S. and Galloway, J. (2003b) *Voices for change: current perception of services for children with palliative care needs and their families*, ACT, Bristol.

Association for Children with Life-threatening or Terminal Conditions and their Families (ACT) Elston, S. (2003c) *Assessment of children with life-limiting conditions and their families: a guide to effective care planning*, ACT, Bristol.

Association for Children with Life-threatening or Terminal Conditions and their Families (ACT) Elston, S. (2004a) *A framework for the development of integrated multi-agency care pathways for children with life-threatening and life-limiting conditions*, ACT, Bristol.

Association for Children with Life-threatening or Terminal Conditions and their Families (ACT) (2004b) *The ACT Charter*, ACT, Bristol.

Association for Children's Palliative Care (ACT) (2007a) *ACT Integrated Palliative Care Pathway Standards: Service Self Assessment Tool*, ACT, Bristol.

Association for Children's Palliative Care (ACT) (2007b) *ACT Transition Care Pathway Standards: Service Self Assessment Tool*, ACT, Bristol.

Bartell, A.S. and Kissane, D.W. (2005) Issues in pediatric palliative care: understanding families, *Journal of Palliative Care*, 21(3): 165–172.

Bluebond-Langner, M. (1978) *The Private Worlds of Dying Children*, Princeton University Press, Princeton, New Jersey.

Brown, M.R. and Sourkes, B. (2006) Psychotherapy in pediatric palliative care, *Child and Adolescent Psychiatric Clinics of North America*, 15: 585–596.

Canadian Hospice Palliative Care Association (CHPCA) (2006) *Pediatric Hospice Palliative Care: Guiding principles and norms of practice*, CHPCA, Ottawa.

Carter, B.S., Howenstein, M., Gilmer, M.J., Throop, P., France, D. and Whitlock, J.A. (2004) Circumstances surrounding the deaths of hospitalized children: opportunities for pediatric palliative care, *Pediatrics*, 114(3): e361–e366.

Collins, J.J. and Frager, G. (2006) Pain and pain relief in pediatric end-of-life care. In Finley, G.A., McGrath, P.J. and Chambers, C.T. (eds.) *Bringing Pain Relief to Children: Treatment Approaches*, Humana Press, Totowa, pp. 59–83.

Collins, J.J., Stevens, M.M. and Cousens, P. (1998) Home care for the dying child, *Australian Family Physician*, 27(7): 610–614.

Collins, J.J., Byrnes, M.E., Dunkel, I.J., Lapin, J., Nadel, T., Thaler, H.T., Polyak, T., Rapkin, B. and Portenoy, R.K. (2000) The measurement of symptoms in children with cancer, *Journal of Pain and Symptom Management*, 19(5): 363–377.

Collins, J.J., Devine, T.D., Dick, G.S., Johnson, E.A., Kilham, H.A., Pinkerton, C.R., Stevens, M.M., Thaler, H.T. and Portenoy, R.K. (2002) The measurement of symptoms in young children with cancer: the validation of the Memorial Symptom Assessment Scale in children aged 7–12, *Journal of Pain and Symptom Management*, 23(1): 10–16.

Craig, F., Abu-Saad, H. Benini, F., Kuttner, L., Wood, C., Ferraris, P.C. and Zernikow, B. EAPC Taskforce Steering Group, (2007) IMPaCCT: standards for paediatric palliative care in Europe, *European Journal of Palliative Care*, 14(3): 109–114.

Dangel, T. (2002) The status of paediatric palliative care in Europe, *Journal of Pain and Symptom Management*, 24(2): 160–165.

Dean, M., Harris J-D., Regnard, C. and Hockley, J. (2006) *Symptom Relief in Palliative Care*, Radcliffe Publishing, Oxford.

Department of Health (2007a) *Palliative Care Services for children and young people in England – An independent review for the Secretary of State for health by Professor Sir Alan Croft and Sue Killen*, The Stationery Office, London.

Department of Health, Cochrane, H., Liyanage, S. and Nantambi, R. (2007b) *Palliative Care statistics for children and young adults*, The Stationery Office, London.

Drake, R., Frost, J. and Collins, J.J. (2003) The symptoms of dying children, *Journal of Pain and Symptom Management*, 26(1): 594–603.

Drake, R., Longworth, J. and Collins, J.J. (2004) Opioid rotation in children with cancer, *Journal of Palliative Medicine*, 7(3): 419–422.

Ellershaw, J. and Ward, C. (2003) Care of the dying patient: the last hours or days of life, *British Medical Journal*, 326: 30–34.

Feudtner, C., Christakis, D.A., Zimmerman, F.J., Muldoon, J.H., Neff, J.M. and Koepsell, T.D. (2002) Characteristics of deaths occurring in children's hospitals: implications for supportive care services, *Pediatrics*, 109(5): 887–893.

Field, M.J and Behrman, R.E. (eds.) (2003) *When Children Die: improving palliative and end-of-life care for children and their families,* Institute of Medicine, National Academy Press, Washington DC.

Frager, G. (1997) Palliative care and terminal care of children, *Child and Adolescent Psychiatric Clinics of North America,* 6(4): 889–909.

Freidrichsdorf, S.J. and Kang, T.I. (2007) The management of pain in children with life-limiting illnesses, *Pediatric Clinics of North America,* 54: 645–672.

Friedrichsdorf, S.J., Menke, A., Brun, S., Wamsler, C. and Zernikow, B. (2005) Status quo of palliative care in pediatric oncology – a nationwide survey in Germany, *Journal of Pain and Symptom Management,* 29(2): 156–164.

Galloway, K.S. and Yaster, M. (2000) Pain and symptom control in terminally ill children, *Pediatric Clinics of North America,* 47(3): 711–747.

Garros, D., Rosychuk, R.J. and Cox, P.N. (2003) Circumstances surrounding end-of-life in a pediatric intensive care unit, *Pediatrics,* 112(5): 3371-e379.

Goldman, A. (1996) Home care of the dying child, *Journal of Palliative Care,* 12(3): 16–19.

Goldman, A. (2000) Symptoms and suffering at the end of life in children with cancer, *New England Journal of Medicine,* 342(26) [Correspondence]: 1997–1999.

Goldman, A., Beardsmore, S. and Hunt, A. (1990) Palliative care for children with cancer – home, hospital, or hospice? *Archives of Disease in Childhood,* 65: 641–643.

Goldman, A., Hain, R. and Liben, S. (eds.) (2006a) *Oxford Textbook of Palliative Care for Children,* Oxford University Press, Oxford.

Goldman, A., Hewitt, M., Collins, G.S., Childs, M. and Hain, R. (2006b) Symptoms in children/young people with progressive malignant disease: United Kingdom Children's Cancer Study Group/Paediatric Oncology Nurses Forum Survey, *Pediatrics,* 117(6): e1179–e1186.

Harding, R. (2006) Palliative care – a basic human right, *id21 insights health,* 8: 1–2.

Harrington Jacobs, H. (2005) Ethics in pediatric end-of-life care: a nursing perspective, *Journal of Pediatric Nursing,* 20(5): 360–369.

Himelstein, B.P. (2005) Palliative care in pediatrics, *Anesthesiology Clinics of North America,* 23: 837–856.

Himelstein, B.P. (2006) Palliative care for infants, children, adolescents and their families, *Journal of Palliative Medicine,* 9(6): 163–181.

Houlahan, K.E., Branowicki, P.A., Mack, J.W., Dinning, C. and McCabe, M. (2006) Can end-of-life care for the pediatric patient suffering with escalating and intractable symptoms be improved? *Journal of Pediatric Oncology Nursing,* 23(1): 45–51.

Hunt, A. (1990) A survey of signs, symptoms and symptom control in 30 terminally ill children, *Developmental Medicine and Child Neurology,* 32: 341–346.

Hutton, N., Jones, B. and Hilden, J.M. (2006) From cure to palliation: managing the transition, *Child and Adolescent Psychiatric Clinics of North America,* 15(3): 575–584.

Hynson, J.L., Gillis, J., Collins, J.J., Irving, H. and Trethewie, S.J. (2003) The dying child: how is care different? *Medical Journal of Australia,* 179(6 Suppl): S20–22.

Jalmsell, L., Kreicbergs, U., Onelov, E., Steineck, G. and Henter, J. (2006) Symptoms affecting children with malignancies during the last month of life: a nationwide follow-up, *Pediatrics,* 117(4): 1314–1320.

Kelly, K.M. (2007) Complementary and alternative medicines for use in supportive care in pediatric cancer, *Support Care Cancer,* 15: 457–460.

Kendall, M., Harris, F., Boyd, K., Sheikh, A., Murray, S.A., Brown, D., Malinson, I., Kearney, N. and Worth, A. (2007) Key challenges and ways forward in researching the 'good death': qualitative in-depth interview and focus group study, *British Medical Journal,* 334: 521, doi:10.1136/bmj.39097.582639.55.

Kersun, L.S. and Shemesh, E. (2007) Depression and anxiety in children at the end of life, *Pediatric Clinics of North America,* 54: 691–708.

Kriecbergs, U., Valdimarsdottir, U., Onelov, E., Henter, J. and Steineck G. (2004) Talking about death with children who have severe malignant disease, *New England Journal of Medicine,* 351(12): 1175–1186.

Kreicbergs, U., Lannen, P., Onelov, E. and Wolfe, J. (2007) Parental grief after losing a child to cancer: impact of professional and social support on long-term outcomes, *Journal of Clinical Oncology,* 25(22): 3307–3312.

Kuttner, L. (2007) Talking with families when their children are dying, *Medical Principles and Practice,* 16(Suppl 1): 16–20.

Levetown, M. (1996) Ethical aspects of pediatric palliative care, *Journal of Palliative Care,* 12(3): 35–39.

Liben, S. and Goldman, A. (1998) Home care for children with life-threatening illness, *Journal of Palliative Care,* 14(3): 33–38.

Mack, J.W. and Wolfe, J. (2006) Early integration of pediatric palliative care: for some children, palliative care starts at diagnosis, *Current Opinion in Pediatrics*, 18(1): 10–14.

McCallum, D.E., Byrne, P. and Breura, E. (2000) How children die in hospital, *Journal of Pain and Symptom Management*, 20(6): 417–423.

McConnell, Y. and Frager, G. (2004) *Module 12: Decision-making in pediatric palliative care*, Ian Anderson Continuing Education Program in End-of Life Care, University of Toronto, Canada, www.cme.utoronto.ca/endoflife/default.html (accessed 15 September 2007).

McCulloch, R. and Collins, J.J. (2006) Pain in children who have life-limiting conditions. *Child and Adolescent Psychiatric Clinics of North America*, 15(3): 657–682.

McGrath, P.J. and Finley, G.A. (1996) Attitudes and beliefs about medication and pain management in children, *Journal of Palliative Care*, 12(3): 46–50.

Mongeau, S. and Liben, S. (2007) Participatory research in pediatric palliative care: benefits and challenges, *Journal of Palliative Care*, 23(1): 5–13.

National Consensus Project for Quality Palliative Care (2004), *Clinical practice guidelines for quality palliative care*, http://www.nationalconsensusproject.org (accessed 1 August 2007).

Poltorak, D.Y. and Benore, E. (2006) Cognitive-behavioral interventions for physical symptom management in pediatric palliative medicine, *Child and Adolescent Psychiatric Clinics of North America*, 15: 683–691.

Ramnarayan, P., Craig, F., Petros, A. and Pierce, C. (2007) Characteristics of deaths occurring in hospitalised children: changing trends, *Journal of Medical Ethics*, 33, 255–260.

Robinson, W.M., Ravilly, S., Berde, C. and Wohl, M.E. (1997) End-of-life care in cystic fibrosis, *Pediatrics*, 100(2): 205–209.

Rourke, M.T. (2007) Compassion fatigue in pediatric palliative care providers, *Pediatric Clinics of North America*, 54: 631–644.

Royal College of Paediatrics and Child Health (2004) *Withholding or Withdrawing Life Sustaining Treatment in Children: A framework in practice*, (2nd edition), Royal College of Paediatrics and Child Health, London.

Russell, C. and Smart, S. (2007) Guided imagery and distraction therapy in paediatric hospice care, *Paediatric Nursing*, 19(2): 24–25.

Santucci, G. and Mack, J.W. (2007) Common gastrointestinal symptoms in pediatric palliative care: nausea, vomiting, constipation, anorexia, cachexia, *Pediatric Clinics of North America*, 54: 673–689.

Sourkes, B., Frankel, L., Brown, M., Contro, N., Benitz, W., Case, C., Good, J., Jones, L., Komejan, J., Modderman-Marshall, J., Reichard, W., Sentivany-Collins, S. and Sunde, C. (2005) Food, toys and love: pediatric palliative care, *Current Problems in Pediatric and Adolescent Health Care*, 35: 350–386.

Vessey, J.A. and Carlson, K.L. (1996) Nonpharmacological interventions to use with children in pain, *Issues in Comprehensive Pediatric Nursing*, 19: 169–182.

Vickers, J.L. and Carlisle, C. (2000) Choices and control: parental experiences in pediatric terminal home care, *Journal of Pediatric Oncology Nursing*, 17(1): 12–21.

Vickers, J., Thompson, A., Collins, G.S., Childs, M. and Hain, R. (2007) Place and provision of palliative care for children with progressive cancer: a study by the Paediatric Nurses' Forum/United Kingdom Children's Cancer Study Group Palliative Care Working Group, *Journal of Clinical Oncology*, 25(28): 4472–4476.

Widger, K.A. and Wilkins, K. (2004) What are the key components of quality perinatal and pediatric end-of-life care? A literature review, *Journal of Palliative Care*, 20(2): 105–112.

Widger, K., Davies, D., Drouin, D.J., Beaune, L., Daoust, L., Farran, P., Humbert, N, Nalewajek, F., Rattray, M., Rugg, M. and Bishop, M. (2007) Pediatric patients receiving palliative care in Canada: results of a multicenter review, *Archives of Pediatrics and Adolescent Medicine*, 161(6): 597–602.

Wolfe, J., Grier, H.E., Klar, N., Levin, S.B., Ellenbogen, J.M., Salem-Schatz, S., Emanuel, E.J. and Weeks, J.C. (2000) Symptoms and suffering at the end of life in children with cancer, *New England Journal of Medicine*, 342(5): 326–333.

World Health Organization (1998) *Cancer Pain Relief and Palliative Care in Children*, World Health Organization, Geneva.

World Health Organization (2006) *Definition of palliative care*, http://www.who.int/cancer/palliative/definition/en/ (accessed 17 November 2007).

Wrede-Seaman, L. (2005) *Pediatric Pain and Symptom Management Algorithms for Palliative Care*, Intellicard Inc, Yakima, Washington.

Wusthoff, C.J., Shellhaas, R.A. and Licht, D.J. (2007) Management of common neurologic symptoms in pediatric palliative care: seizures, agitation and spasticity, *Pediatric Clinics of North America*, 54: 709–733.

Zaki, B.I. (2005) Palliative and pain medicine: radiation oncology, *Techniques in Regional Anesthesia and Pain Management*, 9: 177–183.

CHAPTER 10

Management of Painful Procedures

Elizabeth Bruce

Introduction

The management of procedural pain in children is slowly improving, but is still far from ideal. Children have described the pain of a needle as one of the worst experiences of being in hospital (Doorbar and McClarey 1999). Despite this, in a recent survey of five paediatric emergency departments, only 38% of respondents used pharmacological interventions prior to insertion of an intravenous cannula (Bhargava and Young 2007). This chapter discusses the management of procedural pain in children, highlighting the importance of planning and preparation in the assessment stage and discussing the evidence for the various pharmacological and non-drug interventions that can be used to manage procedural pain. The use of sedation is not covered in this chapter, as the focus is on the management of *painful* procedures. However, the importance of assessing whether analgesia, sedation, anxiety reduction or a general anaesthetic is required is discussed.

> Information on the safe, effective sedation of children for procedures can be found in other documents such as the Scottish Intercollegiate Guidelines Network (SIGN 2004) sedation guidelines. Available from: http://www.apagbi.org.uk/docs/sign58.pdf.

10.1 Assessment

The key to the effective management of painful procedures is preparation, planning and the provision of information. A thorough assessment is essential to determine the amount of pain and fear the procedure is likely to invoke as well as the child's prior experiences of painful procedures. Once this information is gathered, decisions can be made about the most appropriate pain-relieving interventions to use.

There are a number of pain assessment tools that can be used to assess procedural pain (see Chapter 6). Pain should be assessed *before, during and after* the procedure.

Before the procedure: To determine the level of anticipatory pain and fear and the child's current pain status. If the child is already experiencing pain this will make pain and fear during the procedure more likely to occur and harder to manage.

During the procedure: To determine whether interventions to relieve pain and fear are effective. If not, the procedure may need to be stopped and/or new interventions agreed.

After the procedure: To determine what worked well and whether any changes need to be planned to improve any future interventions.

10.1.1 Preparation and information

Preparation and information are essential for the effective management of painful procedures. When planning potentially painful and/or frightening procedures a number of questions should be considered:

1. Why is the procedure being performed and will it need to be repeated?
2. How will the procedure be performed?
3. Where will the procedure be performed?
4. What is the expected intensity and duration of pain?
5. How frightening is the procedure likely to be?
6. How important is it that the child remains still during the procedure?
7. How do parents think they and/or their child might react?
8. What can the parent(s) do to help?
9. Has the child/family been adequately prepared?

Each of these questions will now be addressed in turn.

Why is the procedure being performed and will it need to be repeated?
- Is the procedure essential?
- Will it be carried out by a competent practitioner using the least painful method available?
- If several procedures need to be carried out, can these be grouped together?
- If other tests or procedures are planned under sedation or anaesthesia, could the procedure be delayed until then?
- Is the child being subjected to repeated or unnecessary procedures?
- Have the child and family been given information about why and how the procedure will be carried out?

How will the procedure be performed?
For example:

- When obtaining a blood sample, venepuncture by a skilled practitioner is both less painful and more reliable than a heel prick (Shah and Ohlsson 2004).
- The use of longer needles and pressure to the area afterwards reduces the pain of an intramuscular injection (Schechter et al. 2007).
- Skin glue is less painful than sutures for wound closure (Farion et al. 2001).
- When infiltrating with local anaesthetic solution, buffering with bicarbonate, warming the solution and injecting slowly using a small-gauge needle may reduce pain (Zempskey et al. 2004).

Where will the procedure be performed?
- The child should be involved in this decision if possible.
- It is advisable to avoid carrying out procedures by or in the child's bed so that that this remains a *safe place*.

- Some children find it more comforting to be somewhere familiar.
- If the area chosen does not have a bed or access to oxygen and suction, the use of analgesic drugs such as opioids and nitrous oxide, which can cause sedation, should be avoided until an appropriate venue can be arranged.

Practice point

Give hospitalised children a predictable *safe* time when procedures will not be done.
  Avoid painful routes such as intramuscular injection when giving pain relief.

What is the expected intensity and duration of pain?

- Knowledge regarding how much pain is expected and for how long will help health-care professionals plan the most effective interventions to manage this.
- For short procedures, quick, short-acting drugs should be used and one or two different non-drug interventions will usually be sufficient.
- For longer procedures, it is important that the drugs used are longer acting or able to be titrated. Non-drug interventions will need to last for the duration of the procedure. It is therefore advisable to have a range of different interventions available that can be used interchangeably.
- For longer procedures, identify points at which it would be possible to take a break, if necessary.
- For more painful procedures, a wider range of pharmacological and non-drug interventions should be considered.
- If the use of pharmacological and non-drug interventions is unlikely to be effective, anxiolysis, sedation or a general anaesthetic should be considered (Figure 10.1).

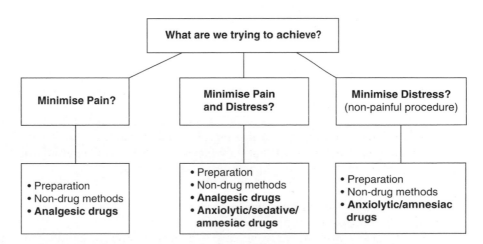

Figure 10.1   Decision-making algorithm (adapted from Penrose and Dowden 2003).

How frightening is the procedure likely to be?

- Fear and other negative emotions such as loss of control affect a child's experience of pain.
- If the child believes that the procedure will cause pain or tissue damage, or they do not understand why the procedure is being performed, this will increase their fear.
- Many children benefit from knowing the types of sensations to expect during the procedure (Royal College of Nursing [RCN] 1999). However, care needs to be taken not to raise children's anxiety through the use of anxiety provoking language.
- Younger children may perceive the procedure as a punishment, which will further exacerbate fear and distress.
- The greater the level of fear and distress, the more likely the child is to experience pain and the less likely they are to remain still during a procedure.
- In a non-random study, children (n = 50) who blamed themselves for their injury anticipated more pain and displayed more behavioural distress during laceration repair (suturing) than children who felt that the injury was not their fault (Langer et al. 2005).
- Age/developmentally appropriate non-drug interventions are essential, as analgesics will manage the *nociceptive* component, but will not reduce the *emotional* component of the painful experience.
- Enabling children to have a degree of control during the procedure (e.g. holding equipment, choosing the plaster or dressing) has been shown to have a positive effect on coping with pain (Hodgins and Lander 1997).

How important is it that the child remains still during the procedure?

- Many procedures require the child to keep fairly still, for example, radiological investigations.
- The greater the likelihood of pain, fear and distress, the more likely the child is to move.
- If the child needs to stay *very* still for a short period, or remain still for a *long period* of time the use of sedation or general anaesthetic should be considered.
- Children should be involved in the decision-making process from an early age and the use of physical restraint should be avoided wherever possible, unless this has been agreed with the child and family (Figure 10.2).

The RCN has written guidelines on the use of restraint on children (RCN 2003). These are available from: http://www.rcn.org.uk/members/downloads/restraining-holding-still-cyp.pdf.

How do parents think they and/or their child might react?

- Obtaining parents' views about how they think they and their child might react during the procedure is an essential part of the planning process.
- Parents may not know how their child will respond if this is their first experience of a medical procedure.

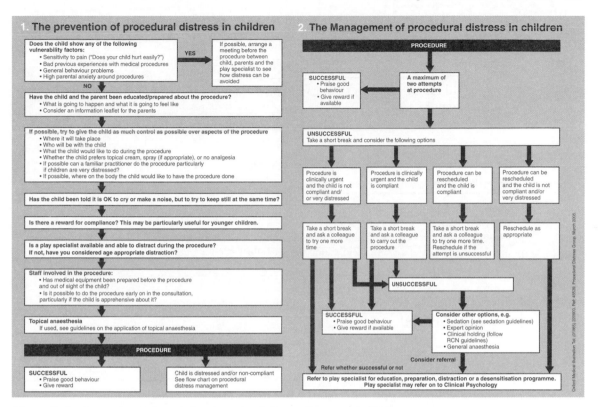

Figure 10.2   Preventing and managing procedural distress (Craze et al. 2005).

What can the parent(s) do to help?

- Children have identified parental presence as the single most important factor that helps them cope with painful and frightening experiences (Woodgate and Kristjanson 1996; Polkki et al. 2003).
- However, if a parent is anxious, this will increase the child's level of anxiety. In an observational study, parents (*n* = 55) experienced an increase in blood pressure, heart rate and anxiety during their child's venepuncture. These responses were predictive of higher levels of child behavioural distress during the procedure (Smith et al. 2007).
- If the parents simply offer reassurance and sympathy this does not help the child and is associated with increased behavioural distress (Kleiber et al. 2001; Langer et al. 2005; Smith et al. 2007).
- Maternal *pain-promoting language* (reassurance, empathy, apology, mild rebuke) *increases* children's reports of pain, while *pain-reducing language* (distraction, humour, encouraging coping behaviours) *decreases* children's reports of pain (Chambers et al. 2002).
- It is therefore important that parents as well as children are given adequate information before the procedure.
- Parents should be encouraged to be present, if possible, but should not be made to feel guilty if they are unable to stay.

If parents intend to be present:

- Their role during the procedure should be planned in advance.
- They should be instructed about coping-promoting behaviours (e.g. distraction, encouragement) and avoid distress-promoting behaviours (e.g. reassurance, sympathy).
- They should be advised not to threaten the child (e.g. *if you don't keep still they'll have to do it again*).
- They should *not* be made to help restrain the child.

Practice point

It is important to educate and reassure the parent, as if they are anxious and think that the procedure will be painful this will influence the child's attitudes and beliefs (Box 10.1).

Children will not always use the coping behaviours they have been taught unless they are encouraged to do so by a parent or nurse during the procedure (Cohen et al. 2002).

Some guidelines to help parents prepare their children for painful procedures are provided in Box 10.1.

BOX 10.1

Helping children cope with pain: what helps and what doesn't help

Things people can do to help with the pain

- **Having a parent or other special person present**. Children feel more secure with their parents there.
- **Simple, accurate information** about what is going to happen. Explain things slowly, in small bits, and repeat as often as needed.
- Children should be helped to **ask questions and express feelings**.
- **Giving a child some control** over treatment. For example, a child who decides whether to sit in a chair or a lap for an injection will probably feel less pain than a child who has no choice.
- **Deep and steady breathing** can help reduce pain and allow the child some control.
- **Distracting the child** from the pain. Talking, video games, breathing exercises, blowing bubbles, television, music, pop-up books, reading and being read to are all distractions.
- **Use the child's imagination** to change from being anxious and frightened to being relaxed and calm Focusing the child's attention on a familiar past activity, or telling or reading a favourite story can help.
- **Use suggestions** for pain relief such as, 'Let the pain just drain away down and out of your body into the bed and away … good … that's it, let it go.' Use the child's own language and the child's favourite activities or experiences.
- **Playing/being silly**. Children relax and forget their worries when they play.
- **Relaxation** is useful for adolescents. Special teaching can be given by a psychologist, nurse or other health professional. Relaxation can reduce anxiety, nausea and vomiting and pain.
- **Comforting touch**. This includes stroking, swaddling, holding, rocking, caressing, cuddling and massaging. Cuddling is nature's own pain remedy.
- **Heat, cold and vibration** can relieve pain. Ice wrapped in a cloth eases some disease and procedure pain. Heat is useful for muscle pain. Vibration, either by gentle tapping or some other mechanical method, can block pain.
- **Positive feedback**. Reminding the child 'you are doing great', 'we're nearly finished'.

BOX 10.1 Continued

Things that don't help with the pain and can make it worse

Lying to children about painful procedures.
Ridiculing or making fun of the child by saying things like 'Only babies cry'.
Using needles as a threat. Lies and threats teach children to distrust and be fearful.
False reassurance. Saying 'it won't hurt at all' when you know it will.
Having very high expectations of the child. It's not useful to make expectations so high that children feel stressed by them.
Talking about the feelings too much. Saying 'I know you're worried/scared' may lessen the child's coping ability.
Focusing too much on the pain or potential pain. Saying 'it will really hurt a lot' is a bad idea. Firstly it might not; secondly it encourages children to expect the worst.

Source: McGrath et al. 2003

Has the child/family been adequately prepared?
- Psychological preparation and the provision of information can reduce procedural pain and distress in children as young as three years of age.
- The information provided needs to be age/developmentally appropriate and delivered in a way that the child can understand.
- Play specialists have an essential role in the preparation of children for and supporting them during painful procedures.
- Therapeutic play can be used to explain a procedure in the third person, to familiarise a child with equipment and to work through any fears that the child might have, as well as providing a method of distraction during the procedure.
- Children and families should be given written information in advance of planned procedures. (Boxes 10.2 and 10.3).
- Computer-based teaching programmes can be used to provide information and teach coping skills to school-age children (Franck and Jones 2003).

How healthcare professionals behave when preparing a child and their parents for a painful procedure also needs to be considered. Inappropriate language or behaviour before

BOX 10.2

Information to help parents prepare their child for painful procedures

Pain, Pain, Go Away: Helping children with pain http://www.rch.org.au/anaes/pain/index.cfm?doc_id=6223
WellChild Pain Research Centre. When your child is in pain. Information to help parents help children when they have pain.
Issue 2. Helping your baby cope with painful medical procedures: www.online.wellchild.org.uk/uploads/documents/pain_leaflet-babies.pdf
Issue 4. Helping your child cope with painful medical procedures. Available from: www.online.wellchild.org.uk/uploads/documents/pain_leaflet-procedure.pdf
Intermountain Primary Children's Medical Center (2006) *Let's Talk About…Helping manage your child's pain*: http://intermountainhealthcare.org/xp/public/documents/pcmc/painmanage.pdf

---

BOX 10.3

Information that the child and parent should be given prior to a painful procedure

A review of procedural pain in children by Young (2005) provides some handy hints for managing procedural pain including:

- Give step-by-step information about what will happen during the procedure, including what the child will see, hear and feel.
- Use age/developmentally appropriate language and avoid medical jargon.
- Avoid high anxiety words such as *pain, hurt, cut* and *shot.*
- Use words such as *poking, freezing* and *squeezing* instead.
- Do not suggest that the procedure will definitely hurt.
- Be aware of possible misinterpretations of words and phrases such as *dye* or *put to sleep.*
- Address children's concerns (for example, *taking all my blood*).
- Consider using books describing the procedure that the child can read with the parent.
- Give information before and during the procedure, and be honest.

---

and during the procedure may adversely affect the child and their parents (see advice about the use of language in Box 10.3).

Young (2005) also provides some **handy hints** for managing procedural pain:

- Maintaining a quiet, calm environment
- Not forcing the child to lie down if they do not want to, unless this is completely necessary
- Avoiding stressors such as beeping monitors
- Avoiding long delays between explaining the procedure to the child and performing it
- Avoiding situations in which children can see or hear procedures being performed on other children
- Avoiding the arm of the preferred thumb in thumb-sucking children for venepuncture or cannulation
- Allowing comfort items such as favourite stuffed animals or blankets
- Allowing *time out* if needed, for long procedures, at set times that have been agreed in advance
- Allowing the child to *count down* from 10 to 1 before a brief procedure
- Giving the child a job, such as holding a dressing or plaster
- Giving the child choices where possible to increase their sense of control
- Using automatic lancets for finger pricks and venepuncture in preference to heel lance wherever possible

10.2 Management of Painful Procedures

As with all types of pain, procedural pain is best managed using a multi-modal approach, involving both pharmacological and non-drug interventions. Pain should be prevented wherever possible. Anxiolytics (anti-anxiety drugs) and sedatives may be required to reduce anxiety and keep the child still, but must always be given with analgesia for painful procedures, as they blunt the behavioural response but do not relieve pain.

If pain and fear are well managed the child is more likely to keep still and cope better with subsequent medical procedures. If a significant amount pain and/or fear is likely, or the child needs to remain very still, then the use of sedation, anxiolysis or a general anaesthetic should be considered. When using intravenous or inhaled sedation, with or without analgesia, to sedate a child for a painful or non-painful procedure, this should be carried out by staff experienced in advanced airway management and the care of the unconscious child (SIGN 2004).

10.2.1 Non-drug interventions

Non-drug methods of pain relief are discussed in Chapter 5. The non-drug methods that are particularly useful for the management of procedural pain can be seen in Figure 10.3. A Cochrane review of the effectiveness of cognitive and cognitive-behavioural interventions for the management of needle-related pain in children is summarised in Box 10.4.

10.2.2 Pharmacological interventions

The main drugs used for safe and effective management of procedural pain are local anaesthetics and self-administered nitrous oxide. The different analgesic drugs and the pros and cons of the different local anaesthetics available are discussed in Chapter 4. When using local anaesthetics to manage procedural pain it is important to adhere to the manufacturer's guidelines regarding application and the length of time it takes for the drug to be effective.

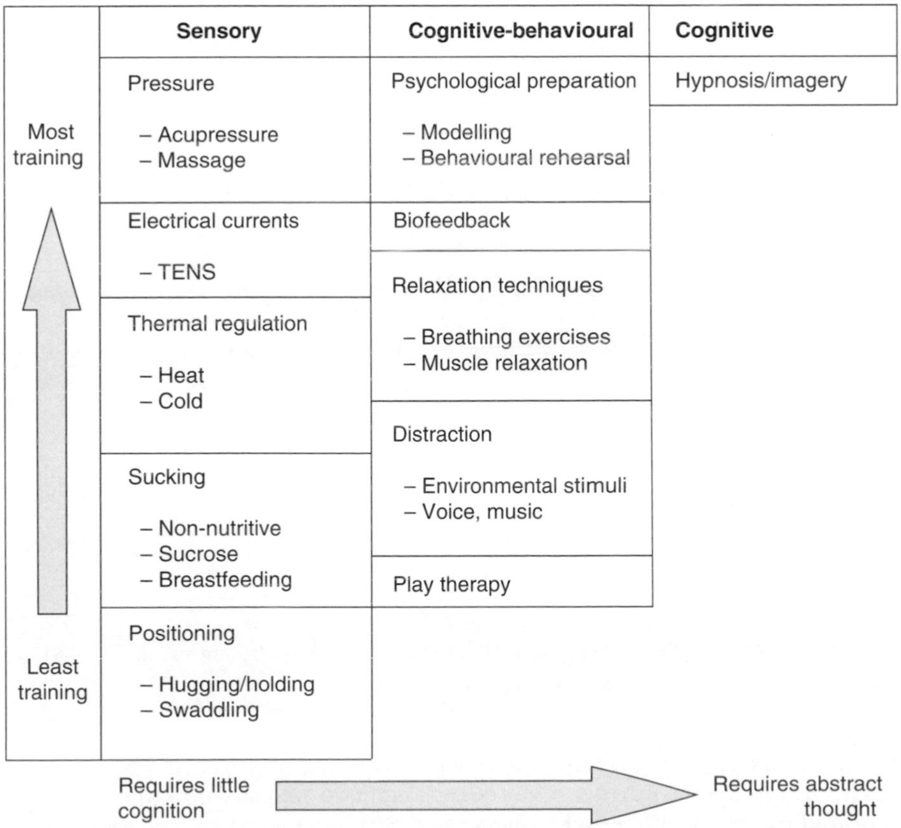

	Sensory	Cognitive-behavioural	Cognitive
Most training	Pressure – Acupressure – Massage	Psychological preparation – Modelling – Behavioural rehearsal	Hypnosis/imagery
	Electrical currents – TENS	Biofeedback	
		Relaxation techniques – Breathing exercises – Muscle relaxation	
	Thermal regulation – Heat – Cold		
		Distraction – Environmental stimuli – Voice, music	
	Sucking – Non-nutritive – Sucrose – Breastfeeding		
		Play therapy	
Least training	Positioning – Hugging/holding – Swaddling		

Requires little cognition → Requires abstract thought

Figure 10.3 Non-drug interventions for procedural pain management (adapted from Vessey and Carlson 1996).

Box 10.4

A review of the effectiveness of cognitive and cognitive behavioural interventions for the management of needle-related pain in children

Psychological interventions for needle-related procedural pain and distress in children and adolescents review of 28 studies (n = 1951; 1039 in treatment, 951 in control groups*):

Sample: healthy children (14 studies), oncology patients (8 studies), children with undiagnosed medical conditions/a range of medical and surgical conditions (5 studies) and healthy children and children with cancer (1 study)

Painful procedure: immunisation (9 studies), venepuncture or finger prick (8 studies), lumbar puncture/bone marrow aspiration (6 studies), intravenous cannulation (4 studies) and intramuscular injection (1 study)

Interventions:

• Distraction (15 studies, 5 of which combined distraction with other interventions; coping skills training and use of a party blower, parent positioning, suggestion and nurse coaching)
• Hypnosis (5 studies)
• Nurse coaching (4 studies, 3 of which involved other interventions)
• Suggestion (3 studies)
• Preparation/procedural information (2 studies)
• Blowing out air, coping skills training, memory alteration, modelling, parent-assisted behavioural intervention, videotape modelling + parent participation, virtual reality distraction (1 study of each intervention)

Findings:

• Distraction (and distraction + suggestion) reduce self-reported pain
• Hypnosis reduces pain and distress
• Combined cognitive behavioural interventions reduce distress
• Nurse coaching and parent positioning (both when combined with distraction) reduce some signs of distress
• There was some evidence to suggest that information/preparation and combined interventions involving distraction are also effective in relieving pain
• Memory alteration reduces diastolic blood pressure

Conclusion: These studies provide *preliminary evidence* but more research involving randomised controlled trials is needed

*39 participants in the treatment group were excluded as they also received EMLA
Source: Uman et al. (2006)

Nitrous oxide

> Nitrous oxide is a potent analgesic and can provide short term pain relief, sedation and reduced anxiety during a wide range of painful procedures (Bruce and Franck 2000).

• Nitrous oxide is an anaesthetic gas with analgesic, sedative and anxiolytic properties.
• The properties of nitrous oxide are thought to be derived either from its action at opioid receptors, N-methyl-D-aspartate (NMDA) receptors, benzodiazepine, or alpha-2-adrenergic receptors (Mason and Koka 1999; Zacny et al. 1999). (See Chapter 2 for more information about these receptors.)

- Nitrous oxide is rapidly absorbed and eliminated, so has a fast onset and offset. Initial analgesia is usually achieved within four to six breaths and thus, if any side effects occur, these will quickly subside once the child stops inhaling the gas.
- A self-administered preparation of 50:50 mix of nitrous oxide and oxygen inhaled via a mask or mouthpiece (Entonox®/Equinox®) is generally considered safest for use by non-anaesthetists in the UK (Bruce and Franck 2000; Pickup and Pagdin 2000).
- Nitrous oxide has been shown to be effective as an analgesic at 30%, 50% and 70% concentrations.
- Nitrous oxide is an anaesthetic gas and has the potential to cause deep sedation, particularly at higher concentrations (70:30 mix of nitrous oxide:oxygen).
- Continuous-flow nitrous oxide, using concentrations up to 70%, has been shown to provide safe, effective analgesia, but this method of administration involves a greater risk of sedation (Gall et al. 2001). This is one reason why nitrous oxide should only be administered by staff who have received specific training.
- It is important that the child is able to co-operate by holding the mask or mouthpiece and breathe the gas themselves, as if the child starts to become sleepy they will stop inhaling the gas.
- If the child is unable to do this, alternative analgesia must be provided, or staff with training in sedation and advanced airway management should be present to supervise the use of continuous-flow nitrous oxide.
- Hospital guidelines and staff training should be available regarding the use of nitrous oxide (an example is provided in Box 10.5).

BOX 10.5

Suggested guidelines for the use of nitrous oxide for procedural pain in children

1. Assess the need for use of nitrous oxide for short painful procedures and determine whether the child is able and willing to inhale the gas. Administer simple analgesics an hour before the procedure. If a high degree of pain is likely, opioid analgesia should also be given as per hospital policy.
2. Ensure that the child has no contra-indications for the use of nitrous oxide. Explain the procedure and the effects of the gas and ensure that the child understands how to use it. Involve the family and play specialist as appropriate. Explain common side effects and ensure that the child understands that alternative analgesia is available if they choose not to inhale the gas.
3. Check the cylinder to ensure it contains the correct mixture: 50:50 nitrous oxide and oxygen has a blue and white cylinder neck. Turn the cylinder on and prime the tubing if necessary. Ensure that the cylinder is at least a quarter full so that it does not run out during the procedure.
4. Show the child the equipment and let them choose whether to inhale the gas through a facemask or mouthpiece. Allow them to practise the technique before the procedure is due to begin.
5. When starting the procedure, ensure that the child has taken at least six to eight breaths before the procedure begins. Encourage the child to breathe normally throughout the procedure and to inform staff if they have any pain.
6. If the child experiences any side effects they should be reassured and if necessary the procedure should be stopped, until they are ready to recommence inhalation.
7. After the procedure, ensure that the patient is comfortable. Clean or discard facemask/mouthpiece as per hospital policy. Document procedure, methods of pain relief used and level of efficacy in the patient's healthcare records.
8. Check levels, switch off cylinder and return equipment to its storage area. Complete any audit forms and order a new cylinder if required.

Source: Bruce and Franck 2000

Adverse effects

Adverse effects are rare, particularly if nitrous oxide is self-administered, and include:

- nausea and vomiting;
- tingling sensations;
- disorientation;
- dizziness;
- a dry mouth.

Several other factors need considering when using nitrous oxide (see also Box 10.6):

- Nitrous oxide can deplete vitamin B_{12} and so repeated or prolonged use should be avoided, as this will affect folate metabolism and DNA synthesis and cause megalo-blastic changes in the bone marrow (Amos et al. 1984; Nunn 1987).
- Children who require the use of nitrous oxide more frequently than every four days should be monitored closely for evidence of megaloblastic changes in red cells, and hypersegmentation of neutrophils (British Oxygen Company 1995b).
- Where repeated use is unavoidable and for at-risk groups (e.g. neutropenic, anaemic or mal-nourished children), supplements should be given to prevent vitamin B_{12} depletion.
- Other considerations include staff and visitor exposure and the need to monitor atmo-spheric levels (Bruce and Franck 2000).

The effectiveness of nitrous oxide analgesia during reduction of fractures has been shown in three studies:

- In a randomised comparison of nitrous oxide and intramuscular (IM) meperidine (pethidine) and promethazine, nitrous oxide was equally effective in reducing pain during the procedure, but had a higher level of patient acceptance and faster recovery period than the IM analgesia and sedation (Evans et al. 1995).
- Self-administered nitrous oxide has been shown to be effective for a range of procedures including fracture reduction (Hennrikus et al. 1995; Evans et al. 1995; Wattenmaker et al. 1990), laceration repair (Burton et al. 1998) and joint injections (Cleary et al. 2002).
- There is limited evidence for the effectiveness of nitrous oxide for other painful procedures. Recent research suggests that neither morphine (100 microgram/kg) nor continuous-flow nitrous oxide is effective when used alone for chest drain removal pain and a combination of interventions is needed (Bruce et al. 2006a,b).

BOX 10.6

Contraindications and cautions to consider for nitrous oxide use

Nitrous oxide expands air-filled cavities, so should not be used in patients with:

- an air embolism
- a pneumothorax
- a middle ear occlusion
- maxillofacial injuries
- gross abdominal distension
- following air encephelography
- severe bullous emphysema
- during myringoplasty
- or any other condition where air might be trapped in the body

Source: British Oxygen Company (1995a)

Simple analgesia

There is limited evidence for the efficacy of paracetamol and non-steroidal anti-inflammatory drugs (NSAIDs) for the management of painful procedures, although Harvey and Morton (2007) suggest they are useful for post-procedure pain.

Opioids

Harvey and Morton (2007) advocate the use of opioids for procedural pain but state that, because of their slow onset of action, sufficient time needs to be allowed from the time of administration to the painful procedure.

Krauss and Green (2000) suggest that fentanyl is the opioid of choice for managing procedural pain because of its faster onset of action, shorter recovery and lack of histamine release.

Morphine (when administered orally or intravenously) has an prolonged duration of action (see Chapter 4) and this, combined with the potential for sedation and respiratory depression, makes it less than ideal for short, painful procedures. If given in combination with sedatives, for example, benzodiazepines or nitrous oxide, this further increases the risk of opioid-related adverse effects (Annequin et al. 2000; Murat et al. 2003). Intranasal and transmucosal (buccal) fentanyl has faster onset and shorter duration of action, but the risk of adverse effects remains. In addition, some children find the intranasal spray unpleasant, particularly if they have not been warned that it may sting.

Several studies have examined the effectiveness of intranasal, transmucosal (buccal) and oral opioids for the management of procedural pain in children:

- Transmucosal fentanyl was more effective than a placebo in children ($n = 48$) undergoing bone marrow aspirate and lumbar puncture (Schechter et al. 1995).
- The effectiveness of transmucosal fentanyl and oral hydromorphone were compared for the wound dressing of children ($n = 14$) by Sharar et al. (1998). The use of oral transmucosal fentanyl resulted in improved pain scores before and improved anxiolysis during wound care.
- Sharar et al. (2002) examined the use of transmucosal fentanyl and oral oxycodone for wound dressing in 22 children. Vital signs, pain scores, anxiety and sedation were comparable in both groups, but the taste of oral transmucosal fentanyl was preferred.
- Intranasal fentanyl was found to provide comparable analgesia to oral morphine in a small randomised double-blind crossover study of analgesia for burns dressings in children ($n = 24$) (Borland et al. 2005).
- Intranasal fentanyl was found to provide comparable analgesia to intravenous morphine in a randomised placebo-controlled trial of analgesia for fracture reduction in 67 children (Borland et al. 2007).
- Intranasal diamorphine spray was compared with intramuscular morphine in children ($n = 404$) with fractures. It provided faster and more effective analgesia in the short term (no difference between the two drugs at 30 minutes) and was preferred by staff and parents (Kendall et al. 2001).

Goldman (2006) summarises the available information on the use of intranasal drug delivery for children in acute illness.

Transmucosal (buccal) and intranasal opioids appear to be effective for the management of procedural pain in children. There is some evidence to suggest that the intranasal and buccal routes are preferred to the oral route of administration of opioids.

Ketamine

The use of ketamine for the management of procedural pain in children is increasing. Ketamine is an anaesthetic agent which provides analgesia, sedation and amnesia (see Chapter 4).

- At low (sub-anaesthetic) doses, ketamine provides effective analgesia for painful procedures and may produce less adverse effects than opioids (Murat et al. 2003; Australian and New Zealand College of Anaesthetists and Faculty of Pain Medicine 2007; Morton 2008).
- Luhmann et al. (2006) compared intravenous ketamine and midazolam with nitrous oxide and a local anaesthetic block in children (*n* = 102) having fracture reduction. Ketamine and midazolam provided comparable analgesia but more adverse effects than nitrous oxide and local anaesthetic.
- Ketamine produces considerably less respiratory depression than opioids but deep sedation and complications can occur with large or repeated doses (Murat et al. 2003).

Morton (2008) summarises the current evidence on the use of ketamine for procedural sedation and analgesis in children in the UK.

Practice point

If two or more sedative agents are used in combination the risk of adverse effects is increased (Murat et al. 2003).

Ketamine, opioids and other analgesic drugs that produce sedation should be administered by staff suitably trained and experienced in sedation and airway management in an environment that is appropriately arranged should an emergency arise (SIGN 2004; Royal Australasian College of Physicians [RACP] 2006a).

10.3 Management of Procedural Pain in Neonates

Neonates are particularly vulnerable to procedural pain due to their inability to communicate and their exposure to multiple painful procedures. There are a number of guidelines and recommendations for the management of procedural pain in neonates (see resource list at the end of this chapter). Box 10.7 provides a summary of the recommendations from one of these guideline statements. For more information on the non-drug interventions for procedural pain management in neonates see Chapter 5.

BOX 10.7

Summary of evidence for the management of procedural pain in neonates
Interventions with evidence of benefit

Level I*
- Sucrose is safe and effective in reducing pain from venepuncture and heel lancing in preterm infants
- Dummies (pacifiers), non-nutritive sucking, rocking are effective in reducing pain responses

BOX 10.7 Continued

Level II**

- Sucrose with pacifiers are effective in reducing pain responses in neonates
- Sucrose and holding are effective in reducing pain responses
- Multisensory stimulation (massage, voice, eye contact and perfume smelling) with oral glucose and sucking is most effective in reducing pain responses to heel lancing in term and preterm infants
- Breast-feeding is effective in reducing pain responses during heel lancing in healthy neonates
- Skin to skin contact is effective in reducing pain responses during heel lancing in healthy neonates
- Automated lancets are superior to conventional lancets (less need for repeat punctures, shorter procedure time, increased volume of blood collected, reduction in haemolysed blood samples)
- A fully retractable automatic lancet is superior to a partially retractable automatic lancet (less pain, less time to perform, fewer punctures, but more expensive)

Interventions with no evidence of benefit or evidence of harm

Level I*

- Midazolam may be associated with a higher incidence of adverse neurological events and longer NICU stay.

Level II**

- EMLA cream, topical amethocaine, lignocaine ointment, oral paracetamol are not effective for heel-lancing pain.
- Warming the heel does not reduce pain or aid blood collection during heel lancing.
- Routine repeated use of sucrose analgesia in preterm neonates, 31 weeks post-conceptual age, may result in poorer neuro-behavioural development.

*Evidence obtained from a systematic review of all relevant RCTs
**Evidence from at least one properly designed RCT

Source: RACP (2006b)

Summary

- It is important to ensure that a procedure is essential and will be carried out by a competent practitioner using the least painful method available.
- Enough time should be allowed to explain the procedure to the child and family and to plan age/developmentally appropriate non-drug interventions that will minimise pain and distress.
- Everyone involved in or present during the procedure must be clear about their role and the role of others.
- Parents can provide considerable comfort and support during painful procedures, but they need to be prepared and supported.
- A combination of pharmacological and non-drug interventions should be employed throughout the procedure.
- Sedation alone must *never* be considered an option for the management of painful procedures, but sedation or general anaesthetic should be considered in combination with analgesia if interventions to manage pain and distress are unlikely to be sufficient.
- Ensure that the child is involved in the procedure as much as possible and feels able to ask for *time out* if needed.
- After the procedure, reassure and praise the child and ensure that they are comfortable and *debriefed*. It is important to determine the opinion of everyone involved regarding

what went well and what could have been done better, as this will help to plan any future procedures.

Useful web resources

Procedural pain guidelines and position statements

American Academy of Pediatrics and American Pain Society (2001) The assessment and management of acute pain in infants, children and adolescents, *Pediatrics* 108(3): 793–93. Available from: http://www.bmc.org/pediatrics/special/PainFree/AssessManagement.pdf

Boston Medical Center Pharmacy and Therapeutics Committee (2002) *Medication Guidelines: Procedural Pain Management in Neonates through Adolescents.* Available from: http://www.bmc.org/pediatrics/special/PainFree/MedGuidelines.pdf

Howard, R., Carter, B., Curry, J., Morton, N., Rivett, K., Rose, M., Tyrrell, J., Walter, S. and Williams, G. (2008) Good Practice in Postoperative and Procedural Pain Management, *Pediatric Anesthesia*, 18: 1–81. http://www.blackwell-synergy.com/toc/pan/18/s1

Royal Australasian College of Physicians, Paediatrics and Child Health Division (2006) *Guideline Statement: Management of Procedure-Related Pain in Children and Adolescents.* Available from: http://www.racp.edu.au/index.cfm?objectid=A4268489-2A57-5487-DEF14F15791C4F22

Royal Australasian College of Physicians (2006) Management of Procedure-Related Pain in Neonates (Guideline Statement), *Journal of Paediatrics and Child Health*, 42: 531–539. Available from: http://www.racp.edu.au/index.cfm?objectid=A4268489-2A57-5487-DEF14F15791C4F22

Scottish Intercollegiate Guidelines Network (SIGN) (2004) *Safe Sedation of Children Undergoing Diagnostic and Therapeutic Procedures. A National Clinical Guideline.* Available from: http://www.apagbi.org.uk/docs/sign58.pdf

---

Other useful resources

Harvey, A.J. and Morton, N.S. (2007) Management of procedural pain in children, *Archives of Disease in Childhood Education and Practice Education*, 92: ep20-ep26.

Krauss, B. and Green, S.M. (2006) Procedural sedation and analgesia in children, *Lancet*, 367: 766–780.

References

Amos, R.J., Amess, J.A.L., Nancekievill, D.G. and Rees, G.M. (1984) Prevention of nitrous oxide induced megaloblastic changes in bone marrow using folinic acid, *British Journal of Anaesthesia* 56: 103–107.

Annequin, D., Carbajal, R., Chauvin, P., Gall, O., Tourniaire, B. and Murat, I. (2000) Fixed 50% nitrous oxide oxygen mixture for painful procedures: a French survey. *Pediatrics* 105(4): E47.

Australian and New Zealand College of Anaesthetists and Faculty of Pain Medicine (2007) *Acute Pain Management: Scientific Evidence*, Updated 2nd edition, Australian and New Zealand College of Anaesthetists, Melbourne.

Bhargava, R. and Young, K.D. (2007) Procedural pain management patterns in academic pediatric emergency departments, *Academic Emergency Medicine*, 14(5): 479–482.

Borland, M.L., Bergesio, R., Pascoe, E.M., Turner, S. and Woodger, S. (2005) Intranasal fentanyl is an equivalent analgesic to oral morphine in paediatric burns patients for dressing changes: a randomised double blind crossover study, *Burns*, 31(7): 831–837.

Borland, M., Jacobs, I., King, B. and O'Brien, D. (2007) A randomized controlled trial comparing intranasal fentanyl to intravenous morphine for managing acute pain in children in the emergency department. *Annals of Emergency Medicine*, 49(3): 335–340.

British Oxygen Company (1995a) *Entonox: The non-invasive Patient Controlled Analgesic: Suggested protocol document*, BOC Ltd, Manchester.

British Oxygen Company (1995b) *Medical Gases Entonox Datasheet*, BOC Ltd, Manchester.

Bruce, E. and Franck, L. (2000) Self-administered nitrous oxide (ENTONOX) for the management of procedural pain, *Paediatric Nursing*, 12 (7): 15–19.

Bruce. E., Franck, L. and Howard, R.F. (2006a) The efficacy of morphine and Entonox analgesia during chest drain removal in children, *Pediatric Anesthesia*, 16: 203–208.

Bruce, E.A., Howard, R.F. and Franck, L.S. (2006b) Chest drain removal pain and its management: a literature review, *Journal of Clinical Nursing*, 15: 145–154.

Burton, J.H., Auble, T.E. and Fuchs, S.M. (1998) Effectiveness of 50% nitrous oxide/50% oxygen during laceration repair in children, *Academic Emergency Medicine*, 5(2): 112–117.

Chambers, C.T., Craig, K.D. and Bennett, S.M. (2002). The impact of maternal behavior on children's pain experiences: an experimental analysis, *Journal of Pediatric Psychology*, 27: 293–301.

Cleary, A.G., Ramanan, A.V., Baildam, E., Birch, A., Sills, J.A. and Davidson, J.E. (2002) Nitrous oxide analgesia during intra-articular injection for juvenile idiopathic arthritis, *Archives of Disease in Childhood*, 86: 416–418.

Cohen, L.L., Bernard, R.S., Greco, L.A. and McClellan, C.B. (2002) A child-focused intervention for coping with procedural pain: Are parent and nurse coaches necessary? *Journal of Pediatric Psychology*, 27(8): 749–757.

Craze, J., Turner, C., Taylor, J., Adam, R., Jacobs, K. et al. (2005) *Guidelines for the Prevention and Management of Procedural Distress*, Multidisciplinary Procedural Distress Group, Oxford Radcliffe Hospital.

Doorbar, P. and McClarey, M. (1999) *Ouch! Sort It Out: Children's Experiences of Pain*, London, RCN Publishing.

Evans, J.K., Buckley, S.L., Alexander, A.H. and Gilpin, A.T. (1995) Analgesia for the reduction of fractures in children: a comparison of nitrous oxide with intramuscular sedation, *Journal of Pediatric Orthopaedics*, 15: 73–77.

Farion, K., Osmond, M.H., Hartling, L., Russell, K., Klassen. T., Crumley. E. and Wiebe. N. (2001) Tissue adhesives for traumatic lacerations in children and adults. *Cochrane Database of Systematic Reviews* 4:CD003326.

Franck, L.S. and Jones, M. (2003) Computer-taught techniques for venepuncture: preliminary findings from usability testing with children and staff, *Journal of Child Health Care*, 7(1): 41–54.

Gall, O., Annequin, D., Benoit, G., VanGlabeke, E., Vrancea, F. and Murat, I. (2001) Adverse events of premixed nitrous oxide and oxygen for procedural sedation in children, *Lancet*, 358: 1514–1515.

Goldman, R.D (2006) Intranasal drug delivery for children with acute illness, *Current Drug Therapy*, 1: 127–130.

Harvey, A.J. and Morton, N.S. (2007) Management of procedural pain in children, *Archives of Disease in Childhood Education and Practice Education*, 92: ep20–ep26.

Hennrikus, W.L., Shin, A.Y. and Klingelberger, C.E. (1995) Self-administered nitrous oxide and a hematoma block for analgesia in the outpatient reduction of fractures in children, *Journal of Bone and Joint Surgery* 77: 335–339.

Hodgins, M.J. and Lander, J. (1997) Children's coping with venepuncture, *Journal of Pain and Symptom Management*, 13(5): 274–285.

Kendall, J.M., Reeves, B.C., Latter, V.S. and Nasal Diamorphine Trial Group (2001) Multicentre randomised controlled trial of nasal diamorphine for analgesia in children and teenagers with clinical fractures, *British Medical Journal*, 322(7281): 261–265.

Kleiber, C., Craft-Rosenberg. M. and Harper, D.C. (2001) Parents as distraction coaches during IV insertion: a randomised study, *Journal of Pain and Symptom Management*, 22(4): 851–861.

Krauss, B. and Green, S.M. (2000) Sedation and analgesia for procedurs in children, *New England Journal of Medicine*, 342(13): 938–945.

Langer, D.A., Chen, E. and Luhmann, J.D. (2005) Attributions and coping in children's pain experiences, *Journal of Pediatric Psychology*, 30(7): 615–622.

Luhmann, J.D., Schootman, M., Luhmann, S.J. and Kennedy, R.M. (2006) A randomized comparison of nitrous oxide plus hematoma block versus ketamine plus midazolam for emergency department forearm fracture reduction in children. *Pediatrics*. 118(4): e1078–1086.

Mason, K. and Koka, B. (1999) Nitrous oxide. In Krauss, B. and Brustowicz, RM. (eds.) *Pediatric Procedural Sedation and Analgesia*, Baltimore, Lippincott, Williams & Wilkins, pp. 83–88.

McGrath, P.J., Finley, G.A., Ritchie, J. and Dowden. S.J. (2003) *Pain, pain, go away: helping children with pain*, 2nd edition. Available from: http://www.rch.org.au/anaes/pain/index.cfm?doc_id=6223 Accessed 10/01/08.

Morton, N.S. (2008) Ketamine for procedural sedation and analgesia in pediatric emergency medicine: a UK perspective, *Pediatric Anesthesia*, 18(1): 25–29.

Murat, I., Gall, O.G. and Tournaire, B. (2003) Procedural pain in children: evidence-based best practice and guidelines, *Regional Anesthesia and Pain Medicine*, 28(6): 561–572.

Nunn, J.F. (1987) Clinical aspects of the interaction between nitrous oxide and vitamin B12, *British Journal of Anaesthesia*, 59: 3–13.

Penrose, S. and Dowden, S.J. (2003) *Medical procedure flow chart* (Unpublished), Children's Pain Management Service, Royal Children's Hospital, Melbourne. (Enquiries: sueann.penrose@rch.org.au)

Pickup, S. and Pagdin, J. (2000) Procedural pain: Entonox can help, *Paediatric Nursing*, 12(10): 33–36.

Polkki, T., Pietila, A-M. and Vehvilamen-Julkunen, K. (2003) Hospitalized children's descriptions of their experiences with postsurgical pain-relieving methods, *International Journal of Nursing Studies*, 40: 33–44.

Royal Australasian College of Physicians (2006a) Management of procedure-related pain in children and adolescents (Guideline Statement), *Journal of Paediatrics and Child Health*, 42: S1–S29.

Royal Australasian College of Physicians (2006b) Management of procedure-related pain in neonates (Guideline Statement), *Journal of Paediatrics and Child Health*, 42: S31–S39.

Royal College of Nursing (1999) *Restraint revisited – rights, risk and responsibility*, London, RCN Publishing.

Royal College of Nursing (2003) *Restraining, holding still and containing children and young people*, London, RCN Publishing.

Schechter, N.L., Weisman, S.J., Rosenblum, M., Bernstein, B. and Conard, P.L. (1995) The use of oral transmucosal fentanyl citrate for painful procedures in children, *Pediatrics*, 95(3): 335–339.

Schechter, N.L., Zempsky, W.T., Cohen, L.L., McGrath, P.J., McMurtry, C.M. and Bright, N.S. (2007) Pain reduction during pediatric immunizations: evidence-based review and recommendations, *Pediatrics*, 119(5) e1184–e1198.

Scottish Intercollegiate Guidelines Network (SIGN) (2004) *Safe Sedation of Children Undergoing Diagnostic and Therapeutic Procedures: A national clinical guideline* SIGN: Edinburgh. http://www. apagbi.org.uk/docs/sign58.pdf (accessed 9 January 2008).

Shah, V. and Ohlsson, A. (2004) Venepuncture versus heel lance for blood sampling in term neonates, *Cochrane Database of Systematic Reviews*, 4:CD001452.

Sharar, S.R., Bratton, S.L., Carrougher, G.J., Edwards, W.T., Summer, G., Levy, F.H. and Cortiella, J. (1998) A comparison of oral transmucosal fentanyl citrate and oral hydromorphone for inpatient pediatric burn wound care analgesia, *Journal of Burn Care Rehabilitation* 19(6): 516–521.

Sharar. S.R., Carrougher, G.J., Selzer, K., O'Donnell, F., Vavilala, M.S. and Lee, L.A. (2002) A comparison of oral transmucosal fentanyl citrate and oral oxycodone for pediatric outpatient wound care, *Journal of Burn Care Rehabilitation*, 23(1): 27–31.

Smith, R.W., Shah, V., Goldman, R.D. and Taddio, A. (2007) Caregivers' responses to pain in their children in the emergency department, *Archives of Pediatric Adolescent Medicine*, 161: 578–582.

Uman L.S., Chambers, C.T., McGrath, P.J. and Kisely, S. (2006) Psychological interventions for needle-related procedural pain and distress in children and adolescents, *Cochrane Database of Systematic Reviews* 18(4):CD005179.

Vessey, J.A. and Carlson, K.L. (1996) Nonpharmacological interventions to use with children in pain, *Issues in Comprehensive Pediatric Nursing*, 19: 169–182.

Wattenmaker, I., Kasser, J.R. and McGravey, A. (1990) Self-administered nitrous oxide for fracture reduction in children in an emergency room setting, *Journal of Orthopaedic Trauma*, 4(1): 35–38.

Woodgate, R. and Kristjanson L. (1996) A young child's pain: How parents and nurses 'take care', *International Journal of Nursing Studies*, 33(3): 271–284.

Young, K.D. (2005) Pediatric procedural pain, *Annals of Emergency Medicine*, 45: 160–171.

Zacny, J.P., Conran, A., Pardo, H., Coalson, D.W., Black, M., Klock, P.A. and Klafta, J.M. (1999) Effects of naloxone on nitrous oxide actions in healthy volunteers, *Pain*, 83: 411–418.

Zempsky, W.T., Cravero, J.P. and Committee on Pediatric Emergency Medicine and Section on Anesthesiology and Pain Medicine (2004) Relief of pain and anxiety in pediatric patients in emergency medical systems, *Pediatrics*, 114: 1348–1356.

CHAPTER 11

Where To From Here?

Alison Twycross and Stephanie J. Dowden

Introduction

Within this chapter the factors contributing to suboptimal pain management practices will be discussed, demonstrating that a multifactorial approach is needed to improve the management of pain in children. Possible solutions will then be presented, which may ensure that children no longer experience unnecessary pain. The management of change will also be discussed and the ethical issues relating to carrying out research with children outlined.

The evidence to guide nurses' pain management practices is readily available, in the form of clinical guidelines (see Chapter 1). However, children's nurses' pain management practices continue to fall short of the ideal (Byrne et al. 2001; Vincent and Denyes 2004; Twycross 2007a) with children still experiencing moderate to severe unrelieved pain postoperatively (Polkki et al. 2003; Health Care Commission 2004; Vincent and Denyes 2004; Johnston et al. 2005).

Indeed the (English) *National Service Framework for Children and Young People* (Department of Health [DH] 2004) states that children's pain management is often suboptimal and stresses the need to provide evidence-based care. This issue has also been highlighted by the International Association for the Study of Pain (IASP) who declared October 2005–October 2006 the *Global Year Against Pain in Children* (Finley et al. 2005).

11.1 Reasons for Suboptimal Practices

Several factors have been suggested as reasons why children's pain is still not managed effectively. These include:

- knowledge deficits;
- incorrect or outdated beliefs about pain and pain management;
- the decision-making strategies used;
- ward culture;
- organisational culture.

11.1.2 Knowledge deficits

Limited theoretical knowledge about managing pain in children has been suggested as one reason children's nurses do not manage pain effectively (Woodgate and Kristjanson

1996; Salantera 1999; Salantera et al. 1999; Simons and Roberson 2002; Simons and MacDonald 2004).

Several studies have examined children's nurses' theoretical knowledge about pain in children:

- Paediatric oncology nurses (*n* = 106) completed a questionnaire, which demonstrated a lack of understanding of basic pharmacological principles in relation to analgesic drugs (Schmidt et al. 1994).
- In Salantera et al.'s (1999) study nurses (*n* = 265) completed a pain management knowledge questionnaire. Gaps were found in nurses' knowledge about managing pain in children in relation to analgesic drugs and non-drug methods of pain relief.
- Salantera and Lauri (2000), using the same questionnaire, found knowledge deficits among final year student nurses (*n* = 73), particularly in relation to analgesic drugs and pain assessment.
- The *Pediatric Nurses' Knowledge and Attitudes Regarding Pain Survey* was completed by nurses (*n* = 274) in Manworren's (2000) study. The mean score for the questionnaire was only 66%, with knowledge deficits apparent in many areas including pain assessment, the pharmacology of analgesic drugs, the use of analgesic drugs, and non-drug methods.
- Nurses (*n* = 67) completed an adapted *Nurses' Knowledge and Attitudes Regarding Pain Survey* in Vincent's (2005) study. Nurses had knowledge deficits in relation to non-drug methods of pain relief, analgesic drugs and the incidence of respiratory depression.
- Twycross (2004) used a modified version of Salantera's questionnaire (as part of a larger study) and found that nurses (*n* = 12) had gaps in their knowledge and that these were particularly noticeable in relation to analgesic drugs, non-drug methods and the physiology of pain as well as the psychology and sociology of pain.
- The effectiveness of a paediatric pain education programme for student nurses was explored by Chiang et al. (2006). Student nurses (*n* = 181) attended a four-hour education programme. Data about knowledge and self-efficacy in relation to managing pain in children were collected. Knowledge (*p* < 0.001) and self-efficacy (*p* < 0.001) had all increased a month after the programme, although knowledge about analgesic drugs did not improve.

> Gaps remain in nurses' knowledge about pain in children, and in particular in relation to pain assessment, analgesic drugs and non-drug methods.

Other studies have examined the impact of deficits in nurses' theoretical knowledge on the quality of pain management practices:

- Vincent and Denyes (2004) observed the care of children (*n* = 132), aged 3½ to 17 years, by nurses (*n* = 67) and found that nurses with a better theoretical knowledge about pain were not more likely to administer analgesia.
- No positive relationship between children's nurses' level of knowledge and how well they actually managed pain was found by Twycross (2007b). Even when the nurses (*n* = 12) had a good level of theoretical knowledge, this appeared not to be reflected in their pain management practices.
- No relationship was found between adult nurses' (*n* = 80) knowledge and patients' ratings of pain and the amount of analgesia administered, although the nurses had moderately good levels of knowledge about pain management (Watt-Watson et al. 2001).

> Gaps in nurses' theoretical knowledge levels do not appear to provide the sole explanation for deficits in pain management practices.

One reason for the limited use of theoretical knowledge in practice could be that due to their knowledge deficits, nurses do not understand the rationale for using specific interventions. Indeed, a review of pain content in pre-registration diploma courses in England found that most child branch curricula included less than 10 hours' education on pain, providing students with little more than a *whistle-stop tour* of pain management (Twycross 2000).

> Gaps in knowledge may mean that nurses do not understand the rationale for pain relieving interventions.

11.1.2 Beliefs about pain in children

Nurses' beliefs about pain and, particularly, the priority nurses attribute to pain management, have also been suggested as reasons for suboptimal pain management practices. Nurses' beliefs about pain management have been examined in several studies:

- Nurses ($n = 20$) seemed to assume (incorrectly) that some pain was to be expected during a hospital stay (Hamers et al. 1994).
- In Woodgate and Kristjanson's (1996) observational study nurses ($n = 24$) were shown to concentrate on technical aspects of care; nurses saw comforting the child as the parent's role.
- Nurses ($n = 13$) were observed to negate (ignore) children's ($n = 16$) pain in Byrne et al.'s (2001) observational study.

Other studies have examined the priority nurses attribute to managing children's pain:

- Nurses who chose pain relief as a priority indicated they would provide more analgesia when presented with clinical scenarios (Burokas 1985; Ross et al. 1991).
- Nurses ($n = 22$) completing a training needs questionnaire about several aspects of nursing attributed a significantly lower priority to pain management than to other aspects of their role (Twycross 1999).
- Twycross (2004) compared data regarding the perceived importance of pain management tasks with observational data relating to individual nurses' ($n = 12$) practices. The importance nurses attributed to the pain management task did not reflect the likelihood of the task being undertaken in practice. Indeed, the perceived importance of a pain management task appeared to bear little relationship to observed practices.

> Outdated and incorrect beliefs about pain management, and not making pain a priority, may be contributing factors but they do not provide a complete explanation for suboptimal pain management practices.

11.1.3 Decision-making strategies

Little is known about how children's nurses make decisions. Twycross and Powls (2006) examined children's nurses' decision-making in relation to both managing pain and caring for children with acute medical conditions and found that:

- Nurses appeared to use an analytical model of decision-making
- All nurses used backward reasoning strategies and collected similar types and amounts of information before making a decision about appropriate nursing care. This is indicative of non-expert decision-making.
- No differences were noted between nurses with five or more years' experience in paediatric surgery and less experienced nurses.
- No differences were apparent between graduate and non-graduate nurses.

An **analytical model** of decision-making is a step-by-step process. For example:

- Gathering information
- Generating hypothesis
- Using the data gathered data to rule the hypothesis in or out
- Deciding on a plan of action from the data gathered/hypothesis generated

Adapted from Elstein et al. (1978)

In **forward reasoning** an individual works forward from a hypothesis to find a problem solution, while in **backward reasoning** an individual works backwards from a hypothesis to evaluate different options or find a solution. Experts are thought to use more forward reasoning while novices tend to use backward reasoning strategies (Lamond et al. 1996).

Further, Hamers et al. (1997) study found that while experienced nurses were most confident and more inclined to administer analgesics than less experienced nurses, expertise (that is, years of experience) did not influence the assessment of pain intensity.

Several factors have been identified as affecting children's nurses' decision-making about pain. These are discussed in Chapter 1.

Suboptimal decision-making strategies might explain, at least in part, why children continue to experience unrelieved pain. Further research is needed about the factors affecting children's nurses' decision-making.

11.1.4 Ward culture

Ward culture may also be an important factor in relation to pain management practices. This relates particularly to nurses, and other healthcare professionals, who have a tendency to learn through role modelling and professional socialisation.

Role modelling
Evidence that nurses copy the behaviours of more senior staff has been found in several studies:

- Novice nurses (*n* = 15) in Taylor's (1997) study commented that 'they just followed the [more experienced] nurse's lead'.

- Student nurses (n = 99) interviewed by Fitzpatrick et al. (1996) discussed modelling their practices on those of more experienced nurses.
- In Twycross' (2004) study two participants indicated that they had learnt about pain management by observing/working with more senior staff, and another participant reported that she had had no formal education 'except what I picked up as I've gone along'.

If nurses learn by copying the behaviours of role models, the quality of their practice will depend on the practices of the role model. If role models have, for example, poor pain assessment skills or use limited non-drug methods of pain relief and merely administer analgesic drugs when a child complains of pain, the novice nurse is likely to develop a similar approach. Thus, even if a nurse has a good level of theoretical knowledge, this is unlikely to be applied in practice.

> Junior staff modelling their pain management practices on those of more senior staff who have suboptimal practices offers another explanation as to why pain management practices remain poor.

Professional socialisation

Wanting to be part of a social group is part of being human (Furnham 1997; Fincham and Rhodes 1999). When starting a placement or job in a new ward or hospital, nurses, and other health care professionals, undergo a period of socialisation, during which they learn the rules (formal and informal) that guide the behaviour of staff.

- Gray and Smith (1999) found that there were rewards for students (n = 17) for conforming to the norms of the ward, such as the increased likelihood of a good placement and feeling part of the team.
- In Philpin's (1999) study nurses (n = 18), half of who had undergone traditional training and half had received Project 2000 education, were interviewed. The results indicated that if new nurses did not conform to the area's norms they were excluded, shouted at in front of everyone and bullied.
- Neonatal nurses (n = 4) demonstrated a tendency to conform to ward practices rather than what they knew to be research-based best practice (Greenwood et al. 2000).
- In a study examining the effects of occupational socialisation on nurses' (n = 23) moving and handling practice, Kneafsey (2000) found that nurses did not use their theoretical knowledge in practice but rather conformed to ward practices.

A nurse's need to *fit in* may mean that they adopt the ward's (poor) pain management practices, despite having (at least some) theoretical knowledge about how children's pain should be managed and believing that pain management is important. If nurses acting differently to the ward culture are *picked on* this is likely to discourage them from using their own discretion, or from questioning practice.

> Professional socialisation may allow non-evidence-based practices to be perpetuated.

11.1.5 Organisational culture

Organisational culture also needs to be considered in relation to improving pain management practices. This has been identified as key to changing practices (Bucknall et al.

2001; Treadwell et al. 2002; Botti et al. 2004; Jordan-Marsh et al. 2004). Indeed participants in an internet-based project to disseminate information about managing pain in children identified organisational culture as a barrier to changing practices (Bruce and Franck 2005). The impact of introducing an organisational pain management policy on practices was explored by Alley (2001). Nurses' knowledge of pain management and their perceived accountability for pain management were significantly related to knowledge of the organisation's pain management policy.

> The impact of organisational culture on pain management practices needs exploring further.

11.2 The Way Forward

Clearly there is no easy answer to improving the management of pain in children. However, if the factors identified in this chapter are addressed simultaneously, practices may improve. Figure 11.1 provides a pictorial representation of the factors that impact on pain management practices. Strategies for improving practices will be discussed in this section.

11.2.1 Educational issues

There will always be a need to educate nurses about pain management. However, there is increasing evidence that nurses are not using their theoretical knowledge in practice (Watt-Watson et al. 2001; Vincent and Denyes 2004; Dihle et al. 2006; Twycross 2007b). A review of literature in this context by Twycross (2002) found that:

- nurse education does not appear to be preparing nurses to manage pain in the clinical area;
- nurses continue to have educational deficits about pain management;
- not all educational interventions result in improvements in pain management practices.

As discussed earlier, several studies have found evidence that gaps in nurses' theoretical knowledge may mean that they do not understand the rationale for pain relieving

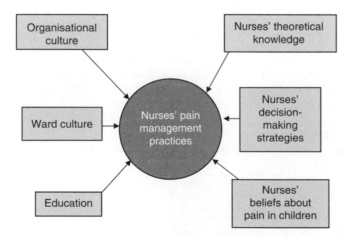

Figure 11.1   Factors influencing pain management practices.

interventions (Salantera et al. 1999; Manworren 2000; Twycross 2004; Vincent 2005), which may explain why nurses do not use their knowledge in practice. If this is the case pre- and post-registration courses need evaluating.

> Pre- and post-registration nurse education content needs evaluating to ensure that nurses have a thorough knowledge of pain and understand the rationale for pain-relieving interventions.

There is a need to develop educational initiatives that promote the use of theoretical knowledge in practice. Several educational strategies have been suggested in this context. These include:

- clinical discussion of individual patients and their care (Graffam 1990; Ochieng 1999) and teaching rounds (Studdy et al. 1994; Melby et al. 1997; Segal and Mason 1998);
- using clinical scenarios to allow students to reflect on practice during classroom-based teaching sessions (Lee and Ryan-Wenger 1997; Cioffi 1998; Jones and Sheridan 1999).
- ward-based journal club meetings (Nolf 1995; Kessenich et al. 1997; Khalid and Gee 1999).

Some methods of learning (e.g. *confluent education*) emphasise the importance of integrating left brain knowledge with right brain creativity.

> **Confluent education** emphasises the importance of integrating **learning with the head** with **learning with the heart** (Brown 1990).

These teaching methods may help ensure the integration of theory and practice. The importance of reflection in integrating theory and practice has also been emphasised (Atkins and Murphy 1994; Rolfe 1996).The use of scenario-based or problem-based learning seems to support the integration of theoretical knowledge into practice; however, this needs further research.

> Educational strategies need to be used that incorporate theoretical knowledge into practice.

11.2.2 Supporting decision-making

A review of the decision-making literature provides no definitive answers about ways to improve nurses' decision-making strategies or how to ensure that current best practice guidelines are used when making clinical decisions. One possible method would be the use of a decision-making algorithm. The effectiveness of an algorithm in conjunction with the administration of regular multimodal analgesia was tested by Falanga et al. (2006). When the algorithm was used, children received more analgesia and had lower pain intensity scores. (Algorithms to support clinical decision-making can be found in Chapters 7, 9 and 10.)

Developing and using algorithms from best practice guidelines would remove much of the stress associated with decision-making and would guide nurses through the process in a step-by-step way. This might help ensure that best practice guidelines are adhered to and thus improve pain management practices.

11.2.3 Making pain an organisational priority

An increasing number of research studies have concentrated on the impact of including pain management in an organisation's quality improvement programme (Ferrell et al. 1995; Weissman et al. 1997; Treadwell et al. 2002; Jordan-Marsh et al. 2004). The JCAHO standards (2001) in the USA and the English *National Service Framework for Children, Young People and Maternity Services* (DH 2004) (see Chapter 1) also promote the need for an organisational commitment to pain management. Several ways of ensuring pain is an organisational priority have been identified including:

- setting pain standards;
- regular audit of pain management;
- having a pain management service;
- introducing pain link nurses.

Pain link nurses provide a link between the pain management service and the wards. They are ward-based nurses who, following additional training, act as role models for other staff.
   Pain link nurses enable nurses working in a pain management service to have better links with the wards. Pain link nurses provide educational support and advice on pain-related issues in their ward or department.

A pictorial representation of the strategies required to make pain an organisational priority can be seen in Figure 11.2.

Setting and auditing pain standards

The first step in making effective pain management an organisational priority is to audit current practice against selected best practice guidelines. (See Chapter 1 for a list of national pain standards and guidelines.) These pain management standards should be audited on a regular basis (at least every six months). Following completion of the audit an action plan should be drawn up. Once sufficient time has been given for changes to be implemented, practice should be re-audited. Figure 11.3 outlines the process of auditing pain management practices.

Pain management standards should be audited on a regular basis and an action plan put in place to address areas where improvements are needed.

Pain management services

Another organisational strategy for improving pain management is the development of a pain service. Guidance on the provision of paediatric anaesthetic services by the Royal College of Anaesthetists (RCA) in the UK emphasises the need for a properly staffed and funded acute pain service covering the needs of children (RCA 2001). The RCA recommend that a member of the acute pain service should visit all children's surgical wards every day and see all children having major surgery. This is also supported by the

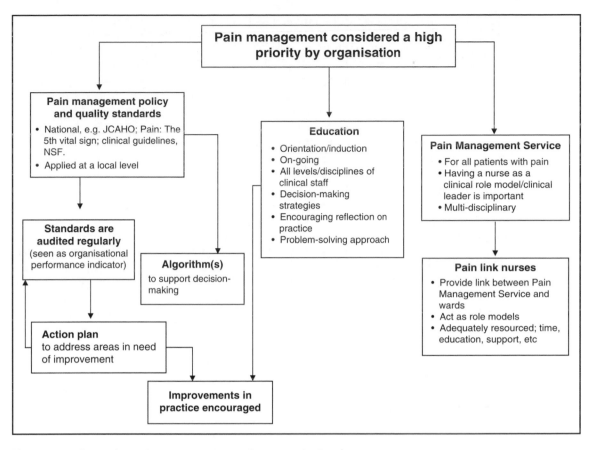

Figure 11.2 Improving pain management practices: organisational aspects.

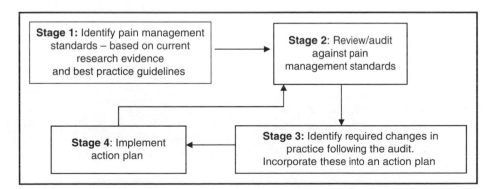

Figure 11.3 Auditing pain management practices.

UNICEF child-friendly hospital initiative, which states that a team should be established whose remit is to establish standards and guidance in the control of pain and discomfort in children (UNICEF 1999). Usually newly established pain services initially only manage acute pain, but as the service develops many expand to include procedural pain, chronic pain and palliative pain management.

A specialist pain management nurse or team visiting the wards each day can provide support to the nurses caring for children in pain. This could reduce the stress associated with decision-making and caring for children in pain and may also increase nurses' confidence regarding pain management. Indeed, a study in Wales found that the introduction of an acute pain service led to considerable improvement in the level of adults' postoperative pain (assessed by visual analogue scores) (Gould et al. 1992). This concurs with the findings of other studies (Stratton 1999; Bardiau et al. 2003; McDonnell et al. 2005).

Pain link nurses

Human sources of information have been shown to be important in changing practices and in the dissemination of research evidence into practice (Thompson et al. 2001; McCaughan 2002). Indeed, facilitators have been described as having a key role in relation to getting evidence into practice (Harvey et al. 2002; Rycroft-Malone et al. 2002). The use of link nurses has been suggested as a way of increasing the application of research in practice both generally (Thompson et al. 2000) and in relation to pain management (Ferrell et al. 1993; McCleary et al. 2004), but such roles need to be resourced adequately.

11.3 Managing Change

If practices are to change, several different strategies need to be implemented simultaneously. Changing behaviour is always a challenge. Improving pain management practices clearly requires more than educating nurses and increasing the priority attributed to pain management by nurses.

When considering strategies for changing nurses' behaviour, the literature relating to changing health behaviours provides some useful suggestions. For change to come about, people have to be ready to change (Prochaska and DiClemente 1983; DiClemente et al. 1991; Prochaska et al. 1992). The stages of change model (Table 11.1) attempts to describe readiness to change and how people move towards making decisions and changing behaviour (Bennett and Murphy 1997; Rollnick et al. 1999; Rutter and Quine 2002). The stages of change model can be used to explain why nurses do not change their practice, even when they have a good level of theoretical knowledge and consider something to be important. Nurses may be in the pre-contemplation, contemplation or preparation stage of change. If nurses are ambivalent about the need to change their pain management practices, they are unlikely to be motivated to do so.

11.4 Researching Children's Pain

There is still limited research regarding children's views about the quality of pain management practices. This is perhaps attributable to the ethical issues that need considering when involving children in research, such as:

- obtaining informed consent for the child;
- determining whether parental consent is required;
- limiting the guarantees of confidentiality;

Table 11.1 The stages of change model

Stage	Description
Pre-contemplation	Not considering the possibility of change, either because they are unaware of the need for change or unwilling to confront the problem.
Contemplation	Aware of the existence of a problem. Seriously considering the possibility of change but feel ambivalent. They see the benefits but feel distressed about the sacrifices involved.
Preparation	Decided on their commitment to change and will make a change in the near future (within three months). Still some ambivalence.
Action	Actually starting to make change in their behaviour. Might be confident in their ability to sustain change at the start.
Maintenance	Attempting to sustain the progress achieved during action. Are likely to be constantly struggling with thoughts about relapsing. Lasts between six months and a lifetime.
Termination	Free from the temptation to return to old behaviours. The new behaviour is more habitual than the old.
Relapse	Not strictly a stage of change, but a possible outcome of action or maintenance. Unsuccessful in their attempt to change. Likely to go back into contemplation and seriously intend to make another attempt at change in the near future.

Source: Prochaska and DiClemente (1983); DiClemente et al. (1991); Prochaska et al. (1992)

- deciding whether payments should be made to children who take part in research;
- protecting children who are research participants;
- monitoring researchers' adherence to ethical codes.

Several organisations have ethical guidelines relating to research with children and young people (Box 11.1).

BOX 11.1

Ethical guidelines relating to undertaking research with children

Royal College of Paediatrics and Child Health (2000) Guidelines for the Ethical Conduct of Medical Research Involving Children. Available from: http://www.rcpch.ac.uk/publications/bpsu/ethics_advice_summary_may_2001.pdf

National Children's Bureau (2003) Guidelines for Research. Available from: http://www.ncb.org.uk/dotpdf/open%20access%20-%20phase%201%20only/research_guidelines_200604.pdf

Medical Research Council (2004) Medical research involving children. Available from: http://www.mrc.ac.uk/Utilities/Documentrecord/index.htm?d=MRC002430

> **BOX 11.1** Continued
>
> Further information about the ethical issues relating to undertaking research with children can be found in:
>
> Gibson, F. and Twycross, A. (2007) Children's participation in research: A position statement on behalf of the Royal College of Nursing's Research in Child Health (RiCH) Group and Children's and Young People's Rights and Ethics Group, *Paediatric Nursing*, 19(4): 14–17.
>
> Twycross, A. (2008) An inter-professional approach to the ethics of undertaking research with children in the United Kingdom, *Nurse Researcher* (in press).

Summary

- Factors that contribute to continuing poor pain management practices include knowledge deficits, incorrect or outdated beliefs about pain and pain management, the decision-making strategies used, ward culture, and organisational culture.
- Improving pain management requires a multifactorial approach encompassing institutional support, attitude shifts, and change leaders (e.g. nurses working in the pain service and pain link nurses in ward areas).
- Issues that need addressing include education, decision-making strategies and organisational practices.
- Educational strategies need to promote the integration of theory and practice as well as ensuring that nurses understand the rationale for pain-relieving interventions.
- Nurses need support in their decision-making about managing children's pain; the use of algorithms may be useful in this context.
- Pain management needs to be an integral part of an organisation's quality improvement programme. This includes setting and auditing standards.
- The use of adequately educated and resourced pain link nurses has also been suggested as a means of providing good role models and of disseminating evidence-based information in a non-threatening way.
- Further research needs to be done to determine other factors that impact on pain management practices.
- Future research should include the views of children about the quality of their pain management.

References

Alley, L.G. (2001) The influence of an organizational pain management policy on nurses' pain management practices, *Oncology Nursing Forum*, 28(5): 867–74.

Atkins, S. and Murphy, K. (1994) Reflective practice, *Nursing Standard*, 22(8): 49–56.

Bardiau, F.M., Taviaux, N.F., Albert, A., Boogaerts, J.G. and Stadler, M. (2003) An intervention study to enhance postoperative pain management, *Anesthesia and Analgesia*, 96(1): 179–185.

Bennett, P. and Murphy, S. (1997) *Psychology and Health Promotion*, Open University Press, Buckingham, UK.

Botti, M., Bucknall, T. and Manias, E. (2004) The problem of postoperative pain: issues for future research, *International Journal of Nursing Practice*, 10(6): 257–263.

Brown, G.I. (1990) *Human Teaching for Human Learning: An Introduction to Confluent Education*, The Gestalt Journal, New York.

Bruce, E. and Franck, L.S. (2005) Using the worldwide web to improve children's pain care, *International Nursing Review*, 52(3): 204–209.

Bucknall, T., Manias, E. and Botti, M. (2001) Acute pain management: implications of scientific evidence for nursing practice in the postoperative context, *International Journal of Nursing Practice*, 7(4): 266–273.

Burokas, L. (1985) Factors affecting nurses' decisions to medicate pediatric patients after surgery, *Heart and Lung*, 14(4): 373–378.

Byrne, A., Morton, J. and Salmon, P. (2001) Defending against patients' pain: a qualitative analysis of nurses' responses to children's postoperative pain, *Journal of Psychosomatic Research*, 50: 69–76.

Chiang, L.C., Chen, H.J. and Huang, L. (2006) Student nurses' knowledge, attitudes, and self-efficacy of children's pain management: evaluation of an education program in Taiwan, *Journal of Pain and Symptom Management*, 32(1): 82–89.

Cioffi, J. (1998) Decision making by emergency nurses in triage assessments, *Accident and Emergency Nursing*, 6: 184–191.

Department of Health (2004) *National Service Framework for Children, Young People and Maternity Services*, The Stationery Office, London.

DiClemente, C.C., Prochaska, J.O., Fairhurst, S.K., Velicer, W.F. and Rossi, J.S. (1991) The process of smoking cessation: an analysis of precontemplation, contemplation and preparation stages of change, *Journal of Consulting and Clinical Psychology*, 59(2): 295–304.

Dihle, A., Bjølseth, G. and Helseth, S. (2006) The gap between saying and doing in postoperative pain management, *Journal of Clinical Nursing*, 5(4): 469–479.

Elstein, A.S., Schulman, L.S. and Sprafka, S.A. (1978*) Medical Problem Solving: An Analysis of Clinical Reasoning*, Harvard University Press, Cambridge.

Falanga, I.J., Lafrenaye, S., Mayer, S.K and Tetrault, J-P. (2006) Management of acute pain in children: safety and efficacy of a nurse-controlled algorithm for pain relief, *Acute Pain*, 8(2): 45–54.

Ferrell, B.R., Grant, M., Ritchey, K.J., Ropchar, L.M. and Rivera, L.M. (1993) The pain resource nurses training program: a unique approach to pain management, *Journal of Pain and Symptom Management*, 8(8): 549–556.

Ferrell, B.R., Dean, G.E., Grant, M. and Coluzzi, P. (1995) An institutional commitment to pain management, *Journal of Clinical Oncology*, 13(9): 2158–2165.

Fincham, R. and Rhodes, P. (1999) *Principles of Organizational Behaviour*, Oxford University Press, Oxford.

Finley, G.A., Franck, L.S., Grunau, R.E. and von Baeyer, C.L. (2005) Why Children's Pain Matters, *Pain: Clinical Updates*, XIII(4): 1–6.

Fitzpatrick, J.M., While, A.E and Roberts, J.D. (1996) Key influences on the professional socialisation and practice of students undertaking different pre-registration nurse education programmes in the United Kingdom, *International Journal of Nursing Studies*, 33(5): 506–518.

Furnham, A. (1997) *The Psychology of Behaviour at Work*, Psychology Press, Hove, UK.

Gould, T.H., Crosby, D.I., Harmer, M., Lloyd, S.M., Lunn, J.N., Rees, G.A.D, Roberts, D.E. and Wenster, J.A. (1992) Policy for controlling pain after surgery: effect of sequential changes in management, *British Medical Journal*, 305(14): 1187–1193.

Graffam, S. (1990) Pain content in the curriculum: a survey, *Nurse Educator*, 15(1): 20–23.

Gray, M. and Smith, L.N. (1999) The professional socialization of diploma of higher education in nursing students (Project 2000): a longitudinal study, *Journal of Advanced Nursing*, 29(3): 639–647.

Greenwood, J., Sullivan, J., Spence, K. and McDonald, M. (2000) Nursing scripts and the organizational influences on critical thinking: report of a study of neonatal nurses' clinical reasoning, *Journal of Advanced Nursing*, 31(5): 1106–1114.

Hamers, J., Abu-Saad, H., Halfens, R.J.G. and Schumacher, J.N.M. (1994) Factors influencing nurses' pain assessment and interventions in children, *Journal of Advanced Nursing*, 20: 853–860.

Hamers, J.P.H., van den Hout, M.A., Halfens, R.J.D., Abu-Saad, H.H. and Heijltjes, A.E.G. (1997) Differences in pain assessment and decisions regarding the administration of analgesics between novices, intermediates and experts in pediatric nursing, *International Journal of Nursing Studies*, 34(5): 325–334.

Harvey, G., Loftus-Hills, A., Rycroft-Malone, J., Titchen, A., Kitson, A., McCormack, B. and Seers, K. (2002) Getting evidence into practice: the role and function of facilitation, *Journal of Advanced Nursing*, 37(6): 577–588.

Health Care Commission (2004) *Patient Survey Report 2004 – Young Patients*, Health Care Commission, London.

Johnston, C.C., Gagnon, A.J., Pepler, C.J. and Bourgault, P. (2005) Pain in the emergency department with one-week follow-up of pain resolution, *Pain Research and Management*, 10(2): 67–70.

Joint Commission for the Accreditation of Healthcare Organizations (2000) *Pain Assessment and Management Standards*, JCAHO, Oakbrook Terrace, Illinois.

Jones, D.C. and Sheridan, M.E. (1999) A case study approach: developing critical thinking skills in novice pediatric nurses, *Journal of Continuing Education in Nursing*, 30(2): 75–78.

Jordan-Marsh, M., Hubbard, J., Watson, R., Deon Hall, R., Miller, P. and Mohan, O. (2004) The social ecology of changing pain management: Do I have to cry? *Journal of Pediatric Nursing*, 19(3): 193–203.

Kessenich, C., Guyatt, G. and DiCenso, A. (1997) Teaching nursing students evidence-based nursing, *Nurse Educator*, 22(6): 25–29.

Khalid, S.K. and Gee, H.A. (1999) A new approach to teaching and learning in journal clubs, *Medical Teacher*, 21: 289–293.

Kneafsey, R. (2000) The effect of occupational socialization in nurses' patient handling practices, *Journal of Clinical Nursing*, 9(4): 585–593.

Lamond, D., Crow, R.A. and Chase, J. (1996) Judgements and processes in care decision in acute medical and surgical wards, *Journal of Evaluation in Clinical Practice*, 2(3): 211–216.

Lee, J.E.M. and Ryan-Wenger, N. (1997) The 'think aloud' seminar for teaching clinical reasoning: a case study of a child with pharyngitis, *Journal of Pediatric Health Care*, 11: 101–110.

Manworren, R.C.B. (2000) Pediatric nurses' knowledge and attitudes survey regarding pain, *Pediatric Nursing*, 26(6): 610–614.

McCaughan, D. (2002) What decisions do nurses make? In Thompson, C. and Dowding, D. (eds.) *Clinical Decision Making and Judgement in Nursing*, Edinburgh, Churchill Livingstone, pp. 95–108.

McCleary, L., Ellis, J.A. and Rowley, B. (2004) Evaluation of the pain resource nurse role: a resource for improving pediatric pain management, *Pain Management Nursing*, 5(1): 29–36.

McDonnell, A., Nicholl, J. and Read, S. (2005) Focus. Exploring the impact of Acute Pain Teams (APTs) on patient outcomes using routine data: can it be done? *Journal of Research in Nursing*, 10(4): 383–402.

Melby, V., Canning, A., Coates, V., Forster, A., Gallagher, A., McCartney, A. and McCartney, M. (1997) The role of demonstrations in the learning of nursing psychomotor skills, *NT Research*, 2(3): 199–207.

Nolf, B. (1995) Teaching tips. Journal club: A tool for continuing education, *Journal of Continuing Education in Nursing*, 26(5): 238–239.

Ochieng, B.M.N. (1999) Use of reflective practice in introducing change on the management of pain in a paediatric setting, *Journal of Nursing Management*, 7: 113–118.

Philpin, S.M. (1999) The impact of 'Project 2000' educational reforms on the occupational socialization of nurses: an exploratory study, *Journal of Advanced Nursing*, 29(6): 1326–1331.

Polkki, T., Pietila, A-M. and Vehvilamen-Julkunen, K. (2003) Hospitalized children's descriptions of their experiences with postsurgical pain relieving methods, *International Journal of Nursing Studies*, 40: 33–44.

Prochaska, J.O. and DiClemente, C.C. (1983) Stages and processes of self-change of smoking: toward an integrative model of change, *Journal of Consulting and Clinical Psychology*, 51(3): 390–395.

Prochaska, J.O., DiClemente, C.C. and Norcross, J.C. (1992) In search of how people change: applications to addictive behaviors, *American Psychologist*, 47(9): 1102–1114.

Rolfe, G. (1996) *Closing the Theory Practice Gap: A New Paradigm for Nursing*, Butterworth-Heinemann, Oxford.

Rollnick, S., Mason, P. and Butler, C. (1999) *Health Behaviour Change*, Churchill Livingstone, Edinburgh.

Ross, R.S., Bush, J.P. and Crummette, B.D. (1991) Factors affecting nurses' decisions to administer PRN analgesic medication to children after surgery: an analog investigation, *Journal of Pediatric Psychology*, 16(2): 151–167.

Royal College of Anaesthetists (2001) *Guidance on the Provision of Paediatric Anaesthetic Services*, Royal College of Anaesthetists, London.

Rutter, D. and Quine, L. (2002) Social cognition models and changing health behaviours. In Rutter, D. and Quine, L. (eds.) *Changing Health Behaviour*, Open University Press, Buckingham, UK, pp. 1–27.

Rycroft-Malone, J., Kitson, A., Harvey, G., McCormack, B., Seers, K. and Estabrooks, C. (2002) Ingredients for change: revisiting a conceptual framework, *Quality and Safety in Health Care*, 11(2): 174–180.

Salantera, S. (1999) Caring for Children in Pain: Nursing Knowledge, Activities and Outcomes. *PhD Thesis, Department of Nursing Science*, University of Turku, Turku, Finland.

Salantera, S. and Lauri, S. (2000) Nursing students' knowledge of and views about children in pain, *Nurse Education Today*, 20: 537–547.

Salantera, S., Lauri, S., Salmi, T.T. and Helenius, H. (1999) Nurses' knowledge about pharmacological and non-pharmacological pain management in children, *Journal of Pain and Symptom Management*, 18(4): 289–299.

Schmidt, K., Eland, J. and Weller, K. (1994) Pediatric cancer pain management: a survey of nurses' knowledge, *Journal of Pediatric Oncology*, 11(1): 4–12.

Segal, S. and Mason, D.J. (1998) The art and science of teaching rounds, *Journal for Nurses in Staff Development*, 14(3): 127–136.

Simons, J. and MacDonald, L.M. (2004) Pain assessment tools: children's nurses' views. *Journal of Child Health Care*, 8(4): 264–278.

Simons, J. and Roberson, E. (2002) Poor communication and knowledge deficits: obstacles to effective management of children's postoperative pain, *Journal of Advanced Nursing*, 40(1): 78–86.

Stratton, L. (1999) Evaluating the effectiveness of a hospital's pain management project, *Journal of Nursing Care Quality*, 13(4): 8–18.

Studdy, S., Nicol, M.J. and Fox-Hiley, A. (1994) Teaching and learning clinical skills, Part 1 – Development of a teaching model and schedule of skills development, *Nurse Education Today*, 14: 186–193.

Taylor, C. (1997) Problem solving in clinical nursing practice, *Journal of Advanced Nursing*, 26(2): 329–336.

Thompson, C., McCaughan, D., Cullum, N., Sheldon, T., Mulhall, A. and Thompson, D. (2001) The accessibility of research-based knowledge for nurses in the United Kingdom acute care settings, *Journal of Advanced Nursing*, 36(1): 11–22.

Treadwell, M.J., Franck, L.S. and Vichinsky, E. (2002) Using quality improvement strategies to enhance pediatric pain assessment, *International Journal for Quality in Health Care*, 14(1); 39–47.

Twycross, A. (1999) Pain management: a nursing priority? *Journal of Child Health Care*, 3(3): 19–25.

Twycross, A. (2000) Education about pain: a neglected area? *Nurse Education Today*, 20: 244–253.

Twycross, A. (2002) Educating nurses about pain management: the way forward, *Journal of Clinical Nursing*, 11: 705–714.

Twycross, A. (2004) *Children's Nurses' Pain Management Practices: Theoretical Knowledge, Perceived Importance and Decision-Making*, Unpublished PhD Thesis, University of Central Lancashire.

Twycross, A. (2007a) Children's nurses' postoperative pain management practices: an observational study, *International Journal of Nursing Studies*, 44(6): 869–881.

Twycross, A. (2007b) What is the impact of theoretical knowledge on children's nurses' postoperative pain management practices? An exploratory study, *Nurse Education Today*, 27(7): 697–707.

Twycross, A. and Powls, L. (2006) How do children's nurses make clinical decisions? Two preliminary studies, *Journal of Clinical Nursing*, 15: 1324–1335.

UNICEF (1999) Global millennium targets: UNICEF child-friendly hospital initiative, *Paediatric Nursing*, 11(10): 7–8.

Vincent, C.V.H. (2005) Nurses' knowledge, attitudes, and practices regarding children's pain, *MCN*, 30(3): 177–183.

Vincent, C.V.H. and Denyes, M.J. (2004) Relieving children's pain: nurses' abilities and analgesic administration practices, *Journal of Pediatric Nursing*, 19(1): 40–50.

Watt-Watson, J., Stevens, B., Garfinkel, P., Streiner, D. and Gallop, R. (2001) Relationship between nurses' pain knowledge and pain management outcomes for their postoperative cardiac patients, *Journal of Advanced Nursing*, 36(4): 535–545.

Weissman, D.E., Griffe, J., Gordon, D.B. and Dahl, J.L. (1997) A role model program to promote institutional changes for management of acute and cancer pain, *Journal of Pain and Symptom Management*, 14(5): 274–279.

Woodgate, R. and Kristjanson L. (1996) A young child's pain: how parents and nurses 'take care', *International Journal of Nursing Studies*, 33(3): 271–284.

Index